GUA SHA

SCRAPING MASSAGE
TECHNIQUES

This book is edited and designed by the Editorial Committee of *Cultural China* series.

Text by Wu Zhongchao
Translation by Cao Jianxin
Design by Wang Wei

Copy Editors: Susan Luu Xiang, Yang Xiaohe
Editors: Wu Yuezhou, Cao Yue
Editorial Director: Zhang Yicong

Senior Consultants: Sun Yong, Wu Ying, Yang Xinci
Managing Director and Publisher: Wang Youbu

ISBN: 978-1-60220-032-6

Address any comments about *Gua Sha Scraping Massage Techniques: A Natural Way of Prevention and Treatment through Traditional Chinese Medicine* to:

Better Link Press
99 Park Ave
New York, NY 10016
USA

or

Shanghai Press and Publishing Development Co., Ltd.
F 7 Donghu Road, Shanghai, China (200031)
Email: comments_betterlinkpress@hotmail.com

Printed in China by Shanghai Donnelley Printing Co., Ltd.

3   5   7   9   10   8   6   4

The material in this book is provided for informational purposes only and is not intended as medical advice. The information contained in this book should not be used to diagnose or treat any illness, disorder, disease or health problem. Always consult your physician or health care provider before beginning any treatment of any illness, disorder or injury. Use of this book, advice, and information contained in this book is at the sole choice and risk of the reader.

Quanjing provides the images on pages 20 (fig. 7) and 25 (fig. 13).

GUA SHA
SCRAPING MASSAGE TECHNIQUES
A Natural Way of
Prevention and Treatment
through
Traditional
Chinese
Medicine

By Wu Zhongchao

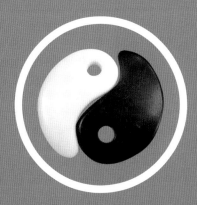

Better Link Press

Contents

PREFACE 9

CHAPTER ONE
Read Your Body's Needs to Expel Toxin 11

1. Eight Indications of Body Toxin 11
Constipation: Intestinal Toxin Expansion 11
Freckles and Spots: Energy and Blood Imbalance 12
Bad Breath: Heat Accumulation in Internal Organs 13
Dull Skin: Toxin Accumulation in Lungs 14
Acne: Damp-Heat Escalation in the Body 14
Obesity: Excessive Fat Accumulation 16
Joint Pain: Cold-Damp Intrusion 16
Excessive Blood Fat: Debris in Blood 17
2. Sources of Body Toxin 18
Accumulation of Metabolites within the Body 18
Main and Collateral Channels Intruded by Toxin 19
Unhealthy Diet and Medicine 20

CHAPTER TWO
Gua Sha Is a Simple and Effective Way of Expelling Toxin 23

1. What is *Sha*? 23
Sha is Toxin 23
The Location of *Sha* Reflects the Nature of the Disease 23
The Appearance of *Sha* Reflects the Severity of the Disease 23
Gua Sha Serves to Expel Toxin 24
2. Scraping Locations 25
Acupoints 26
Reflection Areas 27
Projection Areas 33
Corresponding Areas 34
3. Scraping Tools 35
4. Steps and Methods of *Gua Sha* 37
Choose an Appropriate Place 37
Choose a Comfortable Body Position 37
Choose Locations on the Body 38
Methods of *Gua Sha* 38

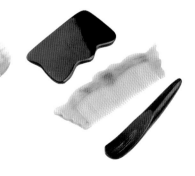

5. Different *Gua Sha* Methods for Different Parts of the Body   43
   The Head   43
   The Face   45
   The Back   45
   The Chest   45
   The Waist   45
   Four Limbs   45
6. Expelling Toxin of Internal Organs through *Gua Sha*   46
   Scraping Methods for Expelling Toxin in the Heart and the Small Intestine   46
   Scraping Methods for Expelling Toxin in the Lungs and the Large Intestine   48
   Scraping Methods for Expelling Toxin in the Liver and the Gallbladder   50
   Scraping Methods for Expelling Toxin in the Spleen and the Stomach   52
   Scraping Methods for Expelling Toxin in the Kidneys and the Bladder   54
7. Diagnostic Principles of *Gua Sha*   56
8. Various Benefits of *Gua Sha*   59
9. Attentions Regarding *Gua Sha*   62

CHAPTER THREE
Use *Gua Sha* to Solve Daily Ailments   65

1. Cold   65
2. Cough   70
3. Fever   72
4. Swollen Sore Throat   74
5. Hypochondriac Pain   76
6. Palpitation and Short Breath   78
7. Dizziness   80
8. Tinnitus   82
9. Headache   84
10. Toothache   86
11. Bad Breath   89
12. Lack of Appetite   91
13. Heat Stroke   93
14. Indigestion   94
15. Hiccups   96
16. Gastrospasm   97
17. Abdominal Distension   98
18. Diarrhea   100
19. Constipation   102
20. Flabby Skin   105
21. Fatigue   106
22. Forgetfulness   108
23. Agitation   110
24. Stiff Neck   112
25. Insomnia   114
26. Acute Conjunctivitis   116
27. Dry Eyes and Eye Strain   118
28. Acne   120
29. Dark Circles   122
30. Puffiness of the Eye Socket   123
31. Chloasma   124
32. Freckles   126
33. Dry Skin   127
34. Dull Complexion   129
35. Skin Itch   130
36. Eczema   131
37. Chilblain   132
38. Cold Hands and Feet   133
39. Neurodermitis   134
40. Urticaria   136
41. Shingles   138
42. Flat Warts   140
43. Facioplegia   142
44. Premature Gray Hair   144
45. Hair Loss   145
46. Aching and Stiff Shoulders and Neck   146
47. Back Waist Pain   148
48. Lower Limb Ache   150

CHAPTER FOUR
Use *Gua Sha* to Detoxify Internal Organs to Prevent and Treat Chronic Diseases 153

1. Hypertension 153
2. Obesity 156
3. Diabetes 158
4. Coronary Heart Disease 160
5. Rheumatic Heart Disease 162
6. Hyperlipemia 164
7. Sequela of Apoplexy 167
8. Chronic Bronchitis 171
9. Chronic Rhinitis 174
10. Allergic Rhinitis 176
11. Presbyopia 178
12. Chronic Pharyngitis 180
13. Chronic Pneumonia 182
14. Asthma 184
15. Chronic Hepatitis 186
16. Fatty Liver 188
17. Chronic Cholecystitis and Cholelithiasis 190
18. Chronic Gastritis 192
19. Chronic Enteritidis 194
20. Peptic Ulcer 196
21. Urinary Incontinence 198
22. Urine Retention 199
23. Chronic Nephritis 200
24. Urinary Calculus 202
25. Gout 204
26. Anaemia 206
27. Hemorrhoids 208

CHAPTER FIVE
Use *Gua Sha* to Expel Wind-Damp and Cold Toxin to Get Rid of Joint Problems 211

1. Cervical Spondylosis 211
2. Scapulohumeral Periarthritis 214
3. Rheumatic Arthritis 216
4. Elbow Joint Pain 219
5. Wrist Pain 220
6. Ankle Joint Pain 221
7. Knee Joint Pain 222
8. Heel Pain 224
9. Lumbar Disc Protrusion 226
10. Lumbar Hyperosteogeny 228
11. Ankylosing Spondylitis 229

CHAPTER SIX
Use *Gua Sha* to Expel Male and Female Diseases 231

1. Premature Ejaculation 231
2. Impotence 233
3. Spermatorrhea 234
4. Prostatitis 236
5. Hyperplasia of Prostate Gland 237
6. Male Infertility 239
7. Female Infertility 240
8. Irregular Menstruation 242
9. Dysmenorrhea 244
10. Amenorrhea 246
11. Abnormal Leukorrhea 248
12. Uterine Prolapse 250
13. Uterine Fibroid 252
14. Chronic Pelvic Inflammation 254
15. Acute Mastitis 256
16. Hyperplasia of Mammary Glands 258
17. Female's Climacteric Syndrome 260

INDEX 262

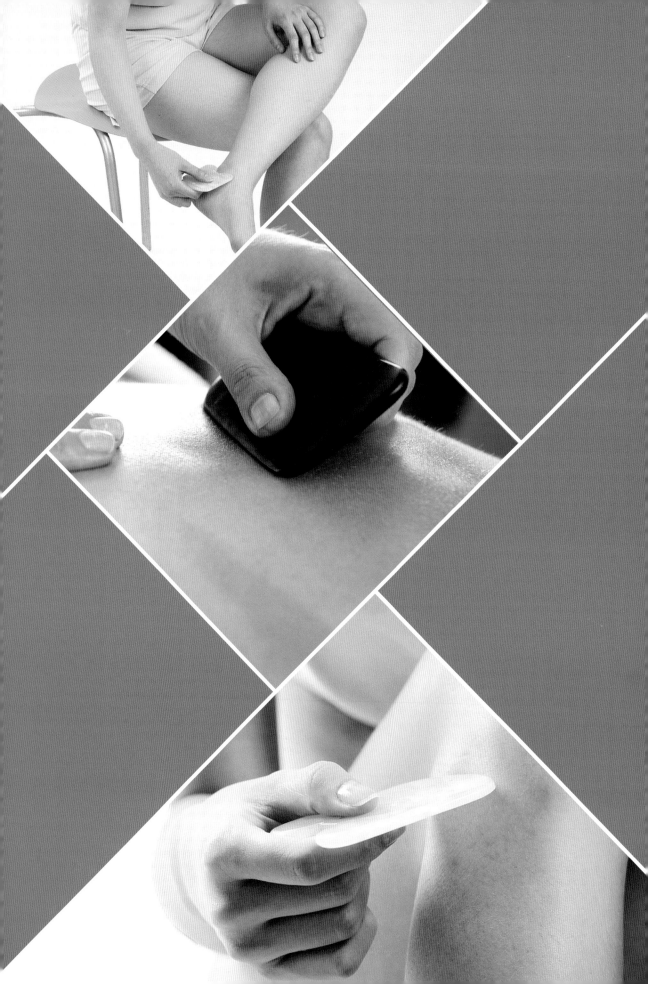

PREFACE

Why do people get sick? Why aren't there long-term cures for diseases? Why are there more and more chronic diseases despite continuous medical treatment?

Along with rapid development of medicine nowadays, the rate of incidence and the rate of mortality of various diseases, such as cancer, cardiovascular diseases, liver diseases, diabetes, and kidney diseases have been rising increasingly. They are related to the changes of the internal and external environments of our bodies. Toxin within our bodies is an important reason for impairing our health and leading to diseases.

What is toxin? It is the substance harmful to human health but cannot be expelled smoothly. It is attached to the tissues and cells of various channels within our bodies. Just like tea stains attached to mugs, it is not easy to be washed off or metabolized, blocking the normal circulation of the vital energy and blood as well as main and collateral channels and resulting in diseases.

Where does toxin come from? Some comes from the body itself. Every day, millions of cells within the human body die and lots of wastes, such as radicals, cholesterol, and lithic acid are generated after the foods are metabolized within the body. They are important sources of the toxin. Some other toxin comes from external environment, such as air pollution, pesticide residues, and chemical medicine, as well as unreasonable diet structure, smoking or excessive alcoholic drinks.

Under normal circumstances, the toxin within the body can be expelled by way of human metabolism. However, too many toxins will lead to accumulation, affecting the circulation of vital energy and blood, interfering with the balance of metabolism, harming the functions of inner organs and speeding up the aging of the human body.

Gua sha is undoubtedly the safest and the most effective way to expel toxin. This is a traditional and natural therapy of Chinese medicine with obvious effects as well as simplicity and convenience. Only a scraping board coupled with lubricants is applied to repeatedly scrape and rub the related acupoints or affected parts, until red spots appear on the skin. These red spots represent the toxin within the body, blocking the circulation of energy and blood and the metabolism of the body. If such toxin cannot be expelled timely, there will be consequently various kinds of diseases, leading to accelerated aging. Therefore, through stimulating the skin, *gua sha* can trigger off the functions of the self-defense system within the human body, expel the accumulated toxin and clean the internal environment of the human body, enhancing the ability of self-adjustment and the ability of resistance against diseases. Persisting in *gua sha* is equal to expelling toxin regularly within the human body. This is not only conducive to dealing with chronic diseases, getting rid of physical pain, raising the function of immunity and the ability of resistance against diseases, but also helping people resist aging and beautify themselves.

The health care and detoxifying therapy of *gua sha* introduced in this book is marked by simplicity, convenience, safety, and flexibility. It is suitable both as an auxiliary physical therapy for patients in the period of recovery and for the daily care of healthy individuals. It is with hope that *gua sha* therapy can be of great help to your health.

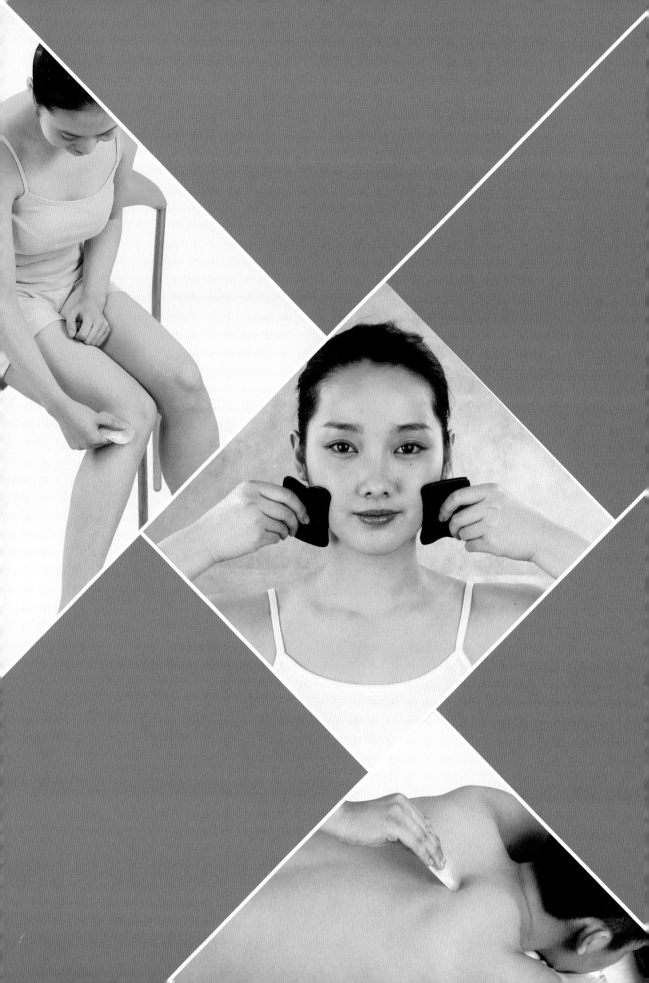

CHAPTER ONE
Read Your Body's Needs to Expel Toxin

Acccording to *The Inner Canon of the Yellow Emperor*, a classic work of traditional Chinese medicine, "All internal elements can surely be observed outside." It means that human ailments will show themselves on the surface of the body. The accumulation of toxin within the body will also appear in various ways. Our careful discovery and timely expulsion can keep the balance of our metabolism and prolong our health.

1. Eight Indications of Body Toxin

The body toxin, when accumulated up to an amount, will show itself in certain ways. The body would remind you to expel toxin when problems occur, such as constipation, bad breath, freckles, unhealthy skin color, acne, obesity, joint pain, and too much blood fat.

Constipation: Intestinal Toxin Expansion

Bowel movement is the most important way for the human body to expel toxin. Usually, the excrement is discharged once every day. Constipation is marked by less than twice or three times a week, or once every two or three days, with small amounts and dryness.

Constipation is harmful in many aspects. Intestines are not only the places for digesting food and absorbing nutrition, but also the places for the concentration of toxin. If the accumulated excrement within intestines cannot be discharged, it will not only add to the burden of intestines, but also enable the toxin to be absorbed twice or many times via the blood and circulate together with blood within the body, seriously polluting the entire body. Its major harm is shown in several aspects as follows:

• Accelerating the aging of the human body: The mood of people with minor constipation will be affected, resulting in the disorder of the functions of gastric and intestinal nerves, discomfort of intestines and stomach, abdominal distention and bitter taste in mouth. People of serious constipation or those with long-term constipation will suffer from the accelerated aging of human tissues and internal organs, finally leading to severe pathological changes.

• Resulting in cancer: Long-term constipation will make carcinogens from germs fermented in intestines irritate the epithelial cell in intestinal mucous membranes, leading to the heteromorphic hyperplasia that is apt to give rise to the cancer.

• Resulting in intestinal necrosis: Hard excrement will block the intestinal cavity, leading to the obstruction of blood circulation due to the pressure on the rectum and the colon and even leading to the excrement-based ulcer. People of serious cases will suffer from intestinal necrosis or intestinal perforation.

• Resulting in angionosis: For people with constipation, the force exerted when the excrement is being discharged will increase abdominal pressure and lead to the attack of cardiovascular diseases, such as angina or myocardial infarction. Therefore, it is rather dangerous for patients of cardiovascular diseases. The incidence of such cases is mostly seen in early morning.

Intestines are both the places for producing toxin and the passages for expelling toxin. As is discovered by scientific research, over half of the immunity system is located within intestines, particularly in the colon. Once the colon fails to operate normally, toxin within the body will be discharged from other channels such as kidneys, skin and breath. Then, in addition to constipation, there will be other problems like body odor, bad breath, unhealthy skin color, skin rash, measles, and freckles. Timely expulsion of toxin can make metabolism smooth and keep human vitality.

Gua Sha Serves to Cure Constipation and Expel Intestinal Toxin
Superficially, constipation results from weakened intestinal functions and slow peristalsis. It is due to the weakness of vital energy and blood, leading to weak intestinal operation. *Gua sha* is a good way to smooth vital energy and blood. Scraping Dachangshu point and Xiaochangshu point on the back, Tianshu point and Guanyuan point on the abdomen as well as Quchi point and Zhigou point on the arm all serve to smooth the vital energy and blood of related channels, effectively improve the intestinal environment, increase intestinal motility, promote bowel movement, and cure such intestinal diseases as constipation (fig. 1). (Scraping to cure constipation can be seen on Page 102.)

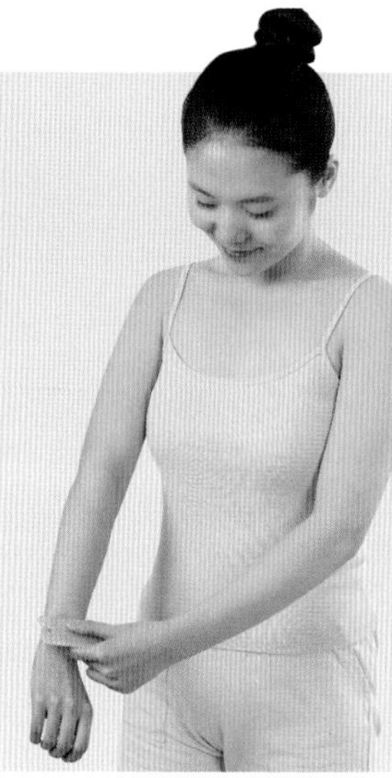

Fig. 1 Scraping Zhigou point serves to relieve constipation.

Freckles and Spots: Energy and Blood Imbalance

Freckles trouble many women and lots of them would try various anti-freckle creams, but fail and make the skin more fragile. In fact, eradication can only be realized when the source of freckles is found.

There are chiefly three reasons for freckles. First, melanin cannot be discharged due to the slow down of metabolism. The second cause is the cumulative harm of the sunlight to the skin. The third reason is imbalanced endocrine due to tension in life and irregular daily routine, leading to the increase of abnormal secretion of the melanin.

From the angle of Chinese medicine, freckles are related with the vital energy and blood in main and collateral channels. The skin is closely associated with inner organs, main and collateral channels as well as vital energy and blood. People would look young with shining and fine skin if the functions of their inner organs are normal with energetic vitality and blood, as well as smoothly functioning main and collateral channels. Otherwise, there will be various problems with the skin, which is related to metabolism. The blockage of vital energy and blood in main and collateral channels tends to be associated with such elements as the cold and damp which are featured by the coldness, condensation and blockage. They would affect the circulation of vital energy and blood, block metabolism, and keep body waste inside, thus leading to the precipitation of melanin, which appears in the form of freckles.

Gua Sha Cleans the Inner Environment Which Is Crucial to Freckle Removal

As it seems, *gua sha* serves to expel toxin only at certain areas, but it mobilizes the vital energy and blood all over the body and promotes their circulation. At the same time, it serves to avoid the precipitation of toxin in blood vessels and the skin. This can not only eradicate the elements for the growth of freckles and speed up the elimination of freckles, but also help maintain the health of blood vessels.

Different areas are scraped depending on different kinds of freckles and spots. For details, please refer to Page 126.

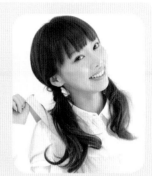

Bad Breath: Heat Accumulation in Internal Organs

Bad breath refers to bad smell in mouth, which is off-putting to others and awkward for yourself. Though a small ailment, bad breath is intolerable. It tends to make one feel hesitated in contacting with other people at a close distance, resulting in a sense of inferiority and blockage of affection and interpersonal communications with others. Bad breath is also likely to be the signal of certain diseases.

People with heavy bad breath can feel it themselves, while some people do not know it until such reaction of disgust is made by other people. In more cases, in order not to hurt one's feeling, people do not point it out, while one with bad breath is not aware of it, too. In fact, it is simple to know whether you have bad breath or not: Cover the mouth and the nose with two palms in a semi-open bowl shape, breathe out between the palms and breathe in with the nose, then you can smell your breath.

Gua Sha Can Remove Bad Breath Caused by Heat in Internal Organs

Such undesirable ways of life as irregular diet or too much spicy food as well as over-fatigue lead to weak gastric functions, which is harmful to proper digestion in intestines and the expelling of food-residues in accumulation, generate toxin in the blood in intestinal walls and harm internal organs to cause diseases. Food residue precipitating in intestines for a long time will give rise to inner heat, produce bad smell, evaporate upwards and lead to bad breath through the mouth, nose and throat.

The cure of bad breath must be based on expelling toxin in blood in intestinal walls and inner organs, restoring normal intestinal and gastric functions so that food-residues precipitating in intestines can be expelled, leading to the eradication of conditions for the existence of bad breath. *Gua sha* is an effective way of expelling accumulated heat and toxin. There will be very good effects if such acupoints as Daling point and Laogong point on the hand, Zusanli point and Neiting point on the shin and the foot are scraped (fig. 2). (Scraping to expel bad breath can be seen on Page 89.)

Fig. 2 Scraping Daling point serves to reduce bad breath.

Dull Skin: Toxin Accumulation in Lungs

At the first thought, people would say that dull and gloomy skin color is due to anaemia, which may be one of the reasons. Undesirable skin is also likely to be related with lungs. If there is toxin in lungs with their functions affected, the skin may be dull with acne, which may also be accompanied by the hair loss.

According to the theories of Chinese medicine, "Lungs are associated with the skin and hair." The so-called "skin and hair" are mentioned in a quite macro-cosmic manner, which are roughly equivalent to skin, hair, sweat glands, glandula sebacea and fingernails with functions of secreting sweat, adjusting breath and resisting intrusion of harmful elements from outside. Through diffusion, lungs spread vital energy and blood all over the body to nourish the skin, hair, and muscles, as well as maintain the normal physiological functions of the hair and skin.

The skin of people with energetic lungs looks soft, smooth and elastic. Since lungs relate to outside environment, the air breathed in would be exchanged in lungs so that various germs from outside would have "close contact" with lungs. People are likely to be infected if they happen to be weak. Such infection would reduce lung functions and lead to the weakness of vital energy in lungs, so the lungs would be weak in spreading vital energy and blood to the skin and hair. Without the nourishment, skin and hair would appear dull, leading to a darkened tone and the hair loss.

Therefore, if the skin is found problematic, one should think about whether it is the problem with lungs, rather than only rely on applying medicinal ointments or going for beauty treatments.

> ### *Gua Sha* Expels Toxin and Enhances Lung Functions
>
> All internal organs are closely associated with main and collateral channels. Therefore, adjusting main and collateral channels serves to adjust inner organs. It is difficult to directly stimulate lungs since they are inside the body. However, some main and collateral channels related to them are tangible on the skin. Scraping the acupoints of related channels can expel body toxin, i.e., toxin that blocks the circulation of vital energy and blood and affects the exchange between nutrients and metabolites, leading to diseases in human tissues and organs. Such expulsion serves to expel toxin in lungs and enhance lung functions.
>
> In terms of adjusting lungs, *gua sha* can be usually conducted along the lung channel. Since lungs match with large intestines in functions, acupoints related to the channel of large intestines can be chosen in coordination, which can achieve better results. For patients suffering from anaemia, acupoints related to the liver channel need to be scraped.

Acne: Damp-Heat Escalation in the Body

Acne, also known as pimples, are constantly seen on the faces of young people. They are caused by too much secretion of oil, the blockage of pores and bacterial infection. According to Chinese medicine, acne is also a result from the toxin as damp-heat in the body. The so-called damp-heat is featured by dampness and heat in the body. Those with acne caused by dampness and heat tend to have more oily skin along with thick and greasy tongues.

Where does damp-heat in the body come from? There are chiefly three causes:
• Improper diet with very spicy, fatty or sweet food. It leads to the accumulation of dampness and heat as well as harm to muscles and skin, resulting in acne. In this case,

dampness and heat tend to accumulate in intestines and stomach, giving rise to bad breath and constipation.

• Five emotions can lead to inner heat, i.e., various kinds of unhealthy moods can give rise to inner heat. Therefore, fluctuating emotions, particularly anger and anxiety, are also very likely to result in acne or make them worse.

• Irregular daily life, such as staying up overnight, can also lead to dampness and heat, or aggravate the acne featured by dampness and heat.

Gua Sha Expels Dampness and Heat and Brings about Nice Skin

Scraping is marked by eliminating heat, expelling toxin, invigorating blood, dispersing stasis, doing away with dampness and sputa. With the toxin of dampness and heat expelled by the scraping, acne can be fundamentally expelled.

Dampness and heat resulting in acne is generally accumulated in lungs. Therefore, scraping can be done in the Lung Channel and Feishu point on the back can be chosen. For those with bad breath, Pishu point, Weishu point, and Dachangshu point can be chosen (fig. 3).

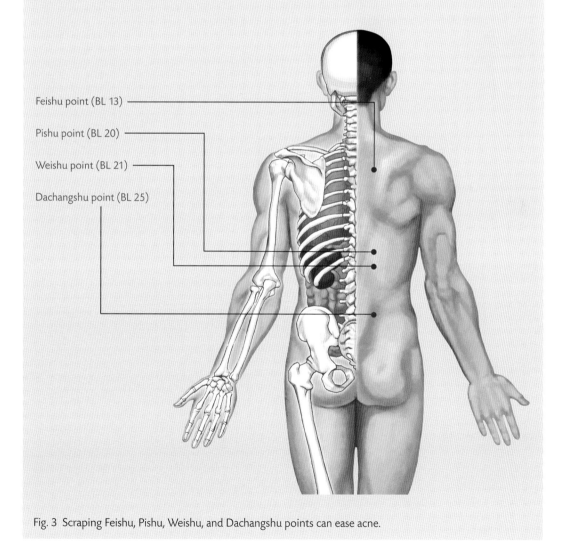

Feishu point (BL 13)

Pishu point (BL 20)

Weishu point (BL 21)

Dachangshu point (BL 25)

Fig. 3 Scraping Feishu, Pishu, Weishu, and Dachangshu points can ease acne.

Obesity: Excessive Fat Accumulation

We often hear such a term as "reducing weight by expelling toxin." In fact, it makes sense by linking "expelling toxin" with "reducing weight," because one of the important reasons for obesity is too much accumulation of toxin in the body.

In nature, obesity is due to the overloading of cells and accumulation of fat, resulting in abnormal metabolism. As compared with healthy people, an obvious high content of blood plasma lipid (including triglyceride, cholesterol and free fatty acid, etc.) takes place in the body of those suffering from obesity, indicating that the disorder of lipid metabolism of different degrees exists in the body of those suffering from obesity. Such lipid, if not metabolized timely, will become garbage that is harmful to health, i.e., toxin as it is often referred to. Too many toxins will aggravate the difficulty of discharge. Therefore, those suffering from obesity will always get half the result with twice the efforts in reducing weight if methods are incorrect.

So, the process of curing obesity is, in nature, one of expelling toxin. Only with toxin expelled and the disorder of lipid metabolism corrected, can obesity be fundamentally cured.

Gua Sha is the Safest and the Most Effective Way of Expelling Fat and Toxin

Scraping has the most direct and obvious impact on the human body, as it can promote metabolism and expel toxin. The human body undergoes metabolism ceaselessly every day. During its course, waste generated would be discharged timely. Scraping can timely bring "garbage" from the metabolism to the body-surface, precipitate it into pores under skin, smooth blood circulation in the body and restore the natural vigor of metabolism.

For those suffering from obesity, the significance of the scraping is not only the expulsion of toxin, but also the adjustment of yin and yang since obesity is a manifestation of the imbalance of yin and yang. Through stimulating some acupoints on related main and collateral channels, scraping enables yin and yang of the human body to reach an ideal state of balance, hence naturally restoring the balance of metabolism.

Stimulating skin via scraping can speed up the burning of fat on the body surface, reducing the accumulation of fat under skin.

Joint Pain: Cold-Damp Intrusion

Pain in the human body mostly occurs in joints with two major reasons. First is over work or sprain due to carelessness. Second cause is intrusion by such exterior evil elements as wind, cold, heat, dampness and dryness, leading to the blockage of vital energy and blood. Pain of these kinds is also called arthromyodynia according to Chinese medicine, with the influence of intrusion by the cold-damp being obvious.

According to Chinese medicine, the cold-damp includes two aspects, i.e., the cold and dampness caused by exterior evil elements and innate cold and dampness. The cold-damp leading to joint pain are mainly caused by exterior evil elements which block the circulation of vital energy and blood, resulting in pain in joints and tendons as commonly seen symptoms.

In daily life, being often exposed to the environment of the cold-damp is an important factor for those suffering from cold-damp and joint pain. For instance, people would suffer from soreness and pain in four limbs due to the intrusion of dampness if they directly sleep on the floor which contains heavy dampness because of the precipitation of water in the air. Moreover, people would suffer from cold-damp if they wear damp clothes, stay in an air-conditioned room with sweat or expose their skin in cold weather, etc. (fig. 4).

Joint pain due to cold-damp is chiefly manifested by joint pain in four limbs, sore and painful neck and shoulders, scapulohumeral periarthritis, sore and painful waist and back, etc. The more the painful areas are and the longer the time is, the heavier the cold-damp is in the body.

***Gua Sha* Can Permeate Main and Collateral Channels and Expel Cold-Damp**

Since joint pain is caused by the blockage of main and collateral channels, as well as the circulation of energy and blood, *gua sha* is a simple and effective way of dredging them.

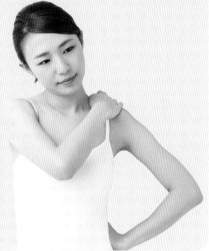

Joint pain relies either on the dredging of main and collateral channels or the stoppage of the intrusion of the cold-damp at their sources. In normal circumstances, the human body is endowed with *wei qi* (defensive energy) which serves to block exterior evil elements. It originates from yang energy. Strong yang energy can nurture inner human organs while preventing exterior evil elements from intruding the human body. Wind, cold, and dampness will take advantage of the human body if yang energy is deficient, resulting in the blockage of vital energy and blood as well as main and collateral channels followed inevitably by joint pain. Therefore, the fundamental way of preventing the cold-damp from intrusion is to invigorate, consolidate, and protect yang energy in the body. Through benign stimulation of skin, *gua sha* enables the human body to be full of yang energy to enhance the body's ability of expelling evil elements. That is how defensive energy is enhanced through *gua sha*.

Fig. 4 Unhealthy habits in daily life cause dampness to enter the body, leading to joint pain.

Excessive Blood Fat: Debris in Blood

Health is marked by the balance of metabolism in the human body and the metabolism of blood fat is a very important link. If metabolism of blood fat is imbalanced, the intake of cholesterol and triglyceride is larger than their discharge, it will lead to the disorder in blood fat metabolism, which is commonly called hyperlipemia.

An important factor affecting blood fat metabolism is the change of the nature of blood, i.e., blood is polluted by toxin. The first manifestation of blood pollution is that blood becomes acidic. In an acidic environment, if fat substances cannot be broke down, they will suspend on or attach to the walls of blood vessels, resulting in hyperlipemia and making the walls of blood vessels thick and lumen narrow, further leading to arteriosclerosis, obstruction of micro-circulation and insufficiency of blood supply.

With the blood becoming acid, substances attached to the walls of blood vessels are more than blood fat. Red blood-cells, blood platelets, toxin and germs are apt to be attached to the walls of blood vessels.

With the blood becoming acid, blood fat and blood sugar will increase. Blood will become thicker and thicker and blood flow will become slower and slower, adding burden to the heart and giving rise to high blood pressure.

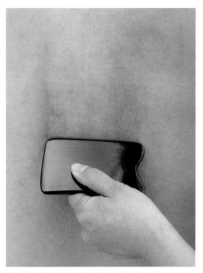

Fig. 5 *Sha* brought about by the scraping helps to judge one's blood situation.

Scraping Can Purify Blood

The appearance and disappearance of *sha* by way of scraping serves to purify blood. This is because blood circulation at the far end (peripheral circulation) is the slowest and the blood vessel there is the finest, apt to form precipitation (stasis and blockage). Scraping serves to directly stimulate this part.

In addition to expelling toxin in blood, scraping can also reflect whether blood is toxic or thick. Fast appearance of *sha* (a short time of scraping with minor force) indicates that blood is thick. Slow appearance of *sha* (a long time of scraping with big force) indicates that blood is sticky. If there is almost no appearance of *sha*, it means that blood is very sticky, and that cupping applied to this part will show black freckles. The appearance of black freckles all over after cupping indicates very sticky blood. Those with this symptom are patients of hyperlipemia (fig. 5).

2. Sources of Body Toxin

Where does toxin in the body come from? Is it due to the internal reason or the external reason? In fact, the generation of toxin is closely associated with our daily habits and the changes of our surrounding environment. For instance, the lack of physical exercise and improper diet can all lead to the accumulation of toxin in the body. In general, toxin in the body comes mainly from three aspects: substances from metabolism, unclean food and the intrusion of exogenous pathogenic factors.

Accumulation of Metabolites within the Body

Our bodies are metabolizing all the time, inevitably leading to the generation of metabolites, which are the sources of most of the toxin in the body.

In normal circumstances, toxin can be expelled timely, keeping the body in metabolic balance. However, the lack of physical exercise will result in the deduction of the mechanism of expelling toxin. These metabolized substances, if attached to the intestinal walls and the walls of blood vessels for a very long time, would be re-absorbed by the body, giving rise to constant accumulation of toxin and harming the body, leading to the decay of memory, fatigue, unhealthy complexion, constipation, and acceleration of aging. Usually, there are several kinds of metabolic waste in the body:

Free radical: Free radical is one of the main elements to cause human aging. An appropriate amount of free radical can prevent human body from being intruded and harmed by chemical substances and other exterior evil substances. However, excessive free radicals will generate a very strong effect of oxidization, intruding and harming human cells and leading to aging and dark skin, etc.

Cholesterol: An appropriate amount of cholesterol is beneficial to the human body.

However, excessive cholesterol will add burden to the liver and increase the amount of cholesterol in blood, causing hyperlipemia, arteriosclerosis and fatty liver, etc.

Accumulated lipid: Too much lipid in blood will make blood thicker. Normal blood flow requires greater pressure, adding burden to the heart and the burden to the walls of blood vessels against pressure (resulting in high blood pressure). Precipitation of lipid on the inner walls of blood vessels obstructs normal blood flow, being apt to result in thrombus.

Accumulated excrement: This is likely to result in diseases of anus and intestines as well as colon cancer. Accumulated excrement is also an important cause of cardiovascular diseases.

Uric acid, lactic acid, and blood stasis are also toxins which should not be overlooked.

Therefore, to avoid the accumulation of metabolites in the body, one should develop the habit of doing physical exercise frequently, since it can maintain and stimulate the normal functions of various human organs, e.g., promoting the function of liver and kidneys, intestinal movement, blood circulation and sweat-expulsion, etc. These are all conducive to expelling toxin from human organs. The lack of physical exercise and the accumulation of various metabolites mentioned above, will threaten health at any time.

Main and Collateral Channels Intruded by Toxin

Toxin in the human body is not only attributed to the garbage generated during body metabolism, but also to exterior elements, i.e., wind, cold, damp, dryness, heat, and fire in Mother Nature. These exterior evil elements, once intruding the human body, will block main and collateral channels and obstruct the circulation of vital energy and blood, leading to diseases.

Wind, cold, heat, damp, dryness and fire are six kinds of climatic phenomena in nature. People would fall ill if they cannot adapt themselves to these six elements when weather changes abnormally or abruptly. Then these six elements would become harmful factors causing illness in the human body, so they are also called "six exopathogens" or "six evils" according to Chinese medicine.

Pathogenic Wind: As a kind of yang malaise, the intrusion of the pathogenic wind will cause openness and discharge of the body surface, which is manifested by sweating. In most cases, pathogenic wind would intrude the upper part of the human body, body surface, muscles and lungs. The nature of wind evil is changeable, resulting in illness in a mobile manner, leading to joint pain in four limbs. Pathogenic wind is also characterized by acuteness and quick changes. For example, rash is itching from time to time and that they move around on the skin, appearing and disappearing at intervals.

Pathogenic Cold: As a kind of yin malaise, pathogenic cold is harmful to yang energy. Due to its condensation and stasis nature, its intrusion is likely to slow down the circulation of vital energy and blood. Stagnation leads to pain. Therefore, pathogenic cold is apt to cause arthralgia.

Pathogenic Heat: As a yang malaise, pathogenic heat often attacks and leads to illness in summer. It is featured by the rise and dispersal of heat that is apt to exhaust body fluid, consume vital energy and depress the spirit. Pathogenic heat attacks mostly together with the pathogenic damp.

Pathogenic Fire: Characterized by heat and upwardness, pathogenic fire is apt to exhaust vital energy and body fluid, intruding the upper part of the body. It tends to harm the liver wind and blood, resulting in various kinds of hemorrhagic diseases. It is also likely to cause distress and carbuncles.

Pathogenic Dryness: Marked by dryness, astringency, purification, and descending, pathogenic dryness is apt to harm body fluid, which is detrimental to the lungs.

Pathogenic Damp: Pathogenic damp is apt to obstruct the circulation of vital energy, harm yang energy, and make the human body feel heavy. Dampness is marked by stickiness and stasis. Consequently, it is difficult to completely cure diseases caused by dampness.

Unhealthy Diet and Medicine

In addition to metabolized garbage in the body and the intrusion of evil elements into the body resulting from wind, cold, damp, dryness, heat and fire in Mother Nature, diet is also an important source of garbage in the body, particularly unhealthy diet. There are several kinds of unhealthy diet:

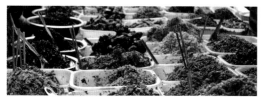
Fig. 6 Pickled food can lead to cancer.

Pickled food: While being processed, pickled food is often added with lots of salt that contains impure substance, such as nitrite, which is likely to generate harmful substances like nitrosamine. Frequent intake of nitrosamine is detrimental to health, even inducing cancer (fig. 6).

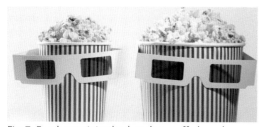
Fig. 7 Food containing lead, such as puffed snacks, can harm the nerve system.

Lead-containing food: Commonly seen lead-containing food includes puffed snacks and canned food. Lead is a heavy metal element with neurotoxins. With lead taken into blood, people will suffer from obstruction of metabolism and harm to tissues and inner organs all over the body, with the harm to the nerve system being the most particularly serious (fig. 7).

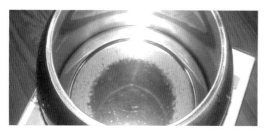
Fig. 8 The scale contains lots of harmful metallic elements.

Scale: Cups, thermos bottles, or water bottles used for a long time will produce scale which contains quite many harmful metal elements such as cadmium, mercury, arsenic and aluminum, etc. If not cleaned timely and thoroughly, they will result in aging due to pathological changes in the systems of digestion, nerves, urination, hematopoiesis, and blood circulation (fig. 8).

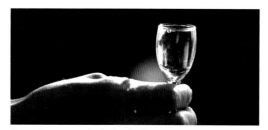
Fig. 9 Excessive alcoholic drinking not only harms the liver, but also increases the incidence of various cancers.

Excessive drinking: Toxic substances, such as alcohol, formaldehyde, methanol, and ethanol will accumulate in the body for those of excessive drinking. They will not only harm the liver, reduce liver ability to expel toxin, but also harm digestive, cardiovascular, and immune systems while increasing the incidence of various cancers (fig. 9).

Medicine: All kinds of medicine that we take would go through detoxification by the liver and kidneys. Abuse of medicine would harm the health of the liver and reduce its ability to expel toxin, resulting in the accumulation of toxin in the body. Long-term intake of certain kinds of medicine, such as sleeping pills, would increase the tolerance of the human body. Medicine residue, when accumulated to a certain amount, would poison people, resulting in the decay of memory, slow reaction, headache, and dizziness. In addition, long-term intake of cathartics and febrifuges can do severe harm to the human body (fig. 10).

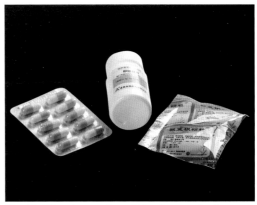

Fig. 10 The abuse of medicine harms the liver, reduces its ability of detoxification and allows toxin to accumulate in the body.

Food additives: To be more attractive in colors and flavors, many snacks and instant foods are applied with pigments and flavoring agents. In order to keep food for a longer time, preservatives are used. Excessive additives in these kinds of food will bring toxin to the human body. Even if the number of additives conforms to the requirements for food safety, long-term intake of such food will inevitably lead to the accumulation of toxin in the body. This toxin accumulation can last for a long time without being observed, so its harm is also long-lasting (fig. 11).

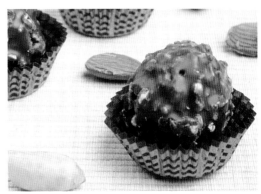

Fig. 11 Snack food contains additive agents which, if taken for a long time, will lead to accumulation of toxin in the body.

Long-term intake of various meats: Many kinds of meats and sea foods are applied with lots of antibiotics in the course of cultivation. Once it enters the human body, the antibiotic residues would interfere with the immune function of the human body, which is detrimental to health. Digestion of meats is a slow process which is apt to result in fermentation and rot in intestines, leading to toxin (fig. 12).

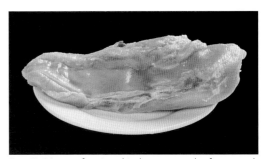

Fig. 12 Meats of various kinds are apt to be fermented within intestines, leading to toxin.

Toxin in the body not only disrupts the normal digestion and absorption, but also does harm to the system of circulation (blood vessels), the system of filtration (liver and kidneys), and the system of digestion (intestines and stomach, etc.).

When we become too weak to resist due to too many toxins, germs and pathogens would enter our bodies. Therefore, if toxins in our body cannot be expelled in time, the defense system of our body will become very weak, being apt to fall ill owing to the climate changes.

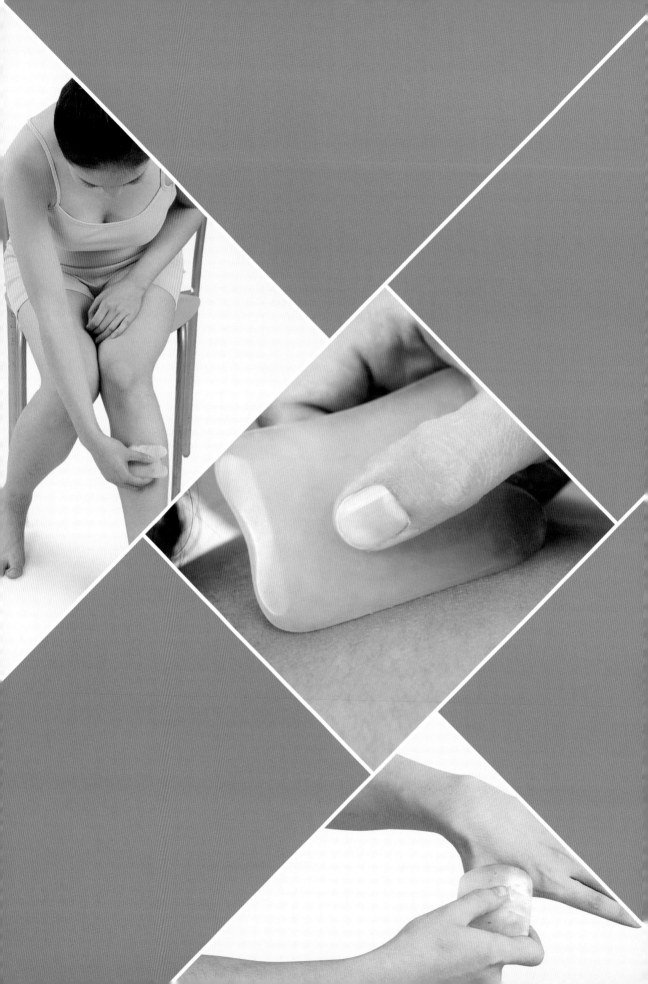

Chapter Two
Gua Sha Is a Simple and Effective Way of Expelling Toxin

Though there are various ways of expelling toxin, some of them result in harm to health, the harm that cannot be healed. *Gua sha* is a safe and effective way of expelling toxin. *Sha* is toxin. With *sha* brought about by scraping, "stasis" in the vital energy and blood in main and collateral channels can be expelled, eradicating toxin in all parts of the body.

1. What Is *Sha* ?

It is a term unique to Chinese medicine, referring to the "stasis" in the vital energy and blood in main and collateral channels. In clinical practice, *sha* stands for red and purplish-red freckles and spots on the skin of the patient brought about by the specially-made scraping plate. *Sha* is also called "*sha* mark."

Sha is Toxin
It can be said that *sha* is the blood stasis and the pathological product separated from micro-circulation. If not expelled timely, it will block the circulation of vital energy and blood, and the exchange between nutrients and metabolites, leading to diseases in human tissues and inner organs. Therefore, according to Chinese medicine, "All kinds of diseases can result in *sha*." The harmful toxin leads to many kinds of diseases while speeding up aging. So, in essence, *sha* itself is the toxin in human body. Consequently, it is also commonly called "toxic *sha*."

Under general circumstances, *sha* brought about by the scraper will gradually disappear in three to five days, or no more than a week. *Sha*, as the toxin expelled from the human body, also reflects the state of diseases in the human body.

The Location of *Sha* Reflects the Nature of the Disease
The locations of *sha* reflect the locations of the disease. *Sha* is apt to appear along the route of main and collateral channels or on the areas of acupoints, suggesting the pathological changes of the functions of inner organs related to corresponding channels. For instance, if *sha* freckles or purple *sha* marks appear at the Xinshu point when the Bladder Meridian on the back is scraped evenly, it indicates that there are abnormal changes in heart functions. Therefore, scraping should be applied as early as possible for health care.

The Appearance of *Sha* Reflects the Severity of the Disease
Different appearances of *sha* (i.e., the form, color, tint and the speed of *sha* appearance) also

reflect the extent of the disease concerned. Dispersed *sha* in light color is equal to minor illness which can be recovered easily. Extensive *sha* in the form of spots and patches in purple blood lumps indicates serious illness, requiring scraping several times for recovery.

Gua Sha Serves to Expel Toxin

According to Chinese medicine, *sha* is the stasis in the vital energy and blood in main and collateral channels. The permeation of *sha* leads to clear main and collateral channels, smooth circulation of vital energy and blood, eliminating diseases as a result. In fact, curing diseases by scraping can also be verified by modern medicine.

The process of the scraping can lead to high hyperemia in partial tissues, stimulate the nerves of blood vessels, enlarge blood vessels, speed up the blood flow and the backflow of the lymph, reinforce the function of phagocytosis and the force of transport, quickly expel the waste and toxin within the body and provide tissues and cells with nutrition, purifying the blood, reducing the state of illness, and promoting recovery.

However, *gua sha* is not directly expelling toxin from under the skin, but taking blood stasis attached to the wall of blood vessels out of the blood vessels and absorbing it into blood vessels again through the blood, finally expelling the waste from urine via circulation all over the body.

The skin looks unpleasing to the eye when *sha* appears, but it will not harm the skin. Instead, it serves to invigorate blood circulation and remove blood stasis, strengthening the circulation of blood in the locations scraped and making skin appear healthier and finer. So, there's no need to worry when *sha* appears.

Gua sha is also a way to check up one's physical condition. With the scraping done, if there is no *sha*, but only ruddiness, local heat and relaxed feeling, it means that the person concerned is healthy, requiring no further scraping so as not to irritate the skin.

Many people can mistake *sha* for blood stasis. Superficially, *sha* looks like ordinary blood stasis. However, they are different, and have very different influences on the human body. Please refer to the table as follows.

Differences between *Sha* and Blood Stasis		
	Sha	Blood stasis
Color	Mostly dark red or purplish red and even bluish black.	Mostly bright red.
Bleeding part	Blood capillary.	Various blood vessels.
Bleeding amount	Light.	Heavy.
Sense of pain	Without or with slight pain.	The pain tends to go beyond forbearance with movement restricted.
Consequence	It can do away with swell and stasis and smooth main and collateral channels. With *sha* dispelled, illness can be eased and even cured.	It harms surrounding tissues, resulting in new pain or obstacle to the movement.
	Sha.	Blood stasis.

2. Scraping Locations

According to the theoretical system of Chinese medicine, main and collateral channels are regarded as the system linking the inside and outside of the human body as well as all inner organs. These channels run through all over the body, connecting internal organs, limbs and joints, smoothing the circulation of vital energy and blood, and nurturing tendons and bones. Roughly speaking, there are 12 channels, including Taiyin Lung Meridian of Hand (LU), Jueyin Pericardium Meridian of Hand (PC), Shaoyin Heart Meridian of Hand (HT), Yangming Large Intestine Meridian of Hand (LI), Shaoyang Sanjiao Meridian of Hand (TE), Taiyang Small Intestine Meridian of Hand (SI), Yangming Stomach Meridian of Foot (ST), Shaoyang Gallbladder Meridian of Foot (GB), Taiyang Bladder Meridian of Foot (BL), Taiyin Spleen Meridian of Foot (SP), Jueyin Liver Meridian of Foot (LR), Shaoyin Kidney Meridian of Foot (KI) as well as Ren Meridian and Du Meridian (fig. 13). Acupoints are special points on the body surface where the transport and transmission of vital energy and blood of human organs as well as main and collateral channels are concentrated. They are mostly distributed along the route of main and collateral channels as well as the places passed through by dense nerve-endings or thick nerve fibers. These points are in close connection with the tissues and organs deep under the skin. Therefore, acupoints are reflecting points of diseases and stimulating points for treatment. There are also extra acupoints on head and neck (EX-HN), on breast and abdomen (EX-CA), on back (EX-B), on upper limbs (EX-UE) and on lower limbs (EX-LE). Stimulation via scraping certain acupoints can effectively mobilize human ability to resist illness, preventing and curing illness. In addition, scraping reflection areas, projection areas, and corresponding areas on the body surface also serve as an effective way to stimulate corresponding inner parts. A concrete introduction to these areas is as follows:

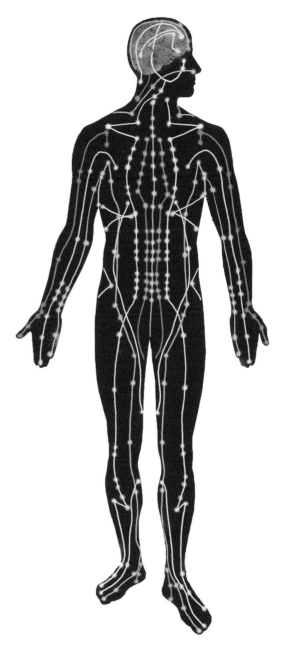

Fig. 13 Meridians and collaterals all over the body and acupoints on them.

Acupoints

Finding acupoints in *gua sha* doesn't need to be as accurate as that for massage, moxibustion and cupping. You only need to find the rough location. But the more accurate the location, the better the effects will be. This requires the methods of locating acupoints, which are divided into two, i.e., body length measurement or physical marks of the body.

Body Length Measurement		
1. Use Thumb Length	**2. Use Middle-Finger Length**	**3. Use Four Fingers Closed Together**
The width of the patient's thumb joint is 1 cun. This is applicable for locating the acupoint on four limbs with vertical cun.	With the patient's middle sections of the bent middle finger as measurement, the distance between two inner crease tips is taken as 1 cun, which is mostly applicable for locating acupoints on four limbs with vertical cun and on the back with horizontal cun.	With the index finger, middle finger, ring finger, and small finger of the patient stretched straight and closed, measure at the level of the large knuckle (the second joint) of the middle finger. The width of the four fingers is 3 cun.

Physical Marks of the Body

1. Use Fixed Marks

These are fixed marks free from the movement of the human body, such as the mouth, ears, nose, eyes, hair, finger and toe nails, breasts, navel as well as various protruding bone joints and cavities. They are ideal for loacting acupoints since they remain unmovable. For instance, Yintang point lies between two eyebrows, Danzhong point lies between two nipples, Tianshu point is 2 cun away from the navel, and Dazhui point lies under the seventh spinous process cervical spine when the patient lower the head (fig. 14).

2. Use Special Postures

This refers to the marks that only appear when corresponding movement takes place, including the appearance of the pore, cavity and wrinkle as the joint, skin and muscle move around, and sometimes the limb movement. For instance, Tinggong point is in a cavity in front of the tragus when the one opens the mouth, and Houxi point can be found at the end of the palm crease when one grips the fist.

3. Use Experience

This is a simple and convenient method accumulated through long-term practice by people. For instance, with the hand drooping vertically, the point touched by the tip of the middle finger is Fengshi point. With two hands crossed naturally and flatly between the thumb and the index finger, the point touched by the tip of the index finger is Lieque point.

Finding the most painful point is another method of locating acupoints, i.e., A'shi point. Acupoints of this sort are generally decided by the kind of diseases, mostly near the place with pathological change, or at a point quite far away from it. A'shi point has no fixed position or name. The place with pain is the location of the point, so it's commonly known as "wherever there is pain, there is an acupoint."

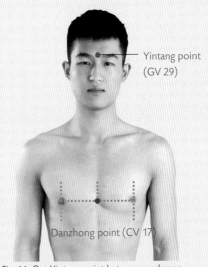

Yintang point (GV 29)

Danzhong point (CV 17)

Fig. 14 Get Yintang point between eyebrows and Danzhong point between two nipples.

Reflection Areas

In a broad sense, reflection areas refer to all areas of reflective effect in any part of the body. However, in Chinese medicine, it usually refers to such reflection areas as the soles, hands, and ears in a narrow sense. Areas of reflection in hands and feet are mentioned in this book (refer to Page 28 to Page 32 for the sketch maps of reflection areas on the hand and the foot).

Back of the Hand

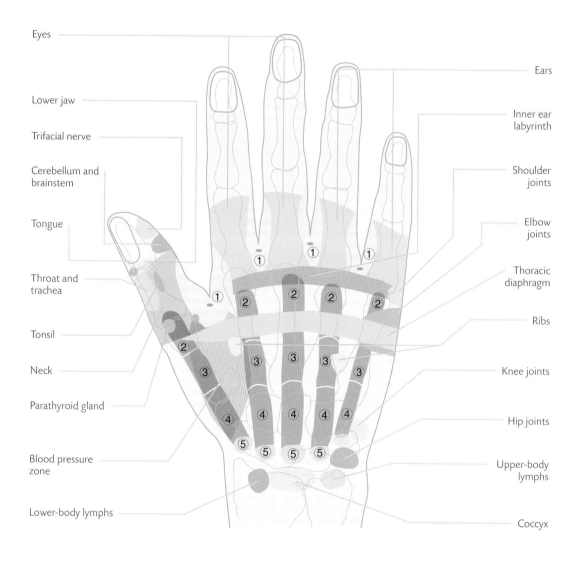

Eyes

Lower jaw

Trifacial nerve

Cerebellum and brainstem

Tongue

Throat and trachea

Tonsil

Neck

Parathyroid gland

Blood pressure zone

Lower-body lymphs

Ears

Inner ear labyrinth

Shoulder joints

Elbow joints

Thoracic diaphragm

Ribs

Knee joints

Hip joints

Upper-body lymphs

Coccyx

① Neck and shoulder ② Cervical vertebra ③ Thoracic vertebra
④ Lumbar vertebra ⑤ Sacrum

Figs. 15–17 Sketch maps of the reflection areas on the hand (pages 28–30).

Palm (Left)

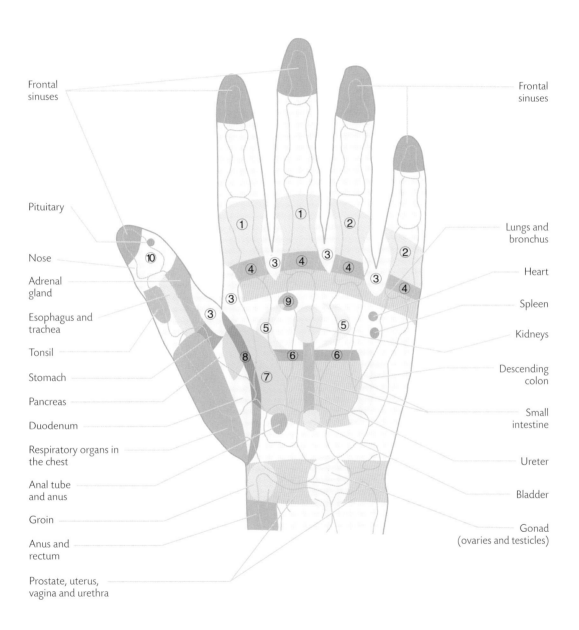

Frontal sinuses

Pituitary

Nose

Adrenal gland

Esophagus and trachea

Tonsil

Stomach

Pancreas

Duodenum

Respiratory organs in the chest

Anal tube and anus

Groin

Anus and rectum

Prostate, uterus, vagina and urethra

Frontal sinuses

Lungs and bronchus

Heart

Spleen

Kidneys

Descending colon

Small intestine

Ureter

Bladder

Gonad (ovaries and testicles)

① Eyes ② Ears ③ Neck and shoulder ④ Trapezius ⑤ Celiac plexus
⑥ Transverse colon ⑦ Spleen, stomach and large intestine ⑧ Thyroid
⑨ Neck ⑩ Brain

The Palm (Right)

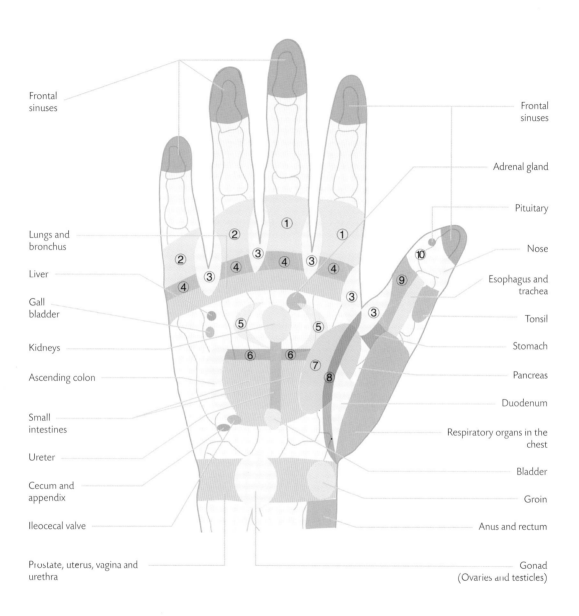

Frontal sinuses

Lungs and bronchus

Liver

Gall bladder

Kidneys

Ascending colon

Small intestines

Ureter

Cecum and appendix

Ileocecal valve

Prostate, uterus, vagina and urethra

Frontal sinuses

Adrenal gland

Pituitary

Nose

Esophagus and trachea

Tonsil

Stomach

Pancreas

Duodenum

Respiratory organs in the chest

Bladder

Groin

Anus and rectum

Gonad (Ovaries and testicles)

① Eyes ② Ears ③ Neck and shoulder ④ Trapezius ⑤ Celiac plexus
⑥ Transverse colon ⑦ Spleen, stomach and large intestine ⑧ Thyroid
⑨ Neck ⑩ Brain

Sole

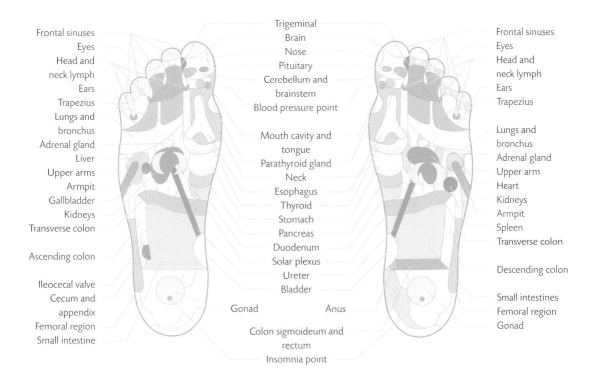

Frontal sinuses
Eyes
Head and
neck lymph
Ears
Trapezius
Lungs and
bronchus
Adrenal gland
Liver
Upper arms
Armpit
Gallbladder
Kidneys
Transverse colon

Ascending colon

Ileocecal valve
Cecum and
appendix
Femoral region
Small intestine

Trigeminal
Brain
Nose
Pituitary
Cerebellum and
brainstem
Blood pressure point

Mouth cavity and
tongue
Parathyroid gland
Neck
Esophagus
Thyroid
Stomach
Pancreas
Duodenum
Solar plexus
Ureter
Bladder

Gonad

Colon sigmoideum and
rectum
Insomnia point

Anus

Frontal sinuses
Eyes
Head and
neck lymph
Ears
Trapezius

Lungs and
bronchus
Adrenal gland
Upper arm
Heart
Kidneys
Armpit
Spleen
Transverse colon

Descending colon

Small intestines
Femoral region
Gonad

Foot Dorsum

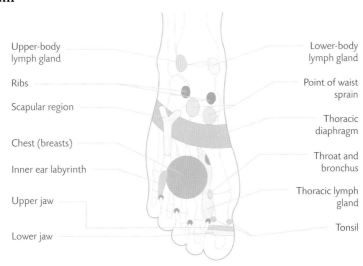

Upper-body
lymph gland

Ribs

Scapular region

Chest (breasts)

Inner ear labyrinth

Upper jaw

Lower jaw

Lower-body
lymph gland

Point of waist
sprain

Thoracic
diaphragm

Throat and
bronchus

Thoracic lymph
gland

Tonsil

Figs. 18–19 Sketch maps of the reflection areas on the foot (pages 31–32).

Lateral Side of the Foot

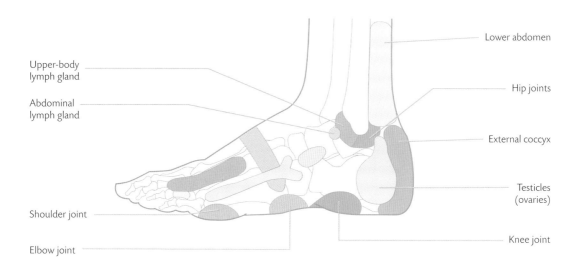

Upper-body lymph gland

Abdominal lymph gland

Shoulder joint

Elbow joint

Lower abdomen

Hip joints

External coccyx

Testicles (ovaries)

Knee joint

Medial Side of the Foot

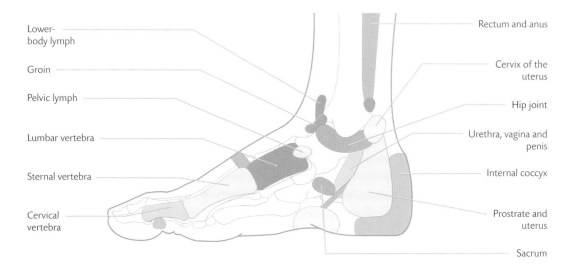

Lower-body lymph

Groin

Pelvic lymph

Lumbar vertebra

Sternal vertebra

Cervical vertebra

Rectum and anus

Cervix of the uterus

Hip joint

Urethra, vagina and penis

Internal coccyx

Prostrate and uterus

Sacrum

Projection Areas

On the front of the body, the projection area on the chest and abdomen corresponds to all inner organs underneath.

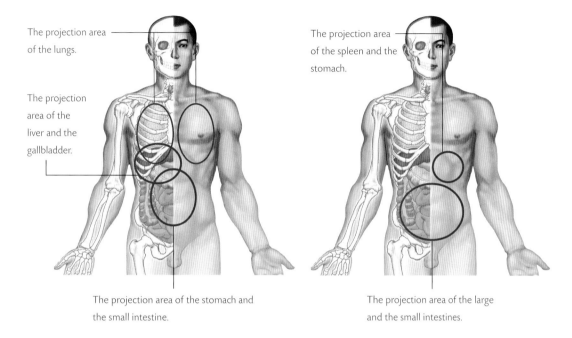

The projection area of the lungs.

The projection area of the liver and the gallbladder.

The projection area of the stomach and the small intestine.

The projection area of the spleen and the stomach.

The projection area of the large and the small intestines.

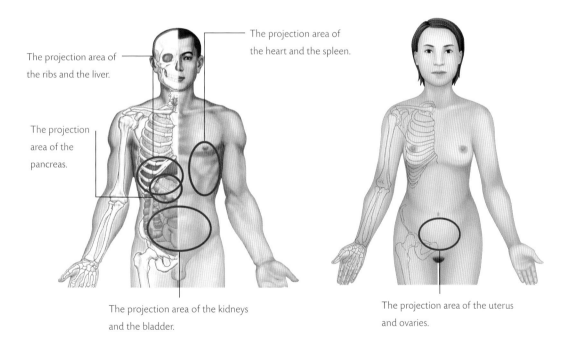

The projection area of the ribs and the liver.

The projection area of the pancreas.

The projection area of the heart and the spleen.

The projection area of the kidneys and the bladder.

The projection area of the uterus and ovaries.

Fig. 20 Sketch maps of the projection areas over the chest and the adomen.

Corresponding Areas

The corresponding areas are the body surface on the back and waist corresponding to inner organs underneath, mostly in the spine areas on the back.

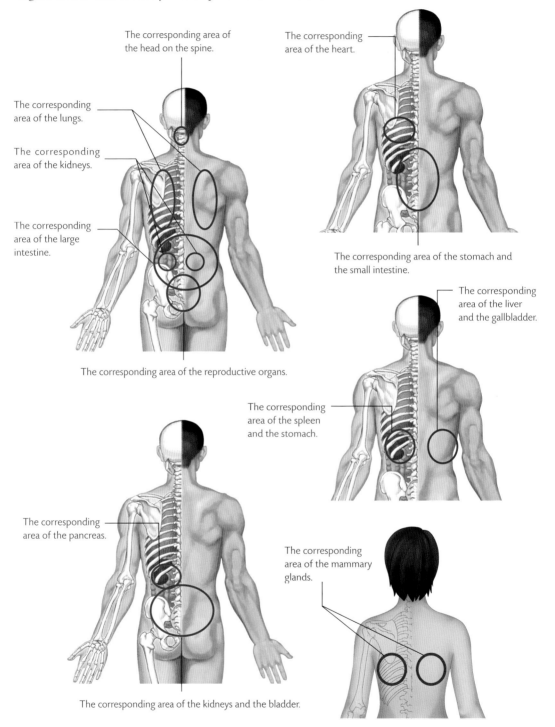

The corresponding area of the head on the spine.

The corresponding area of the heart.

The corresponding area of the lungs.

The corresponding area of the kidneys.

The corresponding area of the large intestine.

The corresponding area of the reproductive organs.

The corresponding area of the stomach and the small intestine.

The corresponding area of the liver and the gallbladder.

The corresponding area of the spleen and the stomach.

The corresponding area of the pancreas.

The corresponding area of the mammary glands.

The corresponding area of the kidneys and the bladder.

Fig. 21 Sketch maps of the corresponding areas on the spine.

3. Scraping Tools

In the past, people often used spoons, copper coins, tender bamboo plates as the scrapers, while using clean water and various kinds of plant oil as lubricants. These tools are simple and available with good effects. However, they are apt to injure skin and that they look coarse for today's people.

Nowadays, holographic scrapers are mostly used. Their edges match perfectly with the anatomic form of each area on the human body, bringing stimulation right to the place while being conducive to increasing the comfort of the scraping. Besides, professional lubricants are now available for the scraping. The combination of the new scraper with the new lubricants makes the scraping more comfortable with more obvious results.

Holographic Scraper

This scraper is oblong with smooth edges and four blunt round angles. Both long sides can scrape the flat areas of the body, while two protruding angles are very suitable for scraping the cavity on the body, as well as for scraping acupoints on the spine and the head.

The holographic scraper is generally made of jade which looks crystal-clear in addition to fine texture, larger density and nice property of heat conduction. The application of the holographic scraper can not only cure and prevent illness, but also nurture yin, reduce inner heat and cultivate mental tranquility. It's better for the operator to keep such a scraper for exclusive use in order to avoid cross-infection (fig. 22).

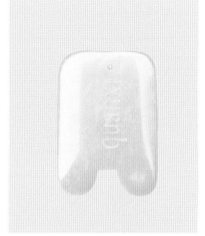

Fig. 22 The holographic scraper for meridians and collaterals.

Multi-Functional Scraping Comb

Its biggest difference from other kinds of scraping plates is that one of its long edges has been designed into thick comb teeth, which is convenient for combing acupoints over the head, without doing harm to the head and the skin. Apart from being used to comb and scrape the head, it can also be applied to the body all over.

This scraper is generally made of buffalo horn, being free from the static electricity. The buffalo horn is also marked by the effect of dispersing blockage in the circulation of vital energy, reduction of heat, expulsion of toxin, invigoration of blood and elimination of stasis. Using it to scrape the body plays a very good role in health care (fig. 23).

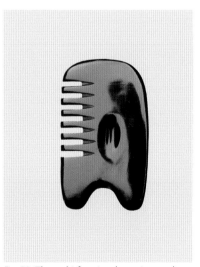

Fig. 23 The multi-functional scraping comb.

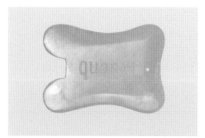
Fig. 24 The jade scraper for beautification.

Jade Scraper for Beauty Care

This kind of scraper has four different edges. The curve of its edges is designed according to the anatomic form of different facial parts. The short curve is suitable for scraping the forehead and the long curve for scraping the face, while two protruding angles are suitable for scraping the lower jaw, the nose bridge and the acupoint around eyes (fig. 24).

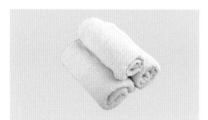
Fig. 25 Clean and soft towels.

Towels or Clean Napkins

Towels or napkins are necessary due to the flow of the scraping oil in the course of the scraping and that the patient has to put on clothes or cover the body with clothes, but the scraping oil tends to remain wet. So, preparing a clean and soft cotton towel or some napkins can save you a lot of trouble (fig. 25).

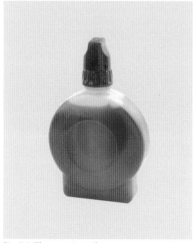
Fig. 26 The scraping oil.

Scraping Oil

As lubricant, the scraping oil is generally made of Chinese herbal medicine featured by reduction of heat, expulsion of toxin, invigoration of blood, elimination of stasis and inflammation, stoppage of pain without toxic and side effect, as well as plant oil with strong penetration and nice lubrication. Chinese herbal medicine is conducive to smoothing main and collateral channels, promoting the circulation of vital energy and blood as well as expelling stasis, while plant oil helps to moisten and protect the skin. The application of the scraping oil can not only lubricate the skin and reduce pain, but also speed up the expulsion of evil substances and prevent infection (fig. 26).

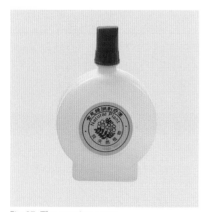
Fig. 27 The scraping cream.

Scraping Cream

It can be used since the liquid scraping oil is apt to flow, making it inconvenient to be applied to the face. The scraping cream is a kind of ointment composed of Chinese herbal medicine with quite nice lubricity. The elements of Chinese medicine in it are mild, with the effect of invigorating blood, dispersing stasis, improving the micro-circulation of the face and nurturing the skin. Please pay attention not to use face-creams for daily-care as the lubricant for the scraping, since most of the elements in them are not natural (fig. 27).

4. Steps and Methods of *Gua Sha*

There are mainly three steps, i.e., choose the body position, choose the scraping areas and operation. However, before and after the scraping, some preparation and follow-up work are needed. For example, the interior environment should be adjusted before the scraping. After the scraping, the patient should drink an appropriate amount of water and pay attention to keeping warm. Concrete methods for scraping also involve many aspects, such as the timing, the extent of force and speed as well as skills by hand.

Choose an Appropiate Place

Before scraping, a suitable environment should be chosen, with an interior environment of fresh air and moderate temperature being the best. The room temperature had better be above 18℃. When the room temperature is too high, the patient should not be exposed to direct cold wind from the air-conditioner or the electric fan.

Choose a Comfortable Body Position

A suitable body position can relax yourself and your muscles, leading to better effects of scraping and the reduction of pain in the course of scraping. The scraper should decide to choose a suitable body position according to the area to be scraped. Generally, there are three kinds of body positions as follows:

Sitting Position

The sitting position is chosen when one scrapes oneself except the waist. If scraping is performed by another person, the patient, except being scraped on the chest and the abdomen, had better face the chair back while sitting with arms placed on the chair back as a supporter (fig. 28).

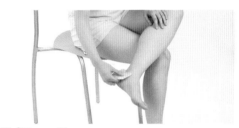
Fig. 28 Sitting position.

Lie on the Back

The patient had better lie on the back when being scraped on such areas as the forehead, the head top, the face, the chest, the abdomen and the front side of lower limbs (fig. 29).

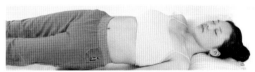
Fig. 29 Lie on the back.

Lie Prostrate

The patient had better lie prostrate when being scraped on such areas as the rear of the head, the shoulders, the back, the waist and the rear side of lower limbs. The abdomen should be cushioned with a soft pillow as a supporter to prevent the waist from falling down, which can lead to the muscle tension in the waist and back and influence the scraping effect or increase pain (fig. 30).

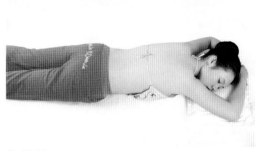
Fig. 30 Lie prostrate.

Choose Locations on the Body

It is very important to choose a correct area for the scraping. The area for the scraping should be judged and chosen according to the physique, symptoms and purpose of treatment of each individual. There are different channels, acupoints or body surface for scraping that are corresponding to different diseases or physical conditions. Concrete scraping areas for specific diseases can be referred to in cases illustrated from Chapter Three to Chapter Six.

With the area for the scraping chosen, expose this area to the full and use napkins to protect clothes near the area to avoid being dirtied. Then, apply scraping oil to this area to start operation (please apply the beauty care cream if the area is on the face) (fig. 31).

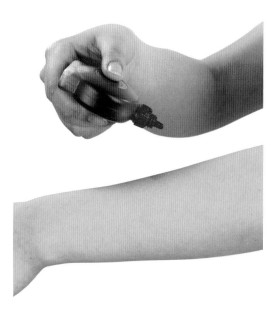

Fig. 31 Apply scraping oil to the area for scraping.

Methods of *Gua Sha*

With the scraper in hand, first use the scraper-rim to smear the skin with scraping oil from bottom upward vertically and evenly. Then, decide on the direction, time, force, speed and techniques of the scraping according to the physique of the patient, the area for scraping and the purpose of scraping. These elements exert a considerable influence on the effect of scraping. A good mastery of points of attention and techniques can enhance the effect of treatment or health care.

Generally, scraping should center on the acupoint. The operator is supposed to move the scraper around within a range of 8 to 15 centimeters as the total length, a range larger than the related acupoint in principle. If the channel to be scraped is quite long, then it can be scraped in sections. There are no strict requirements for scraping order and that the area scraped can be chosen as the case may be. In order to reduce the number of times of taking off and putting on clothes, the operator can start from the upper body to the lower part of the body, from the back and waist to the chest and abdomen, from the torso to four limbs. Besides, the appearance of *sha* and pain in the course of the scraping are normal, with no harm to the health. A good mastery of correct points of attention and techniques can reduce pain while maintaining the curative effect. Points of attention for the scraping are concretely introduced as follows.

The Scraping Direction

Generally, scraping proceeds from top to bottom or from inside to outside many times in the same direction. For example, start from top to bottom when scraping the back, the abdomen and the four limbs (but from the bottom-up if the patient suffers from limb edema, varicosity or visceral ptosis); Start from the neck toward each side of the shoulder-peak when scraping shoulders; Proceed from inside to outside when scraping the ribs and the face.

The Scraping Time

It is usually decided by the physique, scraping area, state of illness and the force applied in the scraping. Generally, it takes no more than 20 minutes each time and the time should be shortened for weak patient as the case may be.

The scraping time can be adjusted according to the speed and the number of times of the scraping. The time can be prolonged as the case may be if the speed of the scraping goes slow. The scraping of each area should stop when pores open slightly or *sha* appears. There will inevitably be pain if the same area is scraped for too long time. If the pain becomes obvious, scraping should stop at once even if there is no appearance of *sha*, and that the operator can turn to a different area (fig. 32).

The interval of the scraping should also be decided according to the physique of the patient and how well the patient has recovered. The criterion is that the partial skin has become normal and that fatigue and the sense of pain when touched have disappeared. Generally, the disappearance of *sha* takes 5 to 7 days on average, and 2 to 3 days as the quickest. The slowest will be about two weeks.

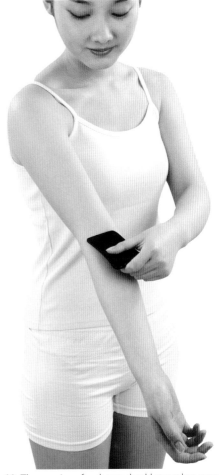

Fig. 32 The scraping of each area should stop when pores open slightly or *sha* appears.

The Scraping Force

Considerable pressure should always be kept in the course of the scraping so as to exert the force of the scraping into deep tissues to produce the curative effect. Only scraping the skin surface will not produce any curative effect, and is likely to cause edema.

However, it does not mean the greater the pressure is, the better the effect will be. Patients of different physique and state of illness should be dealt with as the case may be. If greater force for the scraping is required, the operator should gradually increase the force so that the patient can adapt himself/herself slowly to the force to reduce pain.

The Scraping Speed

Each time, the speed for the scraping should be stable and even with a constant speed. Generally speaking, the quicker the scraping goes, the more painful the patient feels. The slower the scraping goes, the less painful the patient feels.

The Methods of Holding and Using the Scraper

It is very simple to hold the scraper, i.e., hold the scraper in one hand with its bottom rim laid on the center of the palm, while the thumb and the other four fingers bent inward, respectively on the both sides of the scraper (fig. 33). Press downward with the force of the palm center when scraping. There are many ways of using the scraper. However, for the family treatment and health-care, you only need to master several basic ones of them. Commonly-used ways are as follows:

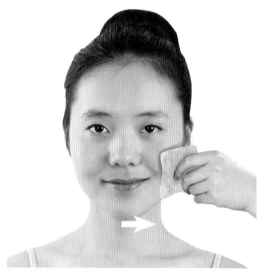

Fig. 33 The method of holding the scraper.

• **Flat-Scraping**

Press the entire surface of a scraper against the skin, and then tilt the scraper with an angle no more than 15 degrees away from the skin surface. The pressing force should be larger than the force pushing forward. This serves to reduce pain and has strong downward penetration force, which is suitable for sensitive areas on the body (fig. 34).

• **Surface-Scraping**

Press the longer side of the scraper against the skin and incline it toward the scraping direction at an angle of 30 to 60 degrees (45 degrees would be best). Then scrape evenly in the same direction. This method is suitable for flat areas on the body (fig. 35).

Fig. 34 Flat-scraping.

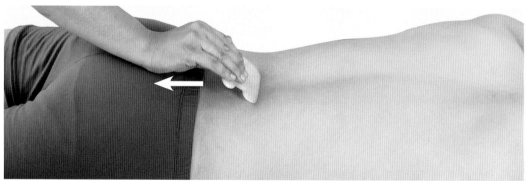

Fig. 35 Face-scraping.

• Angle-Scraping

It is divided into single-angle scraping and dual-angle scraping. As for the single-angle scraping, a corner of the scraper is used to scrape the acupoint from top to bottom at an inclined angle of 45 degrees (fig. 36). This method is often applied to such acupoints as Jianzhen point, Danzhong point and Fengchi point. In dual-angle scraping, the groove of the scraper is directed at the spinous process of the spine, with the two corners on both sides of the groove gently placed between the spinous process of the spine and the processus transversus on both sides at an inclined angle of 45 degrees downward, scraping from top to bottom. This is mostly applied to the spine (fig. 37).

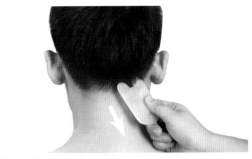

Fig. 36 Single-angle scraping.

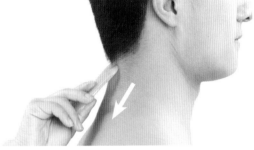

Fig. 37 Dual-angle scraping.

• Sharp-Edge Scraping

Press one corner of the scraping plate at a vertical angle of 90 degrees against the acupoint area. Always attach the scraper to the skin, and rub and scrap it forward and backward, left and right (within a short distance of about 2 to 3 centimeters) with some pressure. This is suitable for reflection areas on the head (fig. 38) (please refer to the map of holographic areas on the head on Page 44).

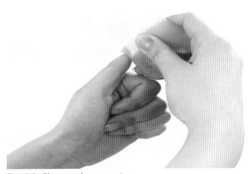

Fig. 38 Sharp-edge scraping.

• Concentrated Pressing

Press the corner of the scraping plate at an angle of 90 degrees against the acupoint and press downward vertically, with the force becoming gradually heavier. Then, lift the plate quickly after a while. This method suits such acupoints as Renzhong and Xiyan (fig. 39).

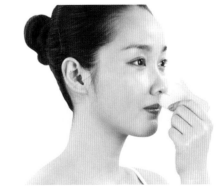

Fig. 39 Concentrated pressing.

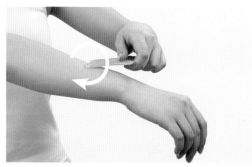
Fig. 40 Flat-pressing and kneading.

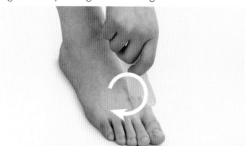
Fig. 41 Vertical-pressing and kneading.

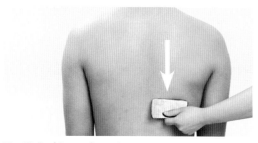
Fig. 42 Pushing and scraping.

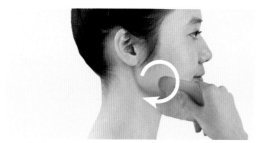
Fig. 43 Angle-kneading.

- **Pressing and Kneading**

This method is divided into flat-pressing and kneading and vertical-pressing and kneading. Flat-pressing and kneading is to press one side of the scraper corner tilting no more than 20 degrees against an appropriate acupoint, followed by slow and gentle kneading in a circular manner (fig. 40). This method usually suits Hegu point, Neiguan point and Zusanli point as well as other areas sensitive to the pain. Vertical-pressing and kneading is to press the scraper against the acupoint with the edge of the scraping plate tilting at angle of 90 degrees, followed by gentle and slow pressing and kneading. This method suits the acupoint in the bone seams and the reflection areas at the radial side of the second palm bone (fig. 41).

- **Pushing and Scraping**

The scraping plate inclines at an angle no more than 45 degrees toward the scraping direction, with the scraping progressing forward inch by inch. Its pressing force is greater than that of the flat-scraping and its speed is slower than that of the flat-scraping (fig. 42).

- **Angle-Kneading**

Use the corner on the thicker side of the scraper to move around in a whirling way near the acupoint on the body surface. The scraping plate should stay unmoved on the skin surface while kneading, but adopt continuous whirls to trigger off the tissue movement under the skin (fig. 43).

The Scraping Techniques

This is divided into reinforcing method and reducing method. Reducing method is applied to the patient of excess syndrome marked by strong physique with red face and ears, excessive evil elements, or the patient in emergency, which requires bigger force and quicker speed during *gua sha*. Reinforcing method should be applied to the patient of deficiency syndrome featured by old age, weakness and pale face, requiring smaller force and slower speed in scraping. In the course of the scraping, if obvious pain, nodules and nodes are found, reinforcing method should first be applied, i.e., slowly scrape and press to reduce pain. For the patient with quite obvious pain, use the flat-scraping method or the pushing and scraping method.

> **Skills to Reduce Pain during *Gua Sha***
>
> To reduce pain in the process of scraping, apart from the mastery of correct scraping methods, adjusting the scraping surface and the angle of the scraper can also reduce pain. As for the scraping surface, the smaller the point of force is, the more painful the patient will feel. On the contrary, enlarging the contact surface of the scraping plate on the skin can reduce pain. In terms of the scraping angle of the scraper, the principle is that it should be conducive to reducing the pain of the patient and making the scraping convenient for the operator. Pain will increase when the tilting angle of the scraping plate with the scraping direction is larger than 45 degrees. Such an angle should be smaller than 15 degrees for the patient sensitive to pain or for the scraped area sensitive to pain. In this way, pain will be obviously reduced.

Keep Warm after Gua Sha

After scraping, use clean napkins or towels to press the area scraped to wipe out remaining oil, put on clothes quickly and drink some warm water to keep warm.

5. Different *Gua Sha* Methods for Different Parts of the Body

Appropriate scraping methods should be chosen according to the anatomic features of different body parts.

The Head

The surface-scraping should be applied over the head since it is covered with hair, without the application of the lubricant. To reinforce the scraping effect, the thin edge or the corner of the scraping plate can be used. Each area can be scraped for about 30 times until the scalp feels heat. Several ways of scraping are concretely introduced as follows:

Taiyang Point

Use the corner of the scraping plate to scrape this acupoint from the front to the back or from up to down (fig. 44).

Both Sides of the Head

Attach the scraping plate vertically to the area between Touwei point and the lower

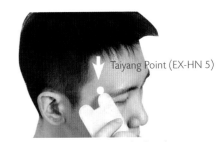

Taiyang Point (EX-HN 5)

Fig. 44 Scraping Taiyang point on the head.

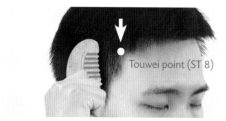

Touwei point (ST 8)

Fig. 45 Scraping Towei point on the head.

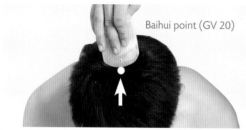

Baihui point (GV 20)

Fig. 46 Scraping Baihui point on the head.

sideburns and scrape all the way from the hairline above the ear to the rear of the hairline (fig. 45).

The Top of the Head

With Baihui point as the border of the top of the head, scrape from the hairline of the forehead to Baihui point or from Baihui point to the hairline from left to right (fig. 46).

The Rear of the Head

Scrape from Baihui point down to the hairline at the rear of the neck from left to right orderly. Fengchi point can also be scraped with the corner of the scraping plate. You can also take Baihui point as the center, and scrape toward all directions.

Reflection Areas on the Head

Scrape the frontal belt of the head top from the front to the rear or vice versa. Scrape the rear belt on the head and the lateral occipital belt from up to down. Scrape the anterior temporal belt and the posterior temporal belt from up to down. Scrape the mid-frontal belt and the lateral-frontal belt from up to down. For health-care, scraping can be done in either up-down or left-right directions. Sharp-edge scraping method is adopted when scraping the reflection areas on the head (fig. 47).

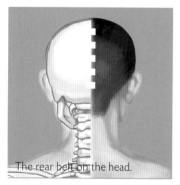

The rear belt on the head.

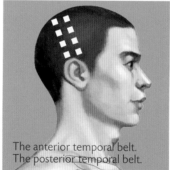

The anterior temporal belt.
The posterior temporal belt.

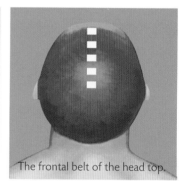

The frontal belt of the head top.

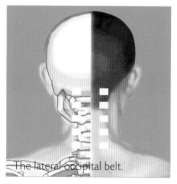

The lateral occipital belt.

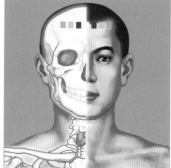

■ The first lateral-frontal belt.
▫ The second lateral-frontal belt.
▪ The third lateral-frontal belt.
The mid-frontal belt.

Fig. 47 Reflection areas on the head.

The Face

Scrape the face from inside to outside according to the direction of facial muscle. Since the appearance of *sha* on the face looks unpleasant, scraping should be gentle and that large-area scraping with heavy force is a taboo. Ask for the permission of the patient before scraping the eyes, mouth, ears and nose for treatment, for it can cause appearance of *sha* in these areas. The force, direction, angle and the number of times for the scraping of the face depends on the convenience of the scraping and the tolerance of the affected part in receiving the scraping (fig. 48).

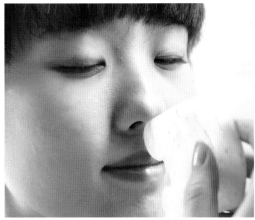
Fig. 48 Scraping acupoints on the face.

The Back

Scrape the back from up to down. Generally, first scrape Du Meridian along the central line on the back and then the Bladder Meridian and Jiaji points. For shoulder problems, scrape from the neck to the acromion on either side respectively (fig. 49).

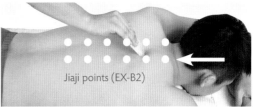
Jiaji points (EX-B2)

Fig. 49 Scraping acupoints on the back.

The Chest

Use the corner of the scraping plate to scrape from Tiantu point to Danzhong point along Ren Meridian at the central line on the chest from up to down. For both sides of the chest, scrape from the anterior median line of Ren Meridian to the left or right along the ribs with the edge of the scraper, pay attention to avoiding the nipples. Scrape the Zhongfu point from up to down with the corner of the scraper (fig. 50).

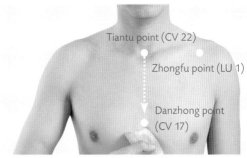
Tiantu point (CV 22)
Zhongfu point (LU 1)
Danzhong point (CV 17)

Fig. 50 Scraping acupoints on the chest.

The Waist

Scrape the waist from up to down with the entire edge or one-third of the edge of the scraper. Scrape from the left side of the waist to its right side in order. For the patient with the visceroptosis, scrape from bottom-up (fig. 51).

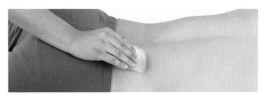
Fig. 51 Scraping acupoints on the waist.

Four Limbs

Scrape four limbs from the near-end to the far-end. For the patient suffering from lower-limb varicosity and lower-limb edema, scrape from the far-end of limbs to the near-end. The force of the scraping should be reduced at the joints or bony parts of the body (fig. 52).

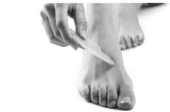
Fig. 52 Scraping acupoints on four limbs.

6. Expelling Toxin of Internal Organs through *Gua Sha*

According to the Chinese medicine, the human body is an organic entity with five major inner organs as the core. These organs are marked by yin and yang respectively. Yin and yang form an integral part and exert influence on one another. For instance, the heart integrates with small intestine, lungs integrate with large intestine, the spleen integrates with the stomach, the liver integrates with the gallbladder, kidneys integrate with the bladder and the pericardium integrates with the tri-*jiao*. Only by having understood these relations can the operator get twice the result with half the efforts in expelling toxin in all inner organs.

Scraping Methods for Expelling Toxin in the Heart and the Small Intestine
Areas to Be Scraped

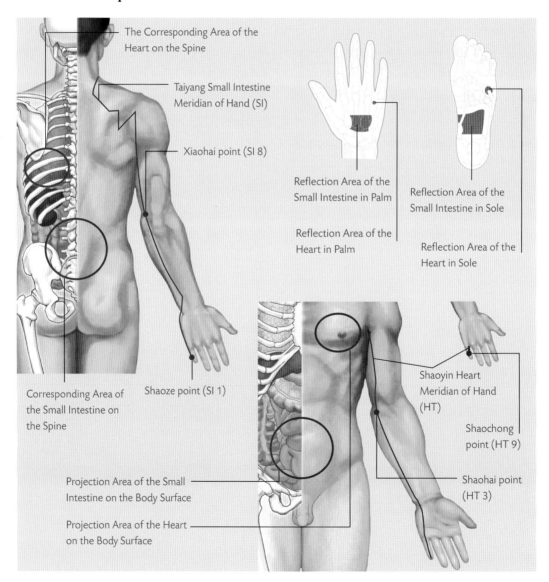

Methods of Scraping

1. Use the surface-scraping to scrape the corresponding area of the heart and the corresponding area of the small intestine on the spine from top to bottom.

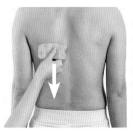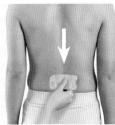

2. Use the surface-scraping to scrape the projection area of the heart and the projection area of the small intestine on the body-surface from top to bottom.

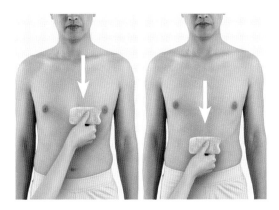

Tips from Chinese Medicine

For the purpose of expelling toxin in inner organs through scraping, once or twice each week will be enough for each organ and that the appearance of *sha* is not a must. The best timeslot for expelling toxin in the heart is between 11:00 a.m. and 13:00 p.m., during which a small nap will be nice for nurturing the heart and expelling toxin at the same time. The following period between 13:00 p.m. and 15:00 p.m. will be the time for expelling toxin in the small intestine. During this period, the patient can eat something as proper supplement of nutrients and do some simple exercise, such as kicking legs, which can stimulate the Small Intestine Meridian for better movement.

3. Use the single-angle kneading to press and knead the reflection area of the heart and the reflection area of the small intestine in palm.

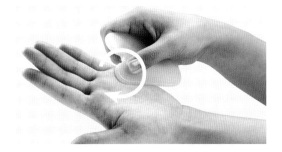

4. Use the surface-scraping to scrape Shaoyin Heart Meridian of Hand and Taiyang Small Intestine Meridian of Hand, with focus on scraping from Shaohai point to Shaochong point, and from Xiaohai point to Shaoze point.

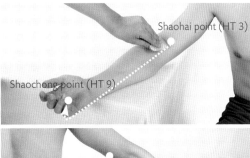

Shaohai point (HT 3)
Shaochong point (HT 9)

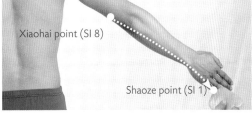

Xiaohai point (SI 8)
Shaoze point (SI 1)

5. Use the single-angle kneading to press and knead the reflection area of the heart and the reflection area of the small intestine in sole.

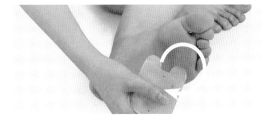

Scraping Methods for Expelling Toxin in the Lungs and the Large Intestine
Areas to Be Scraped

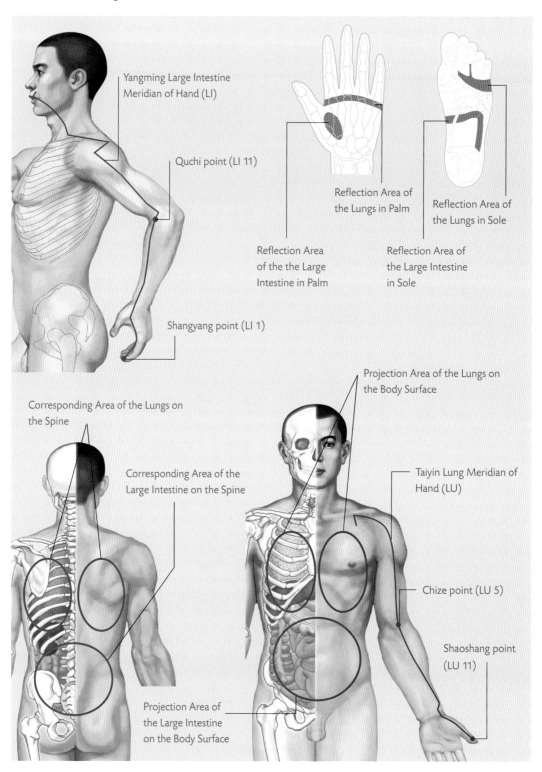

Yangming Large Intestine Meridian of Hand (LI)

Quchi point (LI 11)

Reflection Area of the Lungs in Palm

Reflection Area of the Lungs in Sole

Reflection Area of the the Large Intestine in Palm

Reflection Area of the Large Intestine in Sole

Shangyang point (LI 1)

Projection Area of the Lungs on the Body Surface

Corresponding Area of the Lungs on the Spine

Corresponding Area of the Large Intestine on the Spine

Taiyin Lung Meridian of Hand (LU)

Chize point (LU 5)

Shaoshang point (LU 11)

Projection Area of the Large Intestine on the Body Surface

Methods of Scraping

1. Use the surface-scraping to scrape the corresponding area of the lungs and the corresponding area of the large intestine on the spine from top to bottom.

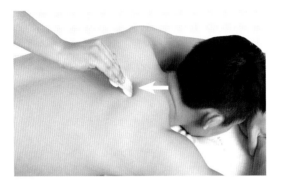

2. Use the surface-scraping to scrape the projection area of the lungs and the projection area of the large intestine on the body surface from top to bottom.

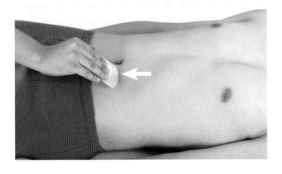

Tips from Chinese Medicine
The time for expelling toxin in lungs is between 3:00 a.m. and 5:00 a.m. in early morning, the period when people should be in deep sleep. People who are apt to cough due to problematic lungs often suffer more in this period. Pressing and kneading the Taiyuan point on Lung Meridian on the inside of the arm can ease the symptom. The time for expelling toxin in Large Intestinal Meridian is the period between 5:00 a.m. and 7:00 a.m. This is the period when people should get up to have bowel movement, which can make the body feel relaxed the whole day.

3. Use the flat-pressing and kneading to press and knead the reflection area of the lungs and the reflection area of the large intestine in palm.

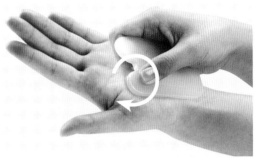

4. Use the surface-scraping to scrape from Chize point to Shaoshang point along the Lung Meridian, and from Quchi point to Shangyang point along the Large Intestine Meridian.

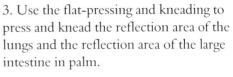
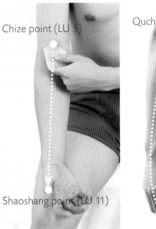
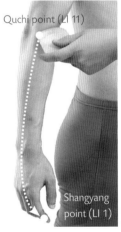

Chize point (LU 5)   Quchi point (LI 11)
Shaoshang point (LU 11)   Shangyang point (LI 1)

5. Use the flat-pressing and kneading to press and knead the reflection area of the lungs and the reflection area of the large intestine in sole.

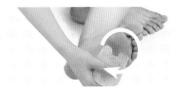

Scraping Methods for Expelling Toxin in the Liver and the Gallbladder
Areas to Be Scraped

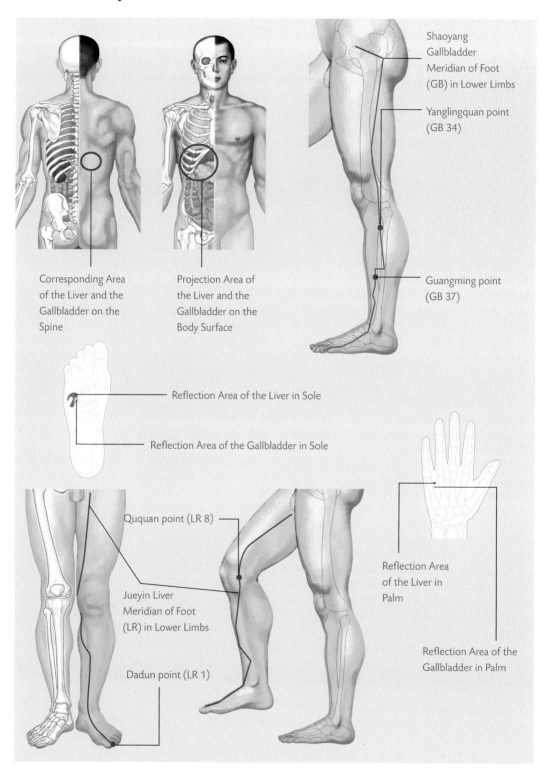

Corresponding Area of the Liver and the Gallbladder on the Spine

Projection Area of the Liver and the Gallbladder on the Body Surface

Shaoyang Gallbladder Meridian of Foot (GB) in Lower Limbs

Yanglingquan point (GB 34)

Guangming point (GB 37)

Reflection Area of the Liver in Sole

Reflection Area of the Gallbladder in Sole

Ququan point (LR 8)

Jueyin Liver Meridian of Foot (LR) in Lower Limbs

Dadun point (LR 1)

Reflection Area of the Liver in Palm

Reflection Area of the Gallbladder in Palm

Methods of Scraping

1. Use the surface-scraping to scrape the corresponding area of the liver and the gallbladder on the spine from top to bottom.

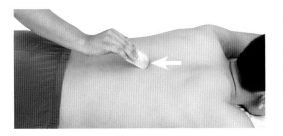

2. Use the surface-scraping to scrape the projection area of the liver and the gallbladder on the body surface from up to bottom.

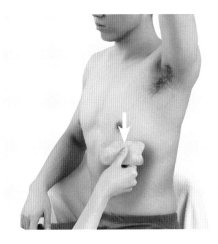

Tips from Chinese Medicine
The period of expelling toxin in the gallbladder is between 23:00 p.m. and 1:00 a.m. at midnight, the period in which yang energy begins to go up. People will be apt to suffer from insomnia if they don't sleep in this period. Long-term insomnia will affect human functions all over the body and further influence functions of the inner organs. The period of expelling toxin in the liver is between 1:00 a.m. and 3:00 a.m. in the early hours, the high time in which the liver produces blood and expels toxin, requiring the guarantee for deep sleep. People with undesirable functions of the liver and the gallbladder must not often stay up late.

3. Use the flat-pressing and kneading to press and knead the reflection areas of the liver and the gallbladder in palm.

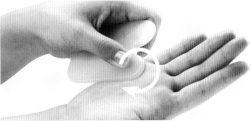

4. Use the surface-scraping to scrape from Yanglingquan point to Guangming point along the Gallbladder Meridian in lower limbs, and from Ququan point to Dadun point along the Liver Meridian.

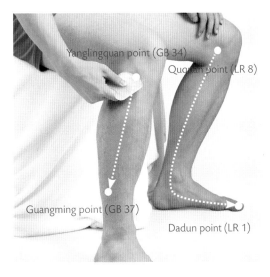

Yanglingquan point (GB 34)
Ququan point (LR 8)
Guangming point (GB 37)
Dadun point (LR 1)

5. Use the flat-pressing and kneading to press and knead the reflection areas of the liver and the gallbladder in sole.

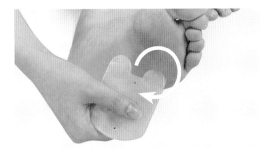

Scraping Methods for Expelling Toxin in the Spleen and the Stomach Areas to Be Scraped

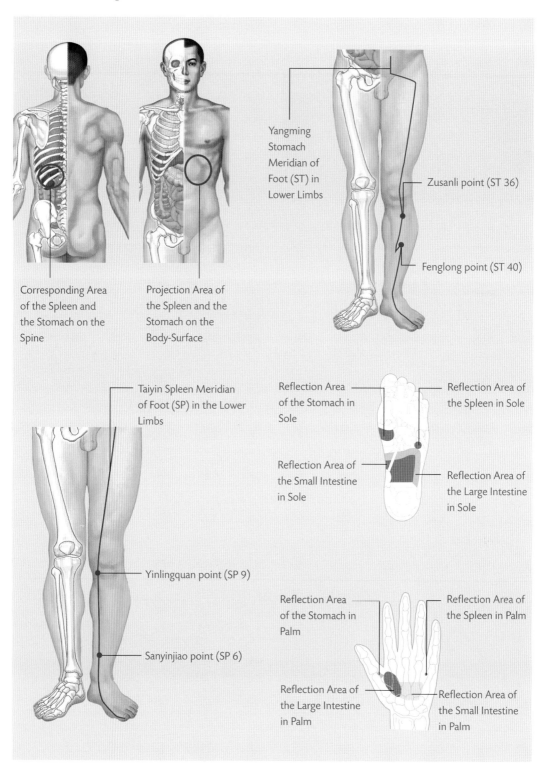

Corresponding Area of the Spleen and the Stomach on the Spine

Projection Area of the Spleen and the Stomach on the Body-Surface

Yangming Stomach Meridian of Foot (ST) in Lower Limbs

Zusanli point (ST 36)

Fenglong point (ST 40)

Taiyin Spleen Meridian of Foot (SP) in the Lower Limbs

Reflection Area of the Stomach in Sole

Reflection Area of the Spleen in Sole

Reflection Area of the Small Intestine in Sole

Reflection Area of the Large Intestine in Sole

Yinlingquan point (SP 9)

Sanyinjiao point (SP 6)

Reflection Area of the Stomach in Palm

Reflection Area of the Spleen in Palm

Reflection Area of the Large Intestine in Palm

Reflection Area of the Small Intestine in Palm

Methods of Scraping

1. Use the surface-scraping to scrape the corresponding area of the spleen and the stomach on the spine from top to bottom.

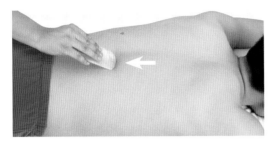

2. Use the surface-scraping to scrape the projection area of the spleen and the stomach on the body surface from top to bottom.

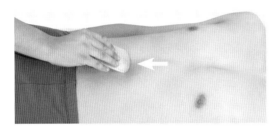

3. Use the flat-pressing and kneading to press and knead the reflection areas of the spleen, the stomach, the small intestine and the large intestoine in palm.

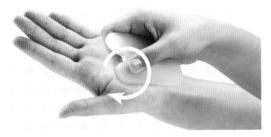

4. Use the surface-scraping to scrape from Yinlingquan point to Sanyinjian point along the Spleen Meridian, and from Zusanli point to Fenglong point along the Stomach Meridian in lower limbs.

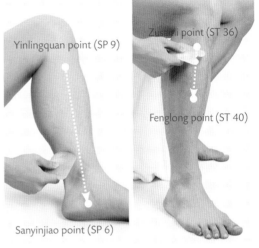

Yinlingquan point (SP 9)
Zusanli point (ST 36)
Fenglong point (ST 40)
Sanyinjiao point (SP 6)

5. Use the flat-pressing and kneading to press and knead the reflection area of the spleen, the stomach, the small intestine and the large intestine in sole.

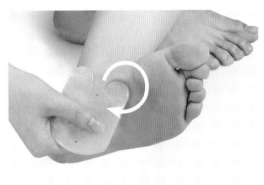

Tips from Chinese Medicine

The period between 7:00 a.m. and 9:00 a.m. in the morning is the time when the energy of Stomach Meridian is in the prime, while the period between 9:00 a.m. and 11:00 a.m. is the time when the energy of Spleen Meridian is in the prime. The stomach absorbs water and grains for digestion while the spleen turns them into vital energy and blood and conveys them all over the body. So, the period between 7:00 a.m. and 9:00 a.m. is the best time for breakfast. A timely and nice breakfast serves to smooth the generation and circulation of the vital energy and blood.

Scraping Methods for Expelling Toxin in the Kidneys and the Bladder
Areas to Be Scraped

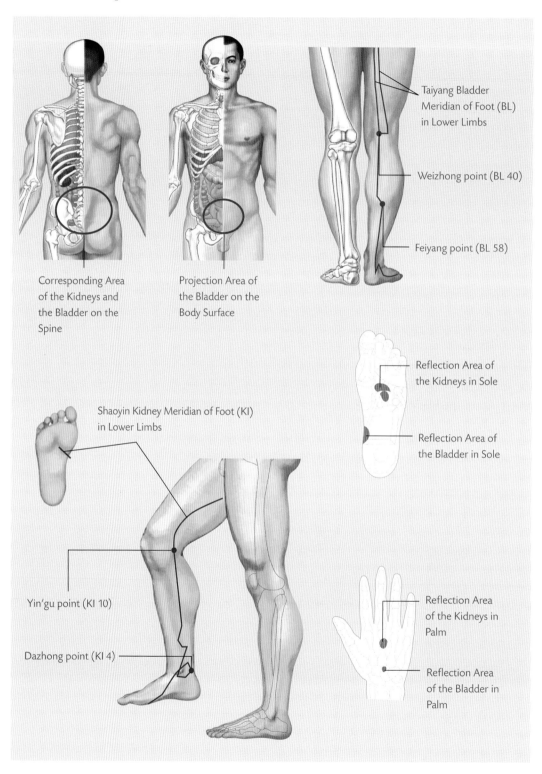

Corresponding Area of the Kidneys and the Bladder on the Spine

Projection Area of the Bladder on the Body Surface

Taiyang Bladder Meridian of Foot (BL) in Lower Limbs

Weizhong point (BL 40)

Feiyang point (BL 58)

Reflection Area of the Kidneys in Sole

Reflection Area of the Bladder in Sole

Shaoyin Kidney Meridian of Foot (KI) in Lower Limbs

Yin'gu point (KI 10)

Dazhong point (KI 4)

Reflection Area of the Kidneys in Palm

Reflection Area of the Bladder in Palm

Methods of Scraping

1. Use the surface-scraping to scrape the corresponding area of the kidneys and the bladder on the spine from top to bottom.

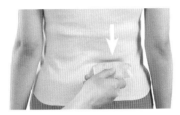

2. Use the surface-scraping to scrape the projection area of the bladder on the body surface from top to bottom.

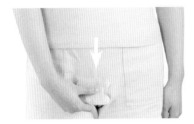

3. Use the flat-pressing and kneading to press and knead the reflection areas of the kidneys and the bladder in palm.

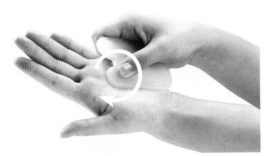

4. Use the surface-scraping to scrape from Yin'gu point to Dazhong point along the Kidney Meridian in lower limbs and from Weizhong point to Feiyang point along the Bladder Meridian.

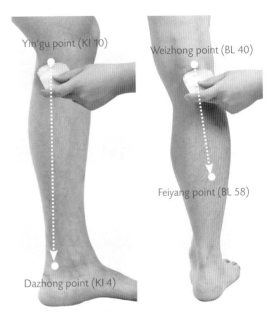

Yin'gu point (KI 10)

Weizhong point (BL 40)

Feiyang point (BL 58)

Dazhong point (KI 4)

5. Use the flat-pressing and kneading to press and knead the reflection areas of the kidneys and the bladder in sole.

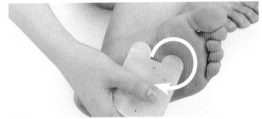

> **Tips from Chinese Medicine**
> The period between 3:00 p.m. and 5:00 p.m. is the time when the energy of Bladder Meridian is in the prime. The bladder chiefly functions as storing water and body fluids, with the water discharged and body fluids kept in the body for circulation. In this period of time, most people are at work, requiring particular attention to the supplement of water to promote the expulsion of garbage in the body, in addition to paying attention to timely discharge of urine. The period between 5:00 p.m. and 7:00 p.m. is the time when the energy of Kidney Meridian is in the prime. After a whole day's work, people would feel extremely tired. Kneading kidney can not only nurture kidneys and help kidneys to expel toxin, but also effectively ease fatigue of the whole day.

7. Diagnostic Principles of *Gua Sha*

Modern medicine has a criterion for identifying diseases, i.e., clinical symptom. A person will not be regarded as a patient for treatment unless the clinical symptom is shown. In fact, this is like mending the fold after the sheep is lost. And those people with potential health problems, if not in a state of attack, are still mistakenly regarded as being healthy.

Many kinds of diseases with no symptoms in the early stage or in the latent period are easily overlooked, resulting in the delay of diagnosis and treatment. Once the clinical symptom crops up, the illness is already very serious. Therefore, early detection and diagnosis are very important for the prevention and treatment of diseases. Scraping therapy of Chinese medicine plays the role of diagnosis ahead of time.

Scraping therapy applies an entirety view of the Chinese medicine, which is to say, the human body itself is an organic integrity. Before the occurrence of illness, any slight change in the body can be reflected at the place corresponding to the acupoint of a related meridian. Scraping therapy can get hold of the information of a certain illness before it takes place and can diagnose the area of the illness within the body before the testing of modern medicine finds any abnormality.

That is to say, any slight change within the body will cause the obstruction in the circulation of vital energy and blood in related meridians and acupoints as well as some corresponding areas whether or not the patient can feel it, and whether or not the result of biochemical or physical check-up is normal. So these small changes in the body can be quickly detected via various abnormal reactions such as the appearance of *sha* or positive reaction.

According to the rules of these reactions, one can discover sub-health status in related meridians and organs, find out the clues hidden in the early stage of illness and make diagnosis of the area of the coming illness ahead of time.

Scraping Therapy Is Both Diagnosis and Treatment

In terms of the scraping therapy, the process of diagnosis is also the course of treatment. In the process of the scraping, the scraper can observe the color and form of *sha* and various abnormal reactions under the scraping plate to judge the patient's physical condition. The appearance of *sha* and the stimulation by scraping at designated area can both play an obvious role in treatment. Therefore, the course of diagnosis is simultaneously the process of treatment. Diagnosis ahead of time through the scraping to predict illness can also offer direction for early-stage treatment.

The Appearance of *Sha* and Health

Sha will appear at the corresponding area on the skin after the scraping is done. These *sha* can be obviously different in shades of color, the form, the number and the range. Different appearances of *sha* reflect different physical status. See the table on the right for details (table 1).

Reaction during Scraping and Health

In addition to different appearances of *sha* after scraping, each person may have different manifestations in receiving the scraping. All this is closely associated with the length of time and the extent of its seriousness regarding the disorder of vital energy and blood in body parts. This can help us judge the state of patient's health and obtain information about certain illnesses. Reactions are categorized in table 2 on Page 58.

Degree of the Appearance of *Sha*	Concrete Appearance of *Sha*	Health Conditions
Dispersed *sha*	*Sha* dots can be light red or red and that there may be *sha* speckles without obvious protrusion.	It indicates good health and the *sha* dots will disappear soon.
Mild appearance of *sha*	Appearance of one or a few light red or red *sha* speckles of generally 1 to 2 centimeters in diameter, without obvious protrusion.	It indicates slight obstruction of micro-circulation and the state of sub-health, but the patient can not feel it.
Moderate appearance of *sha*	Appearance of a few purplish-red or bluish *sha* speckles of about 2 centimeters in diameter, without obvious protrusion or with slight protrusion.	It indicates medium obstruction of micro-circulation of a quite long time and the situation of sub-health or illness, sometimes with symptoms.
Severe appearance of *sha*	Appearance of dark-blue and bluish-black *sha* speckles of more than 2 centimeters in diameter in the form of lumps or blue veins, with obvious protrusion.	It indicates serious obstruction of micro-circulation of a long time and bad health with obvious illness and related symptoms.

Table 1

Sense of Touch	Concrete Manifestations	Indication
Muscle tension	Tense and stiff muscle.	Blockage of vital energy and blood circulation; deficiency of oxygen in meridians, tissues or organs with functions weakened. With excess syndrome (referring to a person whose body is intruded by exogenous pathogenic factors, resulting in the imbalance of functions of inner organs and accumulation of pathological substances within the body).
	Loosened and flaccid muscle.	Blockage of vital energy and blood circulation; deficiency of oxygen in meridians, tissues or organs with functions weakened. With deficiency syndrome (referring to a person with weakness of vital-qi due to congenital deficiency or acquired malnutrition).
Pain	Aching pain.	Deficiency of oxygen due to the blockage of vital energy and blood circulation in meridians, tissues, and organs.
	Distending pain.	Deficiency of oxygen due to the blockage of vital energy in meridians, tissues, and organs.
	Stabbing pain.	Pathological changes are taking place due to long-term stasis of vital energy and blood in meridians, tissues, and organs, but without symptoms at present.
Granular feeling	A feeling of granules without pain.	Pathological changes are taking place due to long-term stasis of vital energy and blood in meridians, tissues, and organs, but without symptoms at present.
	A feeling of granules when touched and with pain.	Deficiency of oxygen in meridians, tissues or organs due to inflammation in certain areas or long-term stasis of vital energy and blood in meridians, tissues, and organs with slight symptoms at present.
Nodules	Nodules without pain.	Long-term stasis of vital energy and blood in meridians, tissues and organs. The bigger and harder the nodules are, the more serious it is. There was inflammation in meridians, tissues, and organs, but without symptoms at present.
	Nodules with pain.	Long-term stasis of vital energy and blood in meridians, tissues, and organs, with symptoms at present.

Table 2

8. Various Benefits of *Gua Sha*

In addition to easing different symptoms by expelling toxin in the body, more importantly, scraping therapy can smooth main and collateral channels, the circulation of vital energy and blood and adjust yin and yang of the body, enhancing immune functions of the body and fundamentally preventing and curing illness. In a word, the benefits of scraping therapy are demonstrated in several aspects as follows:

Relaxing Tendons, Invigorating the Circulation of Blood and Eliminating Pain
The transport of vital energy and blood serves to nurture and warm up the human body. Scraping muscles and skin serves to disperse blood stasis and eliminate blockage. Smooth circulation of vital energy and blood throughout main and collateral channels all over the body can reduce or eliminate pain in related areas.

- **Promoting the Circulation of Vital Energy and Blood**
According to the modern medicine, scraping can lead to blood congestion, expand capillary vessels, and speed up blood circulation in related areas. Stimulation from scraping can adjust the expansion and contraction of blood vessels as well as the permeability of vascular walls through nerves and endocrines as well as enhance blood supply in related areas to improve blood circulation all over the body. The process of bringing about *sha* through scraping is actually a phenomenon marked by gradual expansion of blood vessels followed by the breakage of capillary vessels, the overflow of blood and the formation of speckles in related areas of the skin. Such blood clot (*sha*) will soon disappear to the point of self-hemolysis and form a new stimulin which can reinforce the metabolism in related areas and expel inflammation.

- **Clearing Inner Heat for Detumescence**
Physical pain is sometimes caused by swelling. There is such a principle in the treatment of Chinese medicine as "expulse heat to cure illness." Stimulation through scraping can bring inner heat out to be finally expelled. Elimination of accumulated heat and toxin inside the body serves to stop pain.

- **Relaxing Tendons and Smoothing Meridians**
Related tissues will be on the alert when there is physical pain, featured by contraction, tension, spasm and pain of muscles, which are natural and protective reactions of the human body. Without timely and thorough treatment, the affected tissues will result in adhesion and fibrosis, making spasm and pain worse. Scraping therapy is an effective way of eliminating pain, tension, and spasm of muscles. Its principle is marked by three aspects: First, scraping can reinforce vital energy and blood circulation and increase the temperature in related areas to ease spasm; Second, under the direct stimulation of the scraping plate, threshold of pain will be enhanced in related tissues; Third, muscles under tension or spasm will be relaxed due to scraping, eliminating such tension and spasm so as to remove the pain.

Reinforcing the Immunity Regulation Function to Enhance Body's Disease Resistance

One of the features of the scraping therapy is treatment of illness in addition to building up the physique of healthy people. Building up physique actually refers to the reinforcement of vital-qi, i.e., the reinforcement of immunity, which enhances the body's ability to prevent and resist illness.

- **Strengthening the Body Resistance to Eliminate Pathogenic Factors**

The areas being scraped will be marked by bruise and congestion with *sha*, permeating the space between skin texture and subcutaneous flesh and expelling the wind, cold, phlegm, dampness, blood stasis, heat, and pus in acupoints and corresponding tissues and organs through the skin and hair, which helps to smooth main and collateral channels. Exogenous pathogenic factors would take advantage to intrude when the vital-qi in the body is weakened. The techniques of supplying deficiency and expelling excess, i.e., supply vital-qi and expell malignant elements are basic principles of treatment in Chinese medicine. Patients with excess syndrome should be applied with reducing method marked by larger force and quick speed in scraping. The patient with deficiency syndrome should be applied with reinforcing method marked by smaller force and slow speed in scraping.

- **Promoting Metabolism**

Scraping the skin can reinforce the circulation of blood and lymph and fully nurture muscles and nerve endings so as to promote metabolism all over the body. Smooth metabolism serves to reduce the incidence of illness greatly. Stimulating nerve endings by scraping can reinforce the immune ability of cells and strengthen the body's defense ability.

- **Getting Rid of Sub-Health**

The life of people in modern times is featured by quick rhythm, great pressure and fatigue easily. Long-term pressure and fatigue are likely to result in a number of diseases. Frequent scraping serves to do away with fatigue, reinforce immune functions and prevent pathological changes.

Quickly Cleaning the Internal Environment for Anti-Aging and Beauty Care

The process of scraping can speed up the back flow of blood and lymph, reinforce the function of phagocyte and the force of transport, expel waste and toxin in the body quickly, nurture tissues and cells so as to clean the internal environment of the body, purify blood, smooth the route of transmitting nutrients to the skin to resist aging and beautify skin.

- **Cleaning the Environment within the Body and Purifying Blood**

Decomposition, composition, absorption and energy transformation require coordination of all inner organs and the entire body. The slow down of this process will delay the discharge of metabolites through normal channels, resulting in toxin and affecting blood circulation. Scraping therapy serves to bring out the blood with toxin and make it seep from the capillary vessels with permeability disorder to stay between the skin and muscles, i.e., the appearance of *sha*. This helps the expulsion of toxin in the blood, invigorating blood, dispersing stasis, quickly improving micro-circulation, purifying blood and cleaning the environment within the body.

- **Enabling the Skin Cells to Obtain Nutrients**

The blockage of vital energy and blood in main and collateral channels also blocks the route for skin cells to obtain nutrients, leading to the lack of nutrients in the skin, pale or yellowish face with a lack of glow, dryness and wrinkles. The delay of expelling metabolites will result in such skin problems as darkness, speckles and acne. Scraping therapy can expel blood with toxin out of blood vessels, promote blood circulation, smooth the route for skin cells to obtain nutrients, transport rich nutrients and oxygen continuously to skin tissues and cells, quickly ease the lack of oxygen in related areas, stimulate and reinforce the functions of skin cells.

- **Adjusting the Functions of Inner Organs and Delaying the Aging Process**

The first concern of people over aging lies in the skin. In fact, skin-aging goes together with the aging of inner organs, except that we cannot see inner organs. Scraping therapy seems to improve the face, but it actually adjusts the functions of the inner organs. Normal functions of the inner organs in orderly operation can delay the aging process and make people enjoy prolonged health.

Adjusting Yin and Yang to Cure Chronic Diseases

In normal circumstances, human body is kept with relative balance between yin and yang. There will be such pathological changes as "yin in excess leads to weakness of yang and yang in excess leads to weakness of yin" when the balance between them is disrupted by outer or inner malignant elements. Consequently, there will be such clinical symptoms as "inner heat caused by excessive yang and the inner cold caused by excessive yin."

- **Adjusting Yin and Yang**

The key of scraping therapy for health-care lies in adjusting yin and yang according to the attributes of symptoms, turning the body into the status of "yin and yang in equilibrium" and restoring normal physiological functions to cure illness. As proved by practice, scraping therapy can obviously adjust the functions of inner organs. For instance, for those suffering from intestinal hyperanakinesia, scraping therapy can restrain their intestinal movement and bring their intestinal functions to normal via scraping their abdomen and back. For those suffering from intestinal hypofunction, scraping therapy can bring their intestinal movement to be normal. This shows that scraping therapy can improve and adjust the functions of inner organs and balance of yin and yang of inner organs. Scraping serves to adjust yin and yang in a bidirectional way. For instance, in terms of a person with unstable blood pressure, with related acupoints on his/her body and four limbs scraped, the one of low blood pressure will have his/her blood pressure raised, while the one of high blood pressure will have his/her blood pressure reduced.

- **Curing Chronic Diseases**

Chronic diseases are marked by covert and slow incidence of illness, requiring a slow process for the cure. While expelling pathogenic evils, scraping therapy actually also serves to restore and reinforce the human functions. The application of conventional medical treatment together with scraping therapy can get twice the result with half of the efforts.

Long-term in-take of medicine for some chronic diseases such as metabolic diseases like diabetes and digestive diseases like gastritis will do harm to health, while scraping therapy is very suitable.

9. Attentions Regarding *Gua Sha*

Despite simplicity, safety, and effectiveness, there are some points of attention for scraping therapy. For instance, it is not suitable for some cases to be dealt with by the scraping therapy and that some abnormal situations will occur in the course of scraping. The health of the patient should be taken care of both in the course of and after scraping. Only by paying attention to details can the scraping therapy be made more effective and safer.

Distension and Pain in Related Areas

For some people, there might be swelling and burning sensation in the areas scraped. If such symptoms do not disappear within 24 hours, or there is still obvious pain in the related areas one or two days after the scraping, it means that the time of scraping was too long or the scraping was too much. These symptoms generally will be eased and disappear very soon if the related area is applied with a hot compress 24 hours after scraping.

Dizziness during Scraping

It refers to the symptoms that the patient is featured by fatigue and dizziness, pale complexion, vomit, cold sweat, palpitation and cold limbs. The reasons for these symptoms are mostly due to nervousness, too many areas scraped, heavy force of the operator, empty stomach or excessive fatigue.

If there are signs of dizziness in the course of scraping, the scraping therapy should be stopped at once and the patient should lie on his/her back, covered with quilt or clothes and drink warm or sweet water. For the patient with strong reaction of dizziness, the corner of the scraping plate should be lightly pressed against his/her Renzhong point and that his/her Baihui point and Yongquan point should be scraped by reducing method (see Page 42). If the patient turns better, his/her Neiguan point and Zusanli point should be scraped continuously. The two following points should be paid attention to in order to prevent dizziness during the scraping therapy:

1. The patient should avoid being on an empty stomach and excessive fatigue while receiving the scraping therapy.

2. The operator should should choose a comfortable body-position of the patient and apply proper techniques, with a few but better areas to be scraped with an appropriate amount of time.

Pay Attention to Avoiding Wind and Keeping Warm When Being Scraped

In the course of the scraping therapy, the hair-pores of the patient are open, a state vulnerable to the direct intrusion of malignant elements when it is windy and cold. This will not only affect the curative effect, but also lead to new illness. With the scraping done, the patient should cover the area scraped before going outdoors. If it is the face scraped, the patient is supposed to go outdoors thirty minutes after the scraping is over.

Treatment Is Confined to Only One Kind of Illness Each Time

The principle of treating only one kind of illness should be strictly followed and that the time for the scraping should not be too long. The operator should not try to bring about *sha* in large areas to avoid damaging the vital-qi of the patient. When a number of meridians and acupoints need to be scraped, one can choose alternatively 3 to 4 acupoints each time.

Do Not Insist on Bringing about *Sha*

Whether or not there is the appearance of *sha* in the course of the scraping, as long as hair-pores on the skin are clearly visible, malignant elements can be discharged as an curative effect.

Sha is apt to appear in cases with blood stasis, excess syndrome or heat syndrome, whereas *sha* is not apt to appear in cases with deficiency syndrome, cold syndrome, or for fat people and those who have taken hormone drugs. *Sha* is also not apt to appear under low room temperature. There will be an curative effect as long as the scraping methods and areas scraped are correct for those illnesses and areas even though *sha* is not apt to appear. Insisting on pursuing the appearance of *sha* or excessive scraping will not only exhaust vital-qi, but also lead to soft tissue injury.

Drink a Cup of Hot Water after Scraping

The appearance of *sha* and openness of hair-pores in the course of scraping will lead to the expulsion of malignant elements while exhausting fluid within the body. Therefore, drinking a cup of hot water after the scraping can supplement water, promote metabolism and speed up the expulsion of metabolized substances.

Take Bath 3 Hours after Scraping

The bath is to be taken with the hair-pores closed after the scraping in order to prevent pathogenic wind-cold from intruding the body. Generally, the patient is supposed to take a bath three hours after scraping.

Taboos for the Scraping Therapy

It is not suitable to receive the scraping therapy in seven cases as follows:
• Weak and thin people whose skin is not elastic any more.
• Areas with infectious skin diseases, skin-ulcer, exudation from wound and varicose veins of lower limbs.
• Women in menstruation. The abdomen, waist and lumbosacral area of pregnant women. Other parts of their body should also be scraped cautiously or lightly.
• Eyes, lips, tongue, earholes, nostrils, nipples, navel, vagina, penis and anus are prohibited for scraping.
• Scraping can only be done three months after the recovery of such body parts as infected skin, areas with ulcers and scars, unknown lumps, malignant tumor, acutely damaged ligaments and tendons, new fractures and the scars left over by surgical operation.
• People suffering from haemorrhagic diseases such as thrombocytopenia, leukemia, serious anaemia or hemophilia.
• People suffering from heart failure, renal failure, liver cirrhosis ascites and serious edema all over the body.

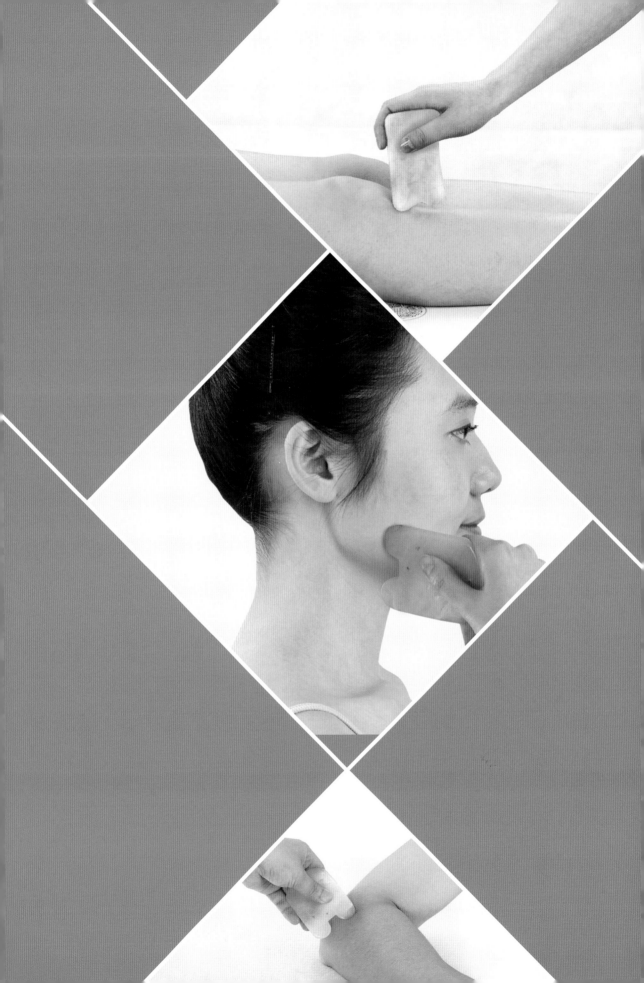

CHAPTER THREE
Use *Gua Sha* to Solve Daily Ailments

It is too troublesome to go to the hospital for some daily ailments, but people really suffer without resorting to medical treatment. Scraping is the best way of dealing with such problems. With areas chosen and techniques applied correctly, one can get rid of ailments while smoothing main and collateral channels and the circulation of vital energy and blood so as to enhance physical resistance.

Cold

Cold is mostly related to the inflammation of the respiratory tract caused by virus or bacterial infection. There are several kinds of cold due to different causes, such as wind-cold, wind-heat and summer-heat and damp. Methods of treatment vary for different kinds of cold. Therefore, scraping therapy should be applied based on the identification of different symptoms.

Cold Caused by Wind-Cold

It often occurs in cold seasons, manifested by the fear of the cold, moderate fever, headache, feeling of heaviness in the body, no sweat, stuffy nose or running nose.

Scraping just once can reduce the symptom of a person with mild symptoms. Scraping can be conducted once every day or once every other day for a person with a little *sha* or without any *sha* after the treatment. Scraping should be conducted after *sha* disappears for a person with lots of *sha* after the treatment.

Recommended Procedures
1. Fengchi Point and Feishu Point
Method: Apply scraping oil. Use the single-angle scraping to scrape Fengchi point from up to down and then use the surface-scraping to scrape Feishu point from up to down and scrape the scapular area downward and outward, until *Sha* appears.

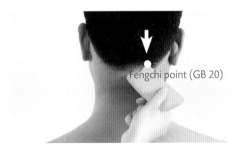

Fengchi point (GB 20)

2. Zhongfu Point
Method: Apply scraping oil. Use the single-angle scraping to scrape Zhongfu point from up to down until *Sha* appears.

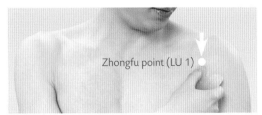

Zhongfu point (LU 1)

3. Shaoshang Point

Method: Apply scraping oil. Scrape Shaoshang point toward the end of the thumb, until *sha* appears.

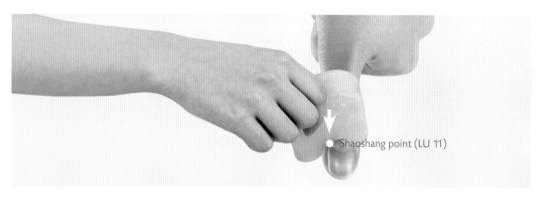

Shaoshang point (LU 11)

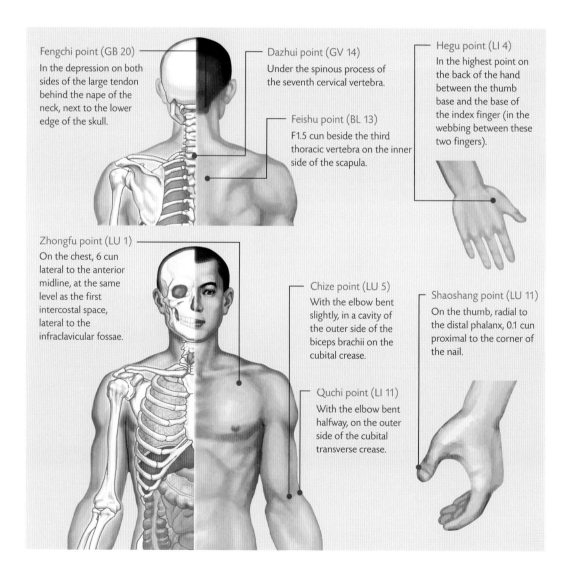

Fengchi point (GB 20)

In the depression on both sides of the large tendon behind the nape of the neck, next to the lower edge of the skull.

Dazhui point (GV 14)

Under the spinous process of the seventh cervical vertebra.

Feishu point (BL 13)

F1.5 cun beside the third thoracic vertebra on the inner side of the scapula.

Hegu point (LI 4)

In the highest point on the back of the hand between the thumb base and the base of the index finger (in the webbing between these two fingers).

Zhongfu point (LU 1)

On the chest, 6 cun lateral to the anterior midline, at the same level as the first intercostal space, lateral to the infraclavicular fossae.

Chize point (LU 5)

With the elbow bent slightly, in a cavity of the outer side of the biceps brachii on the cubital crease.

Shaoshang point (LU 11)

On the thumb, radial to the distal phalanx, 0.1 cun proximal to the corner of the nail.

Quchi point (LI 11)

With the elbow bent halfway, on the outer side of the cubital transverse crease.

Cold Caused by Wind-Heat

It often occurs in spring or at the turn between summer and autumn, which are marked by lots of wind and increasing warmth. Therefore, malignant elements of wind and warmth would cooperate to cause illness, which is generally featured by heavy fever, slight fear of cold, with or without sweat, headache and body pain, stuffy nose, running nose with yellow and turbid discharge, cough, dry and swelling throat, thirst and thick and yellow sputa. Scraping should be marked by the expulsion of the wind, clearing of heat and relief of exterior syndrome.

The symptom of the patient can be turned to wind-heat cold if lots of *sha* appears after the scraping is done, cupping can be adopted as auxiliary treatment. It is likely to be virus infection if the temperature of the patient remains the same or the patient suffers from fever again after the temperature is reduced. In this case, the patient should go to the hospital as soon as possible for check and diagnosis.

Recommended Procedures

1. Dazhui Point

Method: Apply scraping oil. Use the surface-scraping to scrape Dazhui point from up to down, until *sha* appears.

2. Quchi Point and Chize Point

Method: Apply scraping oil. Use the surface-scraping to scrape Quchi point and Chize point from up to down, until *sha* appears.

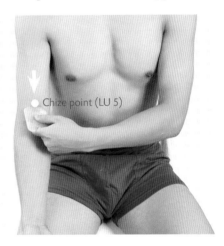

Chize point (LU 5)

3. Hegu Point

Method: Apply scraping oil, and use the single-angle scraping to scrape Hegu point 30 times, until *sha* appears.

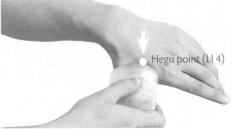

Hegu point (LI 4)

Dazhui point (GV 14)

Cold Caused by Summer-Heat and Damp

It is caused by the intrusion of heat and damp in summer as well as the patient's preference for enjoying the cool and eating cold food. Consequently, summer-heat and damp is contained by the wind-cold, resulting in illness. The symptom is featured by sweating, lingering fever after sweating, dizziness and headache, a sense of oppression in the chest, nausea, yellow and sticky tongue-coating and weak pulse. There will also be such symptoms as cough, sticky sputa and turbid nasal discharge if lungs are intruded by the summer-heat and damp.

Cold caused by summer-heat and damp and cold caused by summer-heat both result from the intrusion of pathogenic heat. However, the difference of the cause and pathogenesis of these two kinds of illness mainly lies in whether or not there is damp. Chinese medicine chiefly resorts to methods of expelling heat and damp to deal with cold caused by summer-heat and damp.

If the patient suffers from fever due to the the combination of the cold and germs or virus infection, medical treatment should be applied as the case may be under the guidance of the doctor when the scraping therapy goes on.

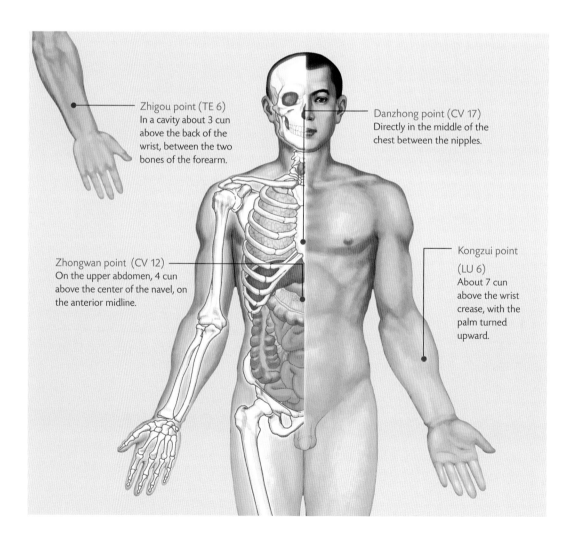

Zhigou point (TE 6)
In a cavity about 3 cun above the back of the wrist, between the two bones of the forearm.

Danzhong point (CV 17)
Directly in the middle of the chest between the nipples.

Zhongwan point (CV 12)
On the upper abdomen, 4 cun above the center of the navel, on the anterior midline.

Kongzui point (LU 6)
About 7 cun above the wrist crease, with the palm turned upward.

Recommended Procedures

1. Danzhong Point and Zhongwan Point

Method: Use the single-angle scraping to scrape Danzhong point on the chest from up to down and then Zhongwan point on the abdomen.

2. Kongzui Point, Zhigou Point and Hegu Point

Method: Use the surface-scraping to scrape Kongzui point on the inside of the upper limb, Zhigou point on the outside of the forearm and Hegu point from up to down.

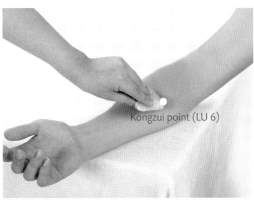

Kongzui point (LU 6)

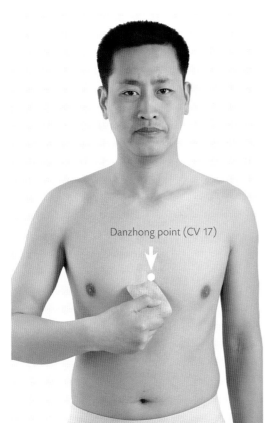

Danzhong point (CV 17)

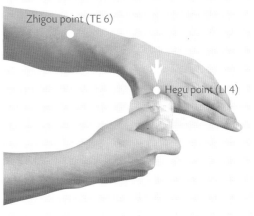

Zhigou point (TE 6)

Hegu point (LI 4)

Therapies to Increase the Curative Effect

The following method of scraping can be applied to any kind of the cold:

• Use the sharp-edge scraping to scrape the mid-frontal belt and the first lateral-frontal belt (see Page 44 for the reflection areas on the head).

• Use the surface-scraping and dual-angle scraping to scrape the corresponding area of head on the spine and the corresponding area of lungs on the spine (see Page 34 for the corresponding areas).

• Use the single-angle scraping to scrape the projection area of throat in front of the neck from up to down and the projection area of weasand at the center of the frontal chest (see Page 33 for the projection areas).

The mid-frontal belt on the head is the corresponding area of the head (including the throat), while the first lateral-frontal belt is the corresponding area of the heart and the lungs. Scraping projection areas of the throat and the weasand is conducive to curing sore throat.

Cough

Cough is one of the main symptoms of lung illness. The acute cough is caused by exterior malignant elements while the chronic one is due to interior factors. The acute cough, if not dealt with properly, will turn into chronic cough which will last long. Chronic cough of old and weak people with inner organs harmed seriously will develop into asthma. In the period of paracmasis, scraping therapy can be used to cure and prevent these two kinds of cough.

If *sha* looks very obvious in the process of the scraping therapy, scraping can be done once every three days. If not obvious, it can be done once a day. A course of scraping treatment is one week in succession. Generally, there will be curative effect within one course.

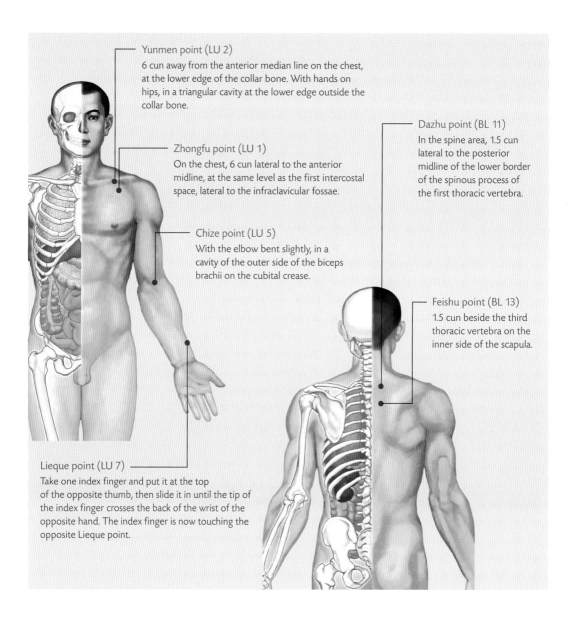

Yunmen point (LU 2)
6 cun away from the anterior median line on the chest, at the lower edge of the collar bone. With hands on hips, in a triangular cavity at the lower edge outside the collar bone.

Zhongfu point (LU 1)
On the chest, 6 cun lateral to the anterior midline, at the same level as the first intercostal space, lateral to the infraclavicular fossae.

Chize point (LU 5)
With the elbow bent slightly, in a cavity of the outer side of the biceps brachii on the cubital crease.

Lieque point (LU 7)
Take one index finger and put it at the top of the opposite thumb, then slide it in until the tip of the index finger crosses the back of the wrist of the opposite hand. The index finger is now touching the opposite Lieque point.

Dazhu point (BL 11)
In the spine area, 1.5 cun lateral to the posterior midline of the lower border of the spinous process of the first thoracic vertebra.

Feishu point (BL 13)
1.5 cun beside the third thoracic vertebra on the inner side of the scapula.

Recommended Procedures

1. Dazhu Point and Feishu Point

Method: Use the surface-scraping to scrape from Dazhu point to Feishu point on both sides from up to down.

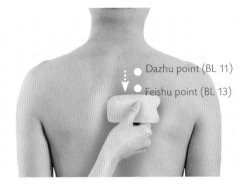

Dazhu point (BL 11)
Feishu point (BL 13)

2. Yunmen Point and Zhongfu Point

Method: Use the single-angle scraping to scrape from Yunmen point to Zhongfu point from up to down.

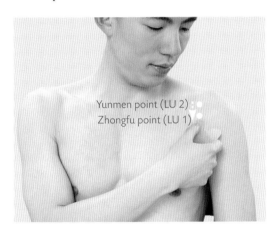

Yunmen point (LU 2)
Zhongfu point (LU 1)

3. Chize Point and Lieque Point

Method: Use the surface-scraping to scrape from Chize poin to Lieque point from up to down on both of the upper limbs.

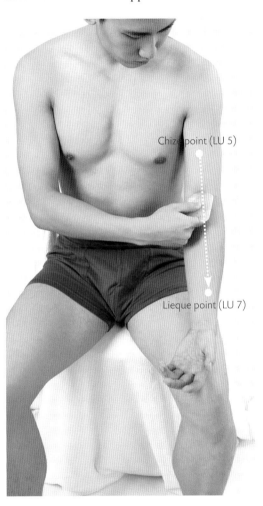

Chize point (LU 5)

Lieque point (LU 7)

Therapies to Increase the Curative Effect

It will produce much better effect for the prevention and cure of cough if the scraping goes together with diet therapy.

- **The diet therapy for the cough caused by wind-cold:** Sliced ginger of ten grams. Immerse it in the boiling water in a pot with a cover for about five minutes, and then add in brown sugar of 15 grams. With this done, drink it while it is hot once every day and then sleep under the quilt for sweating.

- **The diet therapy for the cough caused by wind-heat:** The almond, mulberry leaves and fructus arctii of 9 grams respectively as well as radix platycodi and peppermint leaves of 5 grams respectively are boiled for oral use, twice a day.

- **The diet therapy for chronic cough:** The pear, rock candy, tremella and dried lily are boiled together for oral use. This has a very good curative effect on moistening lungs to relieve cough.

Fever

It means the body temperature is higher than the normal state. According to Chinese medicine, fever can be caused by either exterior elements or interior elements. Fever caused by exterior elements often goes together with the cold, typhia and plague. Fever caused by interior elements is marked by excessive yang, excessive yin, blood deficiency or vital energy deficiency. A number of other diseases such as inflammation and cancer can also lead to fever.

The patient with high fever must lie in bed for rest and move less to reduce the exhaustion of energy and the generation of heat. Paying attention to drinking more water and enjoying nice ventilation to reduce temperature are conducive to lowering down the body temperature.

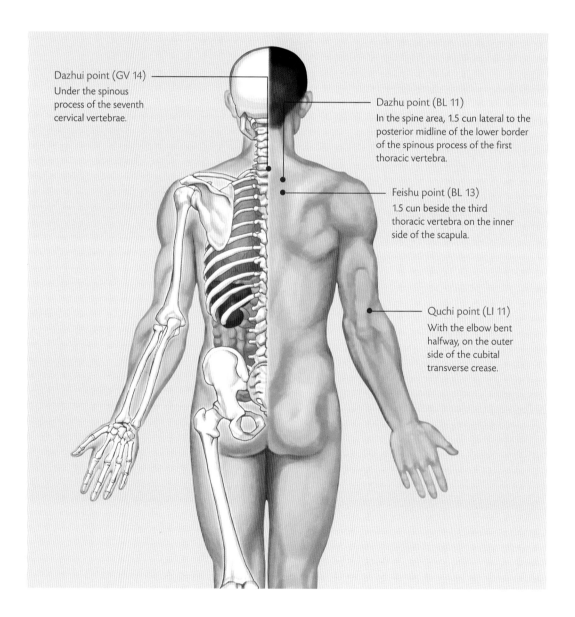

Dazhui point (GV 14)
Under the spinous process of the seventh cervical vertebrae.

Dazhu point (BL 11)
In the spine area, 1.5 cun lateral to the posterior midline of the lower border of the spinous process of the first thoracic vertebra.

Feishu point (BL 13)
1.5 cun beside the third thoracic vertebra on the inner side of the scapula.

Quchi point (LI 11)
With the elbow bent halfway, on the outer side of the cubital transverse crease.

Recommended Procedures

1. Dazhui Point

Method: Use the single-angle scraping to scrape Dazhui point.

2. Dazhu Point and Feishu Point

Method: Use the surface-scraping to scrape from Dazhu point to Feishu point.

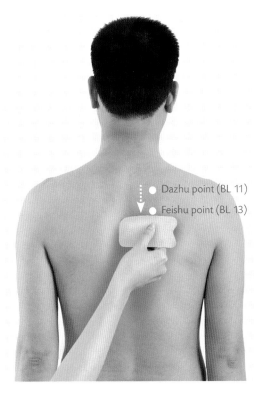

Dazhu point (BL 11)
Feishu point (BL 13)

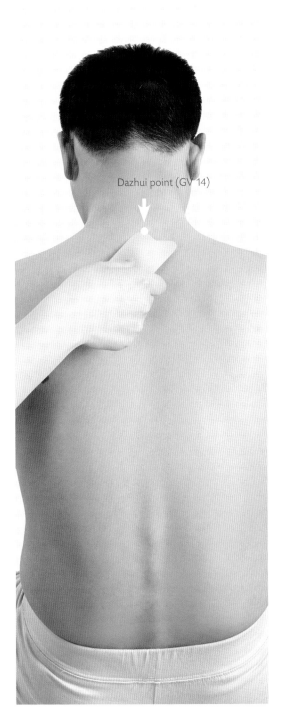

Dazhui point (GV 14)

3. Quchi Point

Method: Use the corner-edge of the scraping plate to scrape Quchi point from up to down until the skin turns red and *sha* appears.

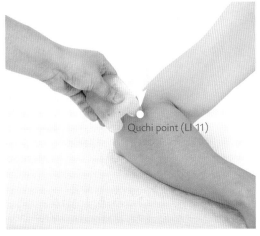

Quchi point (LI 11)

Swollen Sore Throat

It means red swelling and pain in the throat. It is mostly seen in exogenous diseases in the throat, with amygdalitis being the most common. It attacks very quickly, usually lasting for 4 to 6 days. It is apt to become chronic after a number of attacks. Chronic swollen sore throat is likely to induce rheumatic fever and nephritis, requiring more attention.

Acute and chronic amygdalitis, pharyngitis and laryngitis can all be treated with reference to the methods illustrated as follows.

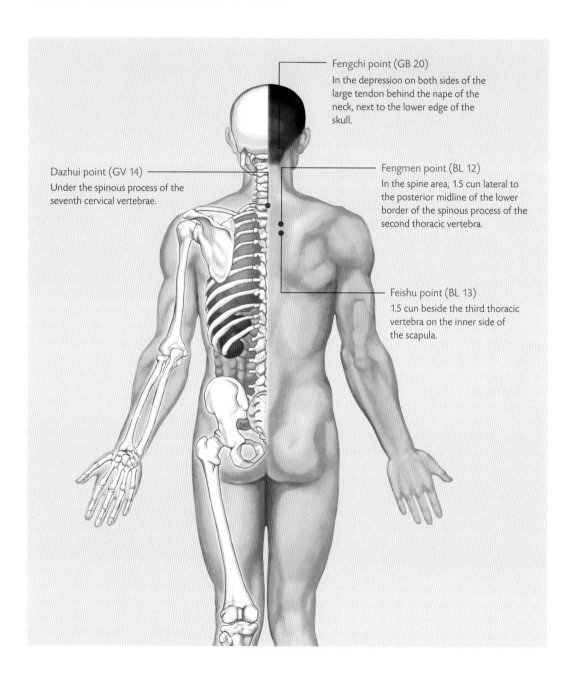

Fengchi point (GB 20)
In the depression on both sides of the large tendon behind the nape of the neck, next to the lower edge of the skull.

Dazhui point (GV 14)
Under the spinous process of the seventh cervical vertebrae.

Fengmen point (BL 12)
In the spine area, 1.5 cun lateral to the posterior midline of the lower border of the spinous process of the second thoracic vertebra.

Feishu point (BL 13)
1.5 cun beside the third thoracic vertebra on the inner side of the scapula.

Recommended Procedures

1. Fengchi Point

Method: Use the single-angle scraping to scrape Fengchi points on both sides in the rear of the head.

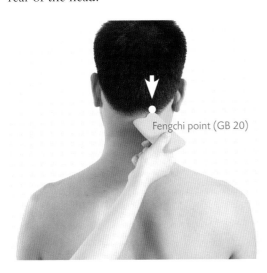

Fengchi point (GB 20)

3. Dazhui Point

Method: Use the surface-scraping to scrape Dazhui point on the back.

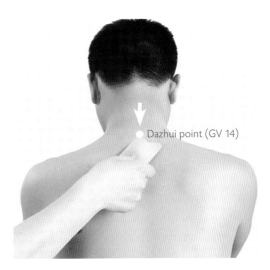

Dazhui point (GV 14)

2. Fengmen Point and Feishu Point

Method: Use the surface-scraping to scrape from Fengmen points to Feishu points on both sides of the Bladder Meridian.

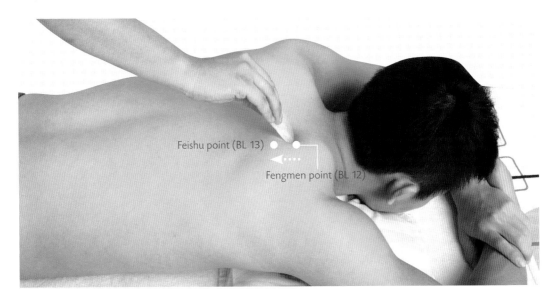

Feishu point (BL 13)

Fengmen point (BL 12)

Therapy to Increase the Curative Effect

Tremella (water-immersed) of 30 grams is boiled under soft fire for 30 minutes. Add chrysanthemum of 5 grams and a little rock candy to be drunk as tea. This serves to deal with deficiency of lung-yin, dry mouth, thick phlegm and swollen sore throat.

Hypochondriac Pain

It is chiefly manifested in the pain on one side or two sides of ribs. According to Chinese medicine, it is mainly due to problems with the liver and gallbladder. Hypochondriac pain can be caused by depression, irregular diet, exhaustion due to long-term illness, excessive fatigue or damp and heat owing to exterior malignant elements.

Scraping therapy can be applied to smooth the vital energy and meridians of liver and gallbladder. Frequent scraping of related areas in daily life can also effectively prevent the occurrence of hypochondriac pain.

Timely medical checkup is required for treatment if hypochondriac pain can not be eased. Hypochondriac pain can be caused by acute and chronic hepatitis, cholecystitis, cholelithiasis, pleurisy and their after-effects.

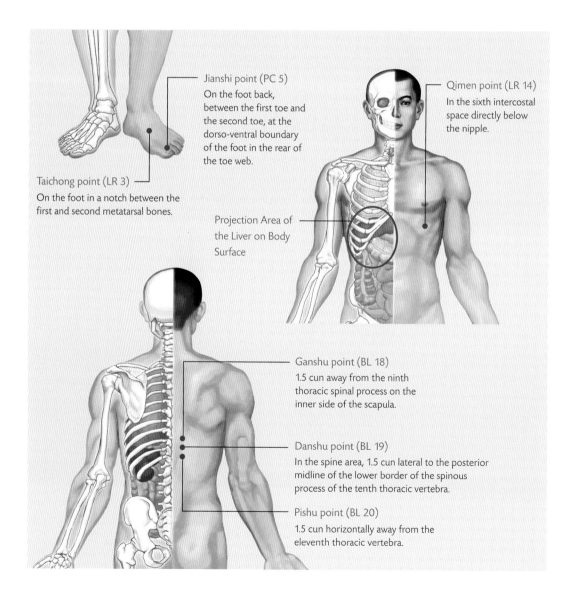

Jianshi point (PC 5)
On the foot back, between the first toe and the second toe, at the dorso-ventral boundary of the foot in the rear of the toe web.

Taichong point (LR 3)
On the foot in a notch between the first and second metatarsal bones.

Qimen point (LR 14)
In the sixth intercostal space directly below the nipple.

Projection Area of the Liver on Body Surface

Ganshu point (BL 18)
1.5 cun away from the ninth thoracic spinal process on the inner side of the scapula.

Danshu point (BL 19)
In the spine area, 1.5 cun lateral to the posterior midline of the lower border of the spinous process of the tenth thoracic vertebra.

Pishu point (BL 20)
1.5 cun horizontally away from the eleventh thoracic vertebra.

Recommended Procedures

1. Projection Area of the Liver on Body Surface

Method: Use the flat-scraping to scrape the projection area of the liver on the right-side of the chest and ribs from inside to outside.

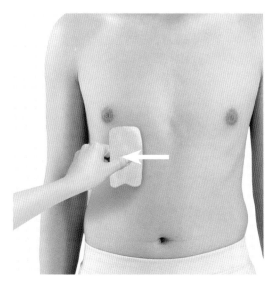

2. Qimen Point and A'shi Point

Method: Use the flat-scraping to scrape Qimen point and A'shi point on the affected area with pain on the chest.

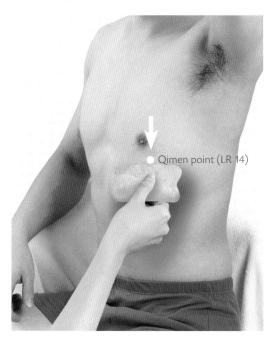

3. Ganshu Point, Danshu Point and Pishu Point

Method: Use the surface-scraping to scrape from Ganshu point, Danshu point to Pishu point on the back from up to down.

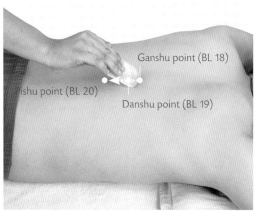

4. Taichong Point and Jianshi Point

Method: Use the angle-scraping to scrape from Taichong point to Jianshi point, until soreness and distension are felt.

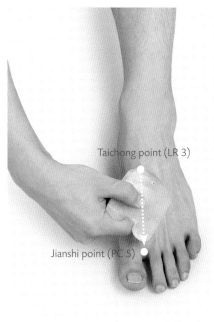

Palpitation and Short Breath

According to Chinese medicine, it is called "pavor" and "trance," taking place in patients with coronary disease, high blood pressure, rheumatic heart disease, pulmonary heart disease, cardiac insufficiency, various kinds of cardiac arrhythmia, anaemia and hyperthyroidism.

Excessive fatigue or excitement can lead to the excitement of supportive nerves, making heart beat fast and raising blood pressure. In a long-term state of excitement or under great pressure, these hormones will continue to secrete, affecting the heart and blood vessels first, resulting in palpitation and short breath.

Palpitation and short breath may be associated with the mood and age or with cardiovascular diseases. Therefore, these warning signals emitted by the body should not be overlooked since they are the pre-warnings of cardiovascular diseases. Timely check-up and treatment can effectively prevent cardiovascular diseases.

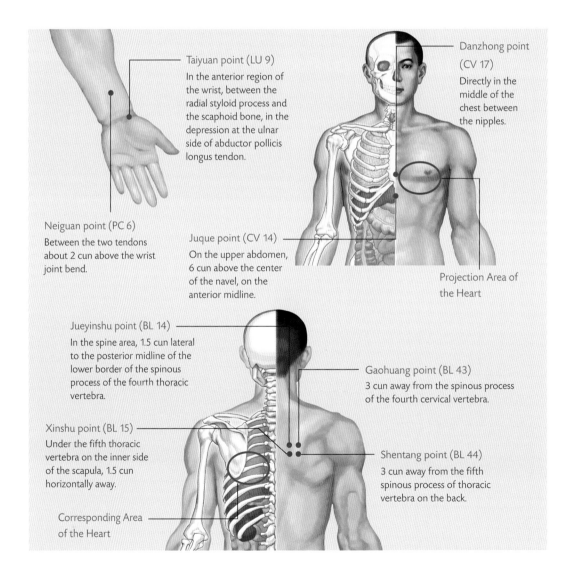

Taiyuan point (LU 9)
In the anterior region of the wrist, between the radial styloid process and the scaphoid bone, in the depression at the ulnar side of abductor pollicis longus tendon.

Danzhong point (CV 17)
Directly in the middle of the chest between the nipples.

Neiguan point (PC 6)
Between the two tendons about 2 cun above the wrist joint bend.

Juque point (CV 14)
On the upper abdomen, 6 cun above the center of the navel, on the anterior midline.

Projection Area of the Heart

Jueyinshu point (BL 14)
In the spine area, 1.5 cun lateral to the posterior midline of the lower border of the spinous process of the fourth thoracic vertebra.

Gaohuang point (BL 43)
3 cun away from the spinous process of the fourth cervical vertebra.

Xinshu point (BL 15)
Under the fifth thoracic vertebra on the inner side of the scapula, 1.5 cun horizontally away.

Shentang point (BL 44)
3 cun away from the fifth spinous process of thoracic vertebra on the back.

Corresponding Area of the Heart

Recommended Procedures

1. Jueyinshu Point, Xinshu Point, Gaohuang Point and Shentang Point

Method: Use the surface-scraping and dual-angle scraping to scrape the corresponding area of the heart on the spine and then use the surface-scraping to scrape Jueyinshu point, Xinshu point, Gaohuang point and Shentang point.

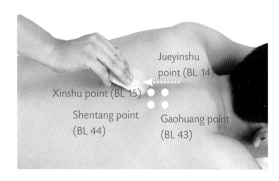

Jueyinshu point (BL 14)
Xinshu point (BL 15)
Shentang point (BL 44)
Gaohuang point (BL 43)

2. Danzhong Point and Juque Point

Method: Use the single-angle scraping to scrape slowly from Danzhong point to Juque point along the central line on the chest, and then use the flat-scraping to scrape the projection area of the heart on the left chest from inside to outside.

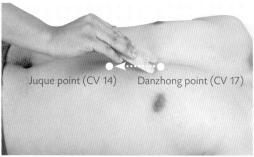

Juque point (CV 14)   Danzhong point (CV 17)

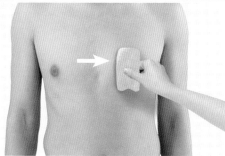

3. Taiyuan Point and Neiguan Point

Method: Use the surface-scraping to scrape Taiyuan point and Neiguan point. The flat-pressing and kneading can also be applied to press and knead Neiguan point.

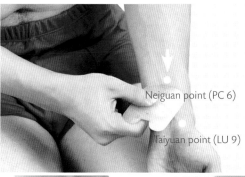

Neiguan point (PC 6)
Taiyuan point (LU 9)

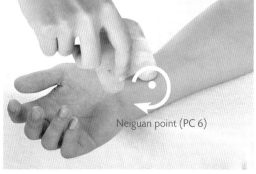

Neiguan point (PC 6)

Therapy to Increase the Curative Effect
When tachycardia and palpitation attack, use the vertical-pressing and kneading to press and knead the reflection area of the heart between the fourth metacarpal bone and the fifth metacarpal bone to ease the symptom.

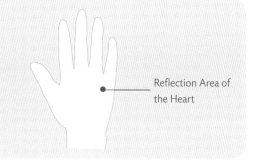

Reflection Area of the Heart

Dizziness

It is chiefly manifested by dizziness and dazzle. The patient of minor case can stop it with eyes closed, whereas the patient with serious case feel whirled like sitting in a car or a boat, being unable to stand up in addition to nausea, vomit, sweating and pale face. He/she may even fall down all of a sudden when it becomes serious.

Auditory vertigo (also called meniere's disease), kinesia, acute labyrinthitis, high blood pressure, hyperlipemia, cerebral arteriosclerosis, anaemia and neurasthenia can also be coupled with dizziness. Therefore, those who often suffer from dizziness should receive timely check-up and treatment in terms of primary diseases.

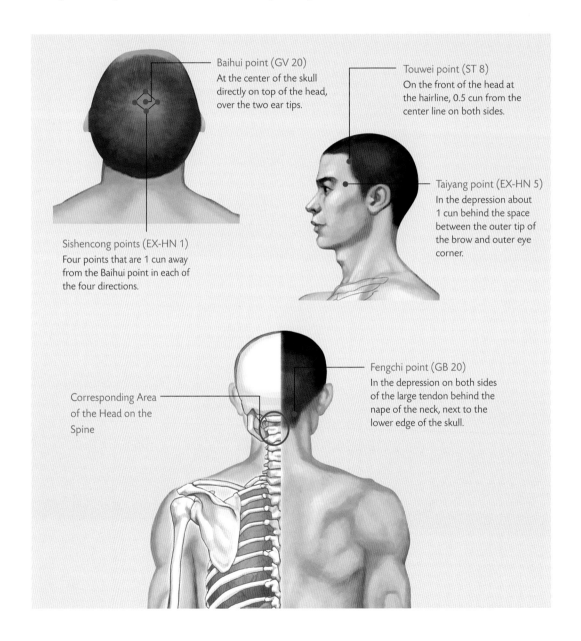

Baihui point (GV 20)
At the center of the skull directly on top of the head, over the two ear tips.

Touwei point (ST 8)
On the front of the head at the hairline, 0.5 cun from the center line on both sides.

Taiyang point (EX-HN 5)
In the depression about 1 cun behind the space between the outer tip of the brow and outer eye corner.

Sishencong points (EX-HN 1)
Four points that are 1 cun away from the Baihui point in each of the four directions.

Corresponding Area of the Head on the Spine

Fengchi point (GB 20)
In the depression on both sides of the large tendon behind the nape of the neck, next to the lower edge of the skull.

Recommended Procedures

1. The Corresponding Area of the Head on the Spine

Method: Use the surface-scraping and dual-angle scraping to scrape the corresponding area of the head on the spine.

3. Baihui Point and Sishenchong Points

Method: Use the surface-scraping to scrape from Baihui point towards Sishencong points.

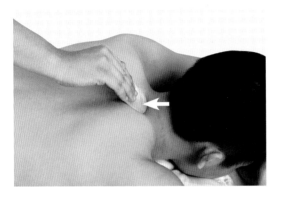

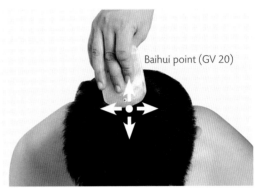

Baihui point (GV 20)

2. Taiyang Point, Touwei Point and Fengchi Point

Method: Use the flat-pressing and kneading to press and knead Taiyang points on both sides and use the single-angle scraping to scrape Touwei point and Fengchi point in the rear of the head.

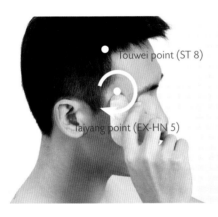

Touwei point (ST 8)

Taiyang point (EX-HN 5)

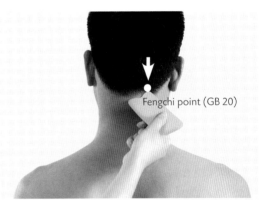

Fengchi point (GB 20)

Health-Care in Daily Life

• People suffering from dizziness should pay attention to the rest and routine life. Excessive fatigue and insufficient sleep are among the inductive factors of dizziness.

• Irritation of the sound and light can also make dizziness worse. Therefore, the bedroom should be quiet without strong light.

• In terms of the diet, eat more light food instead of food of high fat, too salty, sweet or very oily food. Do not smoke, and drink less liquor.

• Such spiritual irritation as depression and anger can lead to excessive rise of liver-yang or endogenous liver-wind, resulting in dizziness. People suffering from dizziness should keep being optimistic and light-hearted in a stable mood, which is very important in preventing the attack of dizziness and reducing the number of attacks of dizziness.

Tinnitus

Some people often feel certain special sounds in ears, but they cannot find the source of these sound nearby. This is called tinnitus. This is a symptom, but not a disease. However, continuous pain in ears and tinnitus are very likely to be symptoms of ear diseases.

According to the Chinese medicine, tinnitus is mainly due to the weakness of kidney energy. Kidneys take charge of bones and generate marrow. Generally speaking, tinnitus is caused by insufficient marrow. Therefore, the treatment of tinnitus through Chinese medicine should be coordinated with tonifying kidneys and benefiting marrow.

Scraping therapy is only applicable to the treatment of tinnitus caused by non-disease factors such as fatigue and deficiency of kidney energy. Tinnitus caused by trauma requires timely medical treatment.

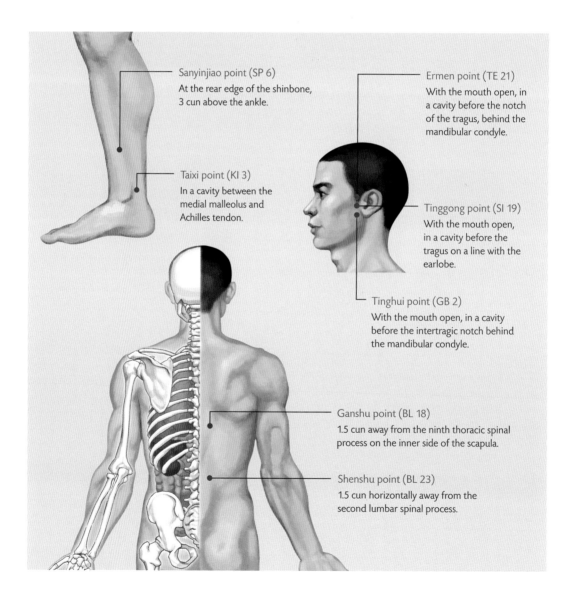

Sanyinjiao point (SP 6)
At the rear edge of the shinbone, 3 cun above the ankle.

Taixi point (KI 3)
In a cavity between the medial malleolus and Achilles tendon.

Ermen point (TE 21)
With the mouth open, in a cavity before the notch of the tragus, behind the mandibular condyle.

Tinggong point (SI 19)
With the mouth open, in a cavity before the tragus on a line with the earlobe.

Tinghui point (GB 2)
With the mouth open, in a cavity before the intertragic notch behind the mandibular condyle.

Ganshu point (BL 18)
1.5 cun away from the ninth thoracic spinal process on the inner side of the scapula.

Shenshu point (BL 23)
1.5 cun horizontally away from the second lumbar spinal process.

Recommended Procedures

1. Ermen Point, Tinggong Point and Tinghui Point

Method: Use the single-angle scraping to scrape Ermen point, Tinggong point and Tinghui point on the head. Since *sha* on the face does not look nice, the techniques applied should be gentle without bringing about *sha*. The scraping should proceed from inside to outside along the direction of muscles, once every day.

3. Ganshu Point and Shenshu Point

Method: Use the surface-scraping to scrape from Ganshu point to Shenshu point on the back from up to down without any stop, until *sha* appears, once every day.

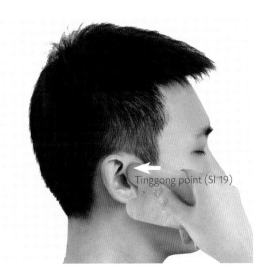

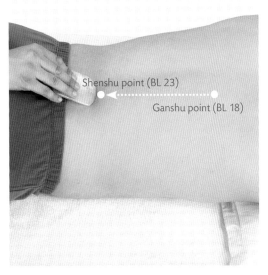

2. Sanyinjiao Point and Taixi Point

Method: Use the flat-scraping to scrape Sanyinjiao point on the inside of the lower limb from up to down without any stop until the skin appears red with the formation of purplish *sha* speckles. Then, use the corner of the scraping plate to scrape Taixi point heavily 30 times, until *sha* appears.

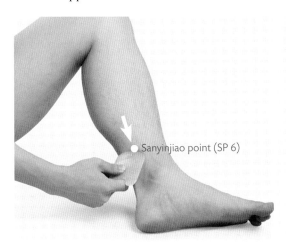

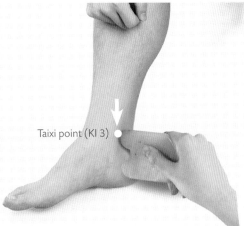

Headache

There are many reasons for headache. Sometimes, it is due to too much psychological pressure or too much tension. Sometimes, it is owing to certain diseases. Headache with the running nose, nasal obstruction or fever is generally caused by the cold. Splitting headache with dizziness and nausea is mostly caused by high blood pressure. Headache with nausea, vomit, difficulty of swallow, murmur and disorder of consciousness is possibly caused by cerebral bleeding or aneurysm. Timely medical check-up is needed if headache fails to be eased and attacks abnormally after the rest and massage. Whatever the reasons are for headache, they are all related to the imbalance and the stasis of vital energy and blood in the head. Therefore, finding out and smoothing the painful region in the head and in the corresponding area of the head through the scraping can quickly ease headache. Headache is mainly caused by the cold and the excessive rising of liver-yang, requiring the scraping of related acupoints and meridians to address both the symptoms and root causes.

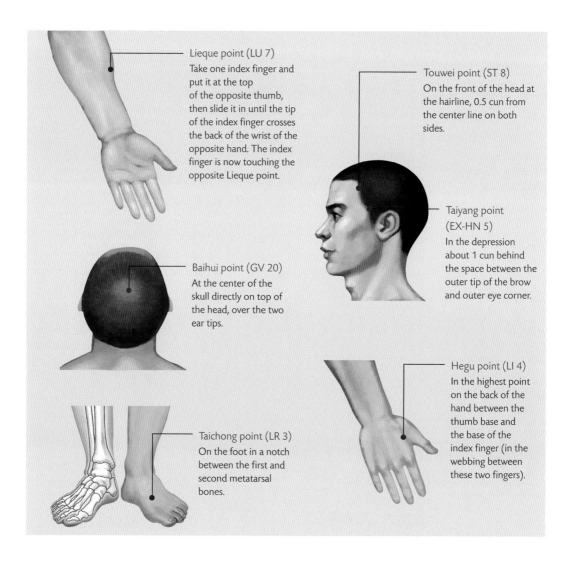

Lieque point (LU 7)
Take one index finger and put it at the top of the opposite thumb, then slide it in until the tip of the index finger crosses the back of the wrist of the opposite hand. The index finger is now touching the opposite Lieque point.

Touwei point (ST 8)
On the front of the head at the hairline, 0.5 cun from the center line on both sides.

Taiyang point (EX-HN 5)
In the depression about 1 cun behind the space between the outer tip of the brow and outer eye corner.

Baihui point (GV 20)
At the center of the skull directly on top of the head, over the two ear tips.

Hegu point (LI 4)
In the highest point on the back of the hand between the thumb base and the base of the index finger (in the webbing between these two fingers).

Taichong point (LR 3)
On the foot in a notch between the first and second metatarsal bones.

Recommended Procedures
1. Touwei Point
Method: Starting from the side of the head with the scraping comb placed vertically on the area between Touwei point at the hair line and the upper part of the ear. Then, scrape from the front to the rear until the edge of the lower hair line of the head side.

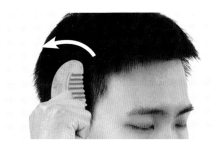

2. Baihui Point
Method: Use the surface-scraping to scrape the head top and the rear of the head, starting from Baihui point to the hair line at the forehead and then from Baihui point to the hair line at the rear of the head. Pay attention to finding the area with pain in the course of the scraping and scrape the painful area emphatically. Scrape each area 20 to 30 times until the scalp feels heat.

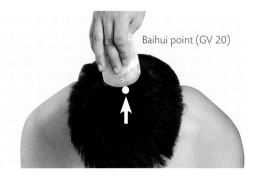

Baihui point (GV 20)

3. Taiyang Point
Method: Use the flat-pressing and kneading to press and knead Taiyang point on both sides, which is suitable for the treatment of various kinds of headache.

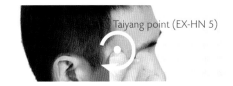

Taiyang point (EX-HN 5)

4. Hegu Point and Lieque Point
Method: Use the flat-pressing and kneading to press and knead Hegu point on both sides of the hand back as well as Lieque point on the wrist, which is suitable for the treatment of headache caused by the cold.

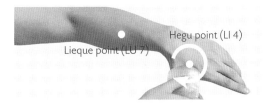

Hegu point (LI 4)

Lieque point (LU 7)

5. Taichong Point
Method: Use the vertical-pressing and kneading to press and knead Taichong point on Liver Meridian behind the big toe and the second toe seam with heavy force. Relax once every 15 seconds of pressing until headache is eased. It is suitable for migraine and pain on the top of the head.

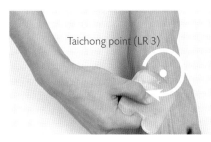

Taichong point (LR 3)

Points of Attention
• The scraping oil is not needed if the head is covered with hair. An appropriate amount of the scraping oil can be applied for the head with a little hair or the head without any hair.

• The side of the head should be emphatically scraped if it is migraine and the pain point should be found.

• Furuncle on the scalp should be avoided.

Toothache

As an ailment of teeth and surrounding tissues, it is the most common symptom among problems in the mouth. Toothache can be caused by the pain in the nearby tissues and illness all over the body. Toothache due to tooth decay, toothache due to deficiency fire and toothache due to excess fire are commonly seen, with toothache due to excess fire frequently caused by stomach fire. Scraping therapy can be applied to both toothache due to deficiency fire and toothache due to excess fire.

Toothache Due to Deficiency Fire

This refers to the toothache due to the flaring up of deficient heat, with such symptoms as chronic and dull pain in teeth from time to time, which aggravates often at night and with loosened teeth and weakness in chewing.

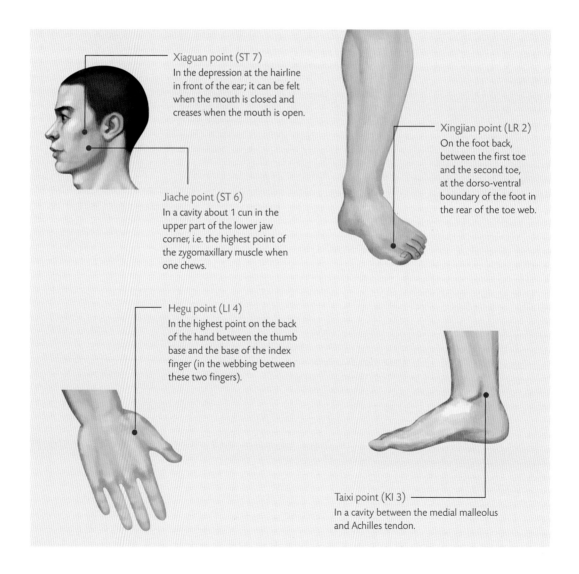

Xiaguan point (ST 7)
In the depression at the hairline in front of the ear; it can be felt when the mouth is closed and creases when the mouth is open.

Xingjian point (LR 2)
On the foot back, between the first toe and the second toe, at the dorso-ventral boundary of the foot in the rear of the toe web.

Jiache point (ST 6)
In a cavity about 1 cun in the upper part of the lower jaw corner, i.e. the highest point of the zygomaxillary muscle when one chews.

Hegu point (LI 4)
In the highest point on the back of the hand between the thumb base and the base of the index finger (in the webbing between these two fingers).

Taixi point (KI 3)
In a cavity between the medial malleolus and Achilles tendon.

Recommended Procedures
Xiaguan Point, Jiache Point, Hegu Point, Taixi Point and Xingjian Point
Apply an appropriate amount of the scraping oil to the area to be scraped. First press and knead Xiaguan point and Jiache point with heavy force. Then, use the flat-pressing and kneading to press and knead Hegu point on the hand until the skin appears red and purplish *sha* speckles appear. Finally, scrape Taixi point and Xingjian point on the feet with the corner of the scraping plate to scrape 30 times with heavy force, until *sha* appears.

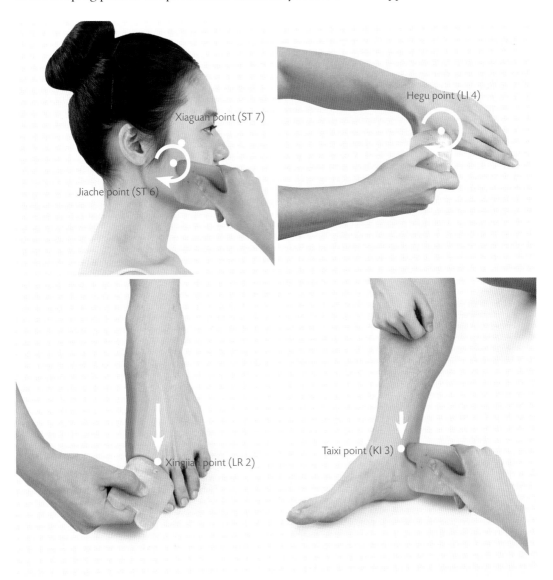

Xiaguan point (ST 7)

Jiache point (ST 6)

Hegu point (LI 4)

Xingjian point (LR 2)

Taixi point (KI 3)

Therapy to Increase the Curative Effect
Soup boiled with green beans and liquorice:100-gram green beans and 15-gram liquorice are boiled for oral use, with residues taken away, twice every day, serving to expel deficiency fire, prevent and cure toothache due to deficiency fire .

Toothache Due to Excess Fire

It is marked by fierce attack of pain, along with the distension of gums (mostly pain in the lower teeth), bad breath, thirst and constipation, mostly due to accumulated inner heat in intestines and stomach.

Recommended Procedures
Xiaguan Point, Jiache Point, Hegu Point, Erjian Point and Neiting Point

Apply an appropriate amount of scraping oil to the area to be scraped. First use the corner of the scraping plate to press and knead Xiaguan point and Jiache point with heavy force. Then, use the flat-pressing and kneading to press and knead Hegu point and Erjian point until the skin appears red and purplish *sha* speckles appear. Finally, scrape Neiting point with the corner of the scraping plate 30 times with heavy force until *sha* appears.

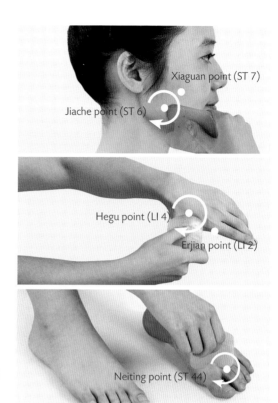

Xiaguan point (ST 7)
Jiache point (ST 6)
Hegu point (LI 4)
Erjian point (LI 2)
Neiting point (ST 44)

Therapy to Increase the Curative Effect

Generally, heat-clearing and fire-clearing drugs are used to reduce inner heat, but it is not effective for the toothache due to excess fire, because fire cannot be dispersed if stasis cannot be expelled. Raw ginger can be used to distribute the inner fire all over main and collateral channels again, eliminating toothache automatically. Generally, chewing a piece of raw ginger of the thumb-size can produce an curative effect in 2 to 3 minutes.

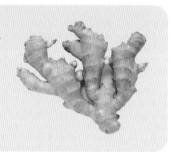

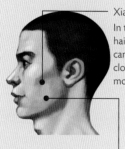

Xiaguan point (ST 7)
In the depression at the hairline in front of the ear; it can be felt when the mouth is closed and creases when the mouth is open.

Jiache point (ST 6)
In a cavity about 1 cun in the upper part of the lower jaw corner, i.e., the highest point of the zygomaxillary muscle when one chews.

Hegu point (LI 4)
In the highest point on the back of the hand between the thumb base and the base of the index finger (in the webbing between these two fingers).

Erjian point (LI 2)
With the fist slightly clenched, on the radial margin of the index finger, in a cavity bordering the dorso-ventral boundary of the hand in front of the second metacarpophalangeal joint.

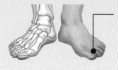

Neiting point (ST 44)
On the dorso-ventral boundary of the foot, in the rear of the toe web between the second and third toe.

Bad Breath

This refers to bad smell from the mouth. According to Chinese medicine, bad breath originates from too much internal fire in the heart and the spleen, with heat accumulated in pericardium meridian for a long time, doing harm to the blood channel. Bad breath can also be caused by rising dampness due to spleen weakness, resulting in heating up the mouth, the tongue and throat. Scraping therapy can help to reduce internal heat in the heart and the stomach, fundamentally expelling bad breath.

People with bad breath had better eat less garlic and onion and some other kinds of irritating food, not smoke and drink alcohol, eat more vegetables, fruit and food of coarse fibers. In daily life, drink an appropriate amount of tea water, which can not only reduce internal heat, but also clean the mouth and improve bad breath.

Recommended Procedures
1. Daling Point and Laogong Point
Method: Use the corner of the scraping plate to scrape, press and knead Daling point and Laogong point, until soreness and distenion are felt.

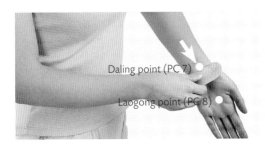

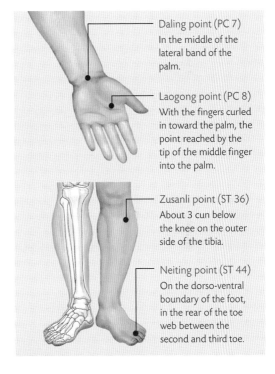

Daling point (PC 7)
In the middle of the lateral band of the palm.

Laogong point (PC 8)
With the fingers curled in toward the palm, the point reached by the tip of the middle finger into the palm.

Zusanli point (ST 36)
About 3 cun below the knee on the outer side of the tibia.

Neiting point (ST 44)
On the dorso-ventral boundary of the foot, in the rear of the toe web between the second and third toe.

2. Zusanli Point and Neiting Point
Method: Use the corner of the scraping plate to press and knead Zusanli point and Neiting point of Stomach Meridian on both sides, until soreness and distension are felt.

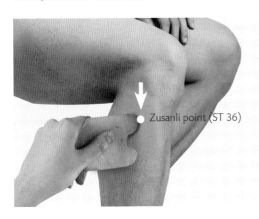

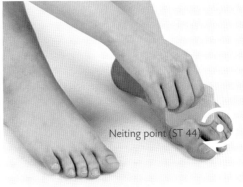

Therapies to Increase the Curative Effect

Tea Therapy

1. Sweet Osmanthus Black Tea

3-gram osmanthus flowers are boiled first and such boiling water is used to brew 5-gram black tea, one dose every day with such water held in the mouth frequently (fig. 53).

2. Sweet Osmanthus and Chrysanthemum Tea

6-gram sweet-scented osmanthus and 6-gram chrysanthemums are boiled together 2 to 3 times, drink one dose every day, which can fresh breath and clear stomach.

3. Green Tea

25-gram green tea is boiled for drinking with tea-leaves chewed, serving to reduce stomach heat.

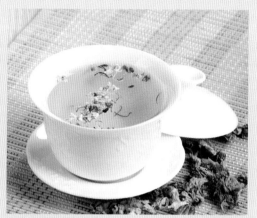

Fig. 53 Sweet osmanthus black tea.

Getting Rid of Other Factors Leading to Bad Breath

1. Avoiding eating certain food:

Avoid eating spicy food. The smell of such spicy food as onion and garlic is apt to stay in the mouth after the meal. Eating too much of these foods will keep the smell longer in the mouth, which cannot be easily done away through tooth-brushing. Smoked sausage, smoked beef and garlic sausage not only have strong smell, but are difficult to be digested, resulting in unpleasant gas in the stomach followed by bad breath.

2. Dealing with decayed tooth timely:

Food residues are apt to be attached to areas of pathological changes such as decayed teeth, residual crowns and roots. Due to the functions of germs in the mouth, food residues would be fermented, leading to bad breath. Bad breath will disappear once the decayed teeth, residual crowns and roots are cured.

3. Treating periodontal diseases:

Bad breath can be caused by periodontal diseases. Particularly, chronic periodontal diseases will lead to blind pouches and produce chronic pyorrhea. Bad breath cannot be expelled unless periodontal disease and blind pouches are done away with. Acute inflammation in the mouth, such as acute peridental abscess and the third molar pericoronitis, etc., will generate some secretion of acute inflammation, resulting in bad breath. With these ailments cured and inflammation expelled, bad breath will disappear.

4. Brushing teeth and rinsing the mouth frequently:

There are crevices amid the teeth of some people. After the meal, some food residues would stay in these crevices and generate bad breath due to the fermentation of germs in the mouth. It is more obvious for old people whose crevices are larger amid the teeth due to physiological atrophy of their periodontal tissues. Therefore, attention should be paid to hygiene in the mouth, i.e., brushing teeth and rinsing the mouth after getting up in the morning and before going to bed to eliminate food residues in the mouth to prevent the occurrence of bad breath.

5. Treating diseases in the digestive tract:

Diseases in the digestive tract and intestines, such as indigestion or the reflux disease of the digestive tract, can bring the smell of food residues in stomach out, leading to bad breath in mouth. Once diseases in the digestive tract are cured, bad breath will disappear.

6. Expelling stomach fire:

The time between 5:00 and 7:00 in the morning is for intestines and stomach to expel toxin. Scraping around the navel during this period can help to expel inner heat in stomach. With stomach fire expelled, gastric distention, constipation, bad breath, oral ulcer, swelling and aching of gum, acne along lips and freckles on the face can all be improved.

Lack of Appetite

As a symptom of frequent occurrence, it is different from food refusal in anorexia, but the lack of desire for food. The spleen is in charge of digestive transformation, adjusting gastric and intestinal functions. The weakness of the spleen and stomach is apt to result in the lack of appetite. Scraping the projection areas of spleen and stomach on the body surface is conducive to adjusting the functions of the spleen and stomach and enhancing appetite.

Apart from the weakness of the spleen and stomach, too much mental stress and fatigue as well as certain diseases can also lead to the lack of appetite. Therefore, the treatment will not be effective until the reason for the lack of appetite is found out.

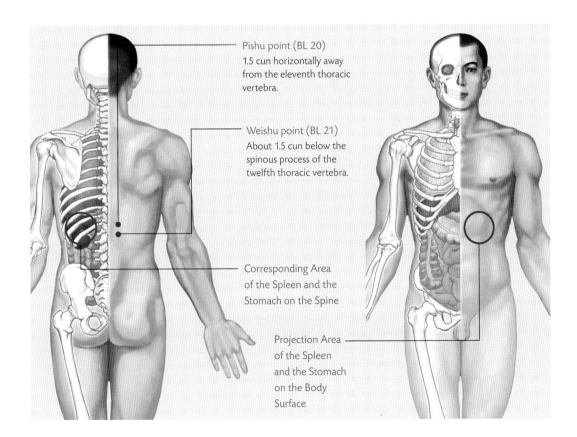

Pishu point (BL 20)
1.5 cun horizontally away from the eleventh thoracic vertebra.

Weishu point (BL 21)
About 1.5 cun below the spinous process of the twelfth thoracic vertebra.

Corresponding Area of the Spleen and the Stomach on the Spine

Projection Area of the Spleen and the Stomach on the Body Surface

Recommended Procedures

1. Corresponding Area of the Spleen and the Stomach on the Spine
Method: Use the surface-scraping and dual-angle scraping to scrape the corresponding area of the spleen and the stomach on the spine from up to down.

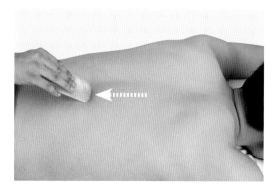

2. Projection Area of the Spleen and the Stomach on the Body Surface
Method: Use the long edge of the scraper to slowly scrape the area with the plate tilting at an angle smaller than 15 degrees from up to down.

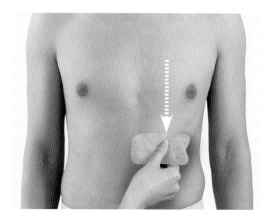

3. Pishu Point and Weishu Point
Method: Use the surface-scraping to scrape Pishu point and Weishu point on both sides of the back until *sha* appears or the pores open slightly.

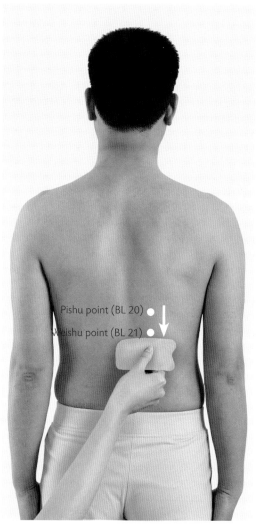

Pishu point (BL 20)
Weishu point (BL 21)

Heat Stroke

This is an acute pathological change because of work or activities under scorching sun or under high temperature, which leads to the intrusion of summer-heat, pathogenic heat accumulation in the body and abnormality of the function for adjusting temperature. Scraping therapy can reduce lung heat, invigorate the head and eyes to prevent heat stroke, and ease the symptoms of heat stroke.

The patient suffering from heat stroke should be quickly moved to a cool and well-ventilated place, given cold drink or light salt brine of 300 to 500 milliliters, along with the medicine of expelling heat. The operator should quickly press and knead Shuigou point (philtrum) of the patient if he/she faints or collapses, until he/she comes round.

Recommended Procedures

1. Fengfu Point, Yamen Point and Dazhui Point

Method: Use the surface-scraping to scrape from Fengfu point to Yamen point on the rear of the head, and scrape Dazhui point from up to down until *sha* appears. This serves to expel inner heat, refresh the mind and the body.

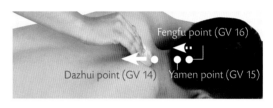

2. Neiguan Point and Hegu Point

Method: Use the corner of the scraping plate to scrape Neiguan point and Hegu point on the forearm, which serves to expel agitation, ease stomach, calm the adverse-rising energy and stop vomiting.

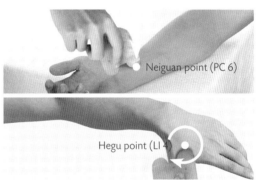

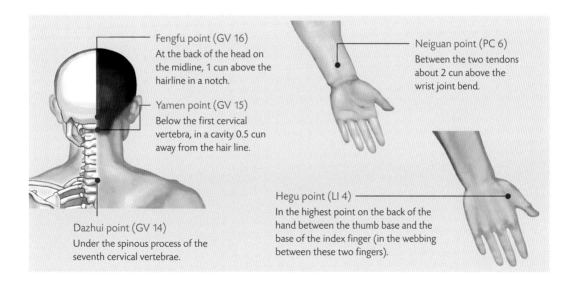

Fengfu point (GV 16)
At the back of the head on the midline, 1 cun above the hairline in a notch.

Yamen point (GV 15)
Below the first cervical vertebra, in a cavity 0.5 cun away from the hair line.

Dazhui point (GV 14)
Under the spinous process of the seventh cervical vertebrae.

Neiguan point (PC 6)
Between the two tendons about 2 cun above the wrist joint bend.

Hegu point (LI 4)
In the highest point on the back of the hand between the thumb base and the base of the index finger (in the webbing between these two fingers).

Indigestion

It is caused by the obstacle of gastric motility, falling into the category of "gastric fullness" and "stomachache." This is due to the in-take of too much fat and sweet food as well as alcoholics, which harmed and overburdened the spleen and stomach for a long time as well as slowed down metabolism. Such illness lies in the stomach, liver and spleen. Therefore, it is advisable to treat the illness by strengthening the spleen and stomach, relieving the depressed liver, promoting digestion and purgation.

People with indigestion should eat less at each meal but eat more frequently, and avoid too much hunger or too much in-take so as to prevent the stomach and intestines from being overburdened. Don't eat cold, hard or spicy food. Don't drink liquor and pay attention to keeping the stomach warm. Eating more coarse grain is conducive to digestion. However, don't eat excessive coarse grain a time or eat too frequently, generally three times a week will be proper. Otherwise, intestines and stomach will feel unbearable and upset.

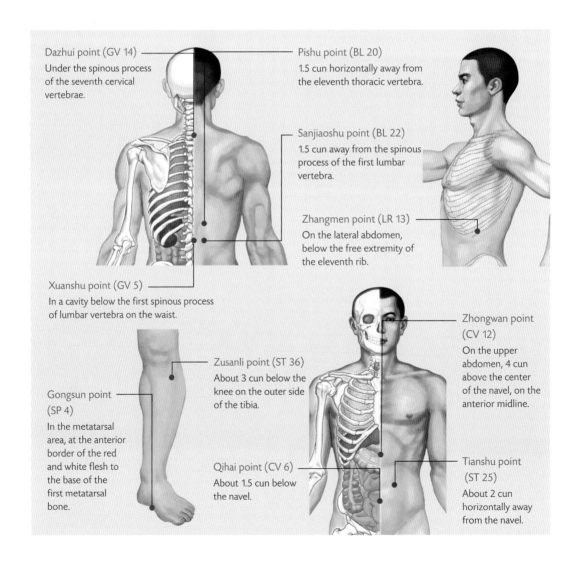

Dazhui point (GV 14)
Under the spinous process of the seventh cervical vertebrae.

Pishu point (BL 20)
1.5 cun horizontally away from the eleventh thoracic vertebra.

Sanjiaoshu point (BL 22)
1.5 cun away from the spinous process of the first lumbar vertebra.

Zhangmen point (LR 13)
On the lateral abdomen, below the free extremity of the eleventh rib.

Xuanshu point (GV 5)
In a cavity below the first spinous process of lumbar vertebra on the waist.

Zhongwan point (CV 12)
On the upper abdomen, 4 cun above the center of the navel, on the anterior midline.

Zusanli point (ST 36)
About 3 cun below the knee on the outer side of the tibia.

Gongsun point (SP 4)
In the metatarsal area, at the anterior border of the red and white flesh to the base of the first metatarsal bone.

Qihai point (CV 6)
About 1.5 cun below the navel.

Tianshu point (ST 25)
About 2 cun horizontally away from the navel.

Recommended Procedures

1. Dazhui Point, Xuanshu Point, Pishu Point and Sanjiaoshu Point

Method: Use the surface-scraping to scrape from Dazhui point to Xuanshu point along Du Meridian on the back from up to down and then scrape both sides of the spine from Pishu point to Sanjiaoshu point along the bladder meridian.

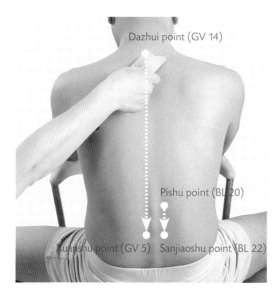

Dazhui point (GV 14)

Pishu point (BL 20)

Xuanshu point (GV 5)   Sanjiaoshu point (BL 22)

2. Zhongwan Point, Qihai Point, Tianshu Point and Zhangmen Point

Method: Use the surface-scraping to scrape from Zhongwan point to Qihai point along Ren Meridian from up to down, as well as Tianshu points on both sides of the Stomach Meridian and Zhangmen points on both sides of the Liver Meridian.

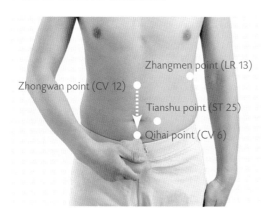

Zhangmen point (LR 13)

Zhongwan point (CV 12)

Tianshu point (ST 25)

Qihai point (CV 6)

3. Zusanli Point and Gongsun Point

Method: Use the flat-scraping to scrape Zusanli point, or use the corner of the scraper to press and knead Zusanli point and Gongsun point.

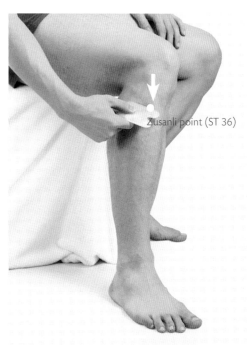

Zusanli point (ST 36)

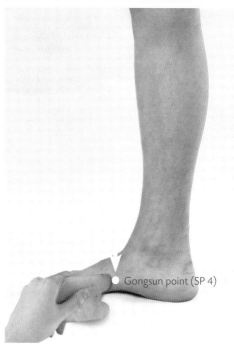

Gongsun point (SP 4)

Hiccups

This is caused by imbalance of gastric and intestinal nerves, or diaphragmatic spasm caused by gastritis or dilatation of the stomach. It can take place all by itself or go together with other kinds of illness. Sudden hiccup occurring in some acute and chronic diseases or in the final phase of some kinds of serious illness mostly foretells the aggravation of the illness.

Frequent hiccup or continuous hiccup are mostly marked by the blockage of vital energy circulation. Scraping from Qihai point to Guanyuan point and pressing Taixi point can help vital energy circulation within the body. Pressing Neiguan point can also relax the spasm of diaphragm and ease acute hiccup.

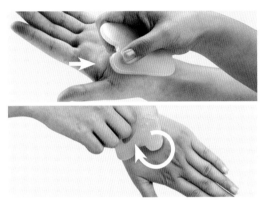

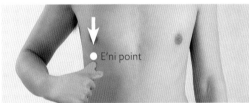

Recommended Procedures
1. Reflection Area of Thoracic Diaphragm on the Hand Back and the Reflection Area of the Stomach in the Palm
Method: Use the vertical-pressing and kneading to press and knead the reflection area of thoracic diaphragm on the hand back and use the single-angle scraping to scrape the reflection area of the stomach in the palm.

2. E'ni Point
Method: Use the single corner of the scraping plate to scrape E'ni point on both sides of the chest.

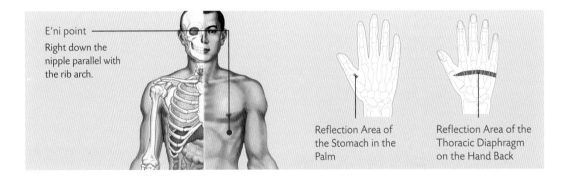

E'ni point
Right down the nipple parallel with the rib arch.

Reflection Area of the Stomach in the Palm

Reflection Area of the Thoracic Diaphragm on the Hand Back

Therapy to Increase the Curative Effect
Thirty grams of fresh ginger is mashed into juice to be mixed with honey and boiled water for oral use, serving to get rid of hiccups.

Gastrospasm

This is mostly caused by the intrusion of the cold into stomach, irregular diet or stasis of liver energy. Scraping therapy can smooth the related meridians, relax the spasm of gastric parietal muscle and promote the blood and vital energy circulation in stomach, easing stomachache.

Scraping the projection area of the stomach on the abdomen and the corresponding area of the stomach on the spine serves to treat those patients who often suffer from gastric spasm. With gastric spasm eased, scraping these areas can adjust gastric functions, and prevent and reduce the occurrence of gastric spasm.

Timely medical treatment and diagnosis are needed if scraping therapy fails to produce any curative effect, the patient often suffers from gastric spasm or for those who suffer from gastric bleeding.

The scraping in stomach area should be conducted half an hour after meal.

Recommended Procedures
1. Reflection Area of the Stomach in the Palm
Method: Use the vertical-pressing and kneading to press and knead the reflection area of the stomach on the radial side of the second metacarpal bone. Look carefully for the point of sensitivity to pain within the area and emphatically press and knead this sensitivity point.

2. Geshu Point and Weishu Point
Method: Use the surface-scraping to scrape from Geshu point to Weishu point from up to down.

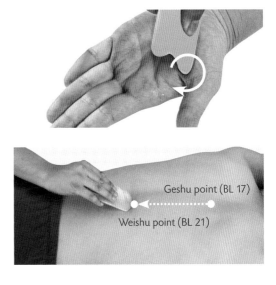

Geshu point (BL 17)

Weishu point (BL 21)

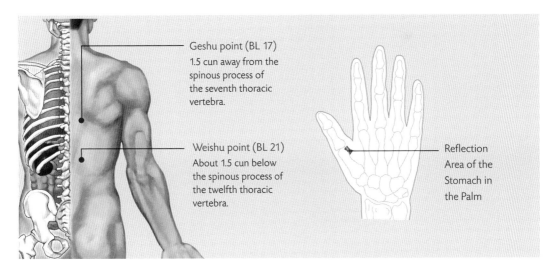

Geshu point (BL 17)
1.5 cun away from the spinous process of the seventh thoracic vertebra.

Weishu point (BL 21)
About 1.5 cun below the spinous process of the twelfth thoracic vertebra.

Reflection Area of the Stomach in the Palm

Abdominal Distension

It is the commonest symptom of abdominal discomfort due to abdominal fullness, which takes place in many kinds of illness. Here, it purely refers to illness of intestinal and gastric functions, excluding such diseases of internal and surgical departments as intestinal obstruction, tumor, liver cirrhosis ascites, intestinal tuberculosis or tuberculous peritonitis.

According to Chinese medicine, it is divided into abdominal distention due to vital energy stasis and abdominal distension due to dyspepsia. The former is mostly caused by depression and blockage of vital energy circulation, whereas the latter tends to be caused by too much drink and food and accumulation of food and indigestion in the stomach.

The patient should go to hospital immediately for diagnosis if abdominal distension exceeds for over three days. If it is due to improper diet, the patient can take some medicine for digestion under the guidance of a doctor.

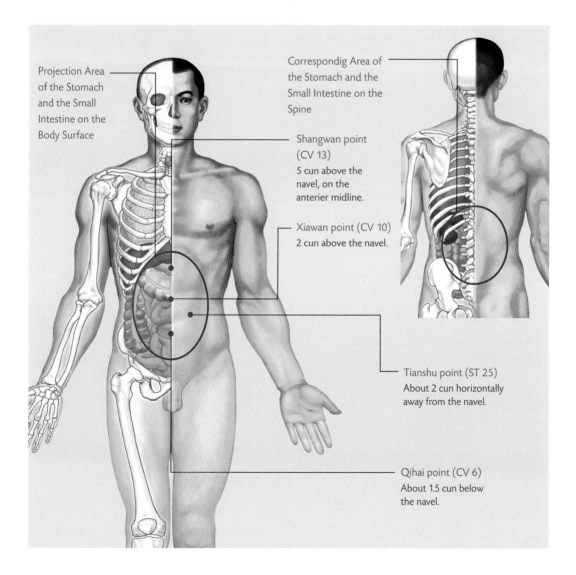

Projection Area of the Stomach and the Small Intestine on the Body Surface

Correspondig Area of the Stomach and the Small Intestine on the Spine

Shangwan point (CV 13)
5 cun above the navel, on the anterier midline.

Xiawan point (CV 10)
2 cun above the navel.

Tianshu point (ST 25)
About 2 cun horizontally away from the navel.

Qihai point (CV 6)
About 1.5 cun below the navel.

Recommended Procedures

1. Projection Area of the Stomach and the Small Intestine on the Body Surface

Method: Use the surface-scraping to scrape the areas from up to down.

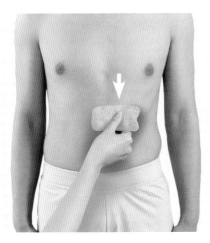

2. Corresponding Area of the Stomach and the Small Intestine on the Spine

Method: Use the surface-scraping and the dual-angle scraping to scrape the area from up to down.

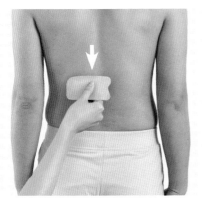

3. Shangwan Point, Xiawan Point, Qihai Point and Tianshu Point

Method: Use the surface-scraping to respectively scrape from Shangwan point to Xiawan point and Qihai point on Ren Meridian. And scrape Tianshu point on Stomach Meridian.

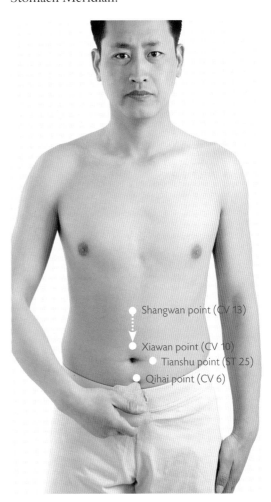

Shangwan point (CV 13)
Xiawan point (CV 10)
Tianshu point (ST 25)
Qihai point (CV 6)

Therapy to Increase the Curative Effect

Kneading the lower abdomen: The patient lies on his/her back and places his/her right palm on the abdomen overlapped with the left palm. Then, use the thenar eminence and the palm root to press against the abdomen, kneading around the navel 50 to100 times clockwise with a light force that the abdomen does not feel painful and uncomfortable from it. Kneading the abdomen can reinforce the functions of intestines and stomach as well as the muscle of abdominal walls, increase the secretion of digestive juice and the movement of stomach and intestines, promote blood circulation and the digestion and absorption of food.

Diarrhea

It is divided into acute diarrhea and chronic diarrhea. The former is mostly caused by intestinal infection, whereas the latter is manifested by diarrhea repeatedly, or diarrhea lasting several months or even several years.

According to the Chinese medicine, diarrhea is caused by the intrusion of the wind-cold, wind-heat, overeating, insufficiency of the spleen, yang deficiency and imbalance between liver and spleen. Germ infection or toxin in food are also important causes. Scraping therapy can adjust gastric and intestinal functions and help to stop diarrhea.

Some patients of diarrhea are accustomed to taking antidiarrheal. In fact, some kinds of diarrhea cannot be stopped randomly, such as infectious diarrhea. Diarrhea caused by infection is a kind of manifestation of self-protection of the human body, through which some toxin can be expelled, which is beneficial to the human body. In this case, on the contrary, the application of the antidiarrheal will cover the state of an illness.

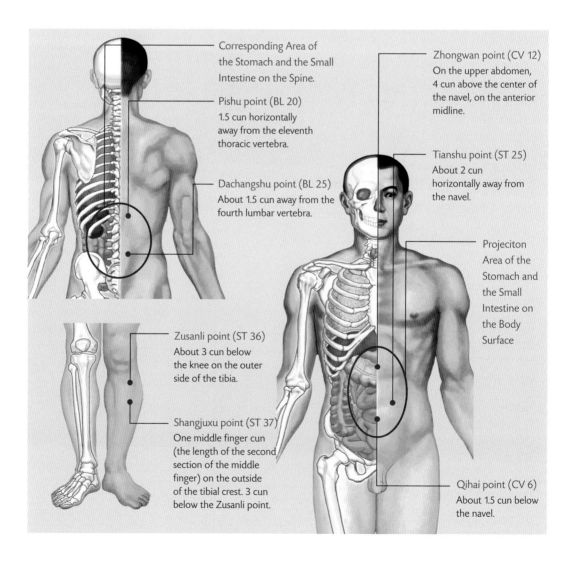

Corresponding Area of the Stomach and the Small Intestine on the Spine.

Pishu point (BL 20)
1.5 cun horizontally away from the eleventh thoracic vertebra.

Dachangshu point (BL 25)
About 1.5 cun away from the fourth lumbar vertebra.

Zhongwan point (CV 12)
On the upper abdomen, 4 cun above the center of the navel, on the anterior midline.

Tianshu point (ST 25)
About 2 cun horizontally away from the navel.

Projeciton Area of the Stomach and the Small Intestine on the Body Surface

Zusanli point (ST 36)
About 3 cun below the knee on the outer side of the tibia.

Shangjuxu point (ST 37)
One middle finger cun (the length of the second section of the middle finger) on the outside of the tibial crest. 3 cun below the Zusanli point.

Qihai point (CV 6)
About 1.5 cun below the navel.

Recommended Procedures

1. Projection Area of the Stomach and the Small Intestine on the Body Surface

Method: Use the surface-scraping to scrape the area from up to down.

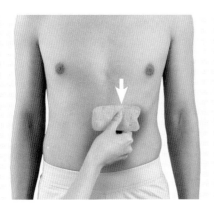

2. Corresponding Area of the Stomach and the Small Intestine on the Spine

Method: Use the surface-scraping and the dual-angle scraping to scrape the area from up to down.

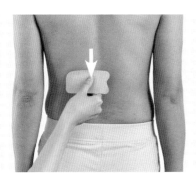

Therapies to Increase the Curative Effect

Use mild moxibustion, direct a burning moxa stick at Tianshu points on both sides (2 cun away from the navel) for 10 to 15 minutes respectively until warmth is felt, two times a day.

As for acute diarrhea, Diji point can be chosen (3 cun below Yinlingquan point), since it specially serves to cure abdominal pain and diarrhea. Direct a moxa stick at this acupoint for 3 to 5 minutes, which is of a particular effect on stopping diarrhea.

3. Pishu Point and Dachangshu Point

Method: Use the surface-scraping to scrape from Pishu point to Dachangshu point on the back from up to down.

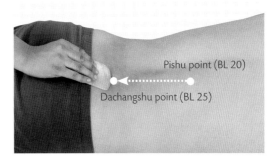

Pishu point (BL 20)
Dachangshu point (BL 25)

4. Zhongwan Point, Qihai Point and Tianshu Point

Method: Use the surface-scraping to scrape from Zhongwan point to Qihai point, and Tianshu points on both sides of the abdomen from up to down.

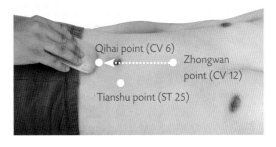

Qihai point (CV 6)
Zhongwan point (CV 12)
Tianshu point (ST 25)

5. Zusanli Point and Shangjuxu Point

Method: Use the surface-scraping to scrape from Zusanli point to Shangjuxu point from up to down.

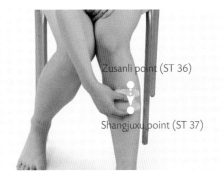

Zusanli point (ST 36)
Shangjuxu point (ST 37)

Constipation

Constipation is often caused by insufficient in-take of water or dietary fiber, tension, abuse of laxative or some intestinal and endocrine diseases. It is a common disease of people in modern times. In particular, office workers often sitting in the chair and seldom moving around under work strain are apt to suffer from constipation. Constipation can also be caused by other kinds of diseases or due to weak spleen-stomach functions, weakness of intestinal movement or internal heat of the body. According to Chinese medicine, the fundamental reasons are attributed to the lack and weakness of essential liquid and deficiency of vital energy and blood as well as excess yang and deficiency of yin. Therefore, scraping to get rid of constipation bases itself chiefly on regenerating body fluid, nourishing blood, supplementing yin and dispersing yang.

The key to the prevention and treatment of constipation lies in changing the habits of life and diet, rather than medication. Eat more fresh vegetables, drink water frequently and have some coarse grain. Doing more exercise and keeping a pleasant mood are conducive to preventing and improving constipation. Long-term abuse of laxative will not improve constipation, but on the contrary irritate intestines and stomach, making such abuse indispensable and doing harm to the body.

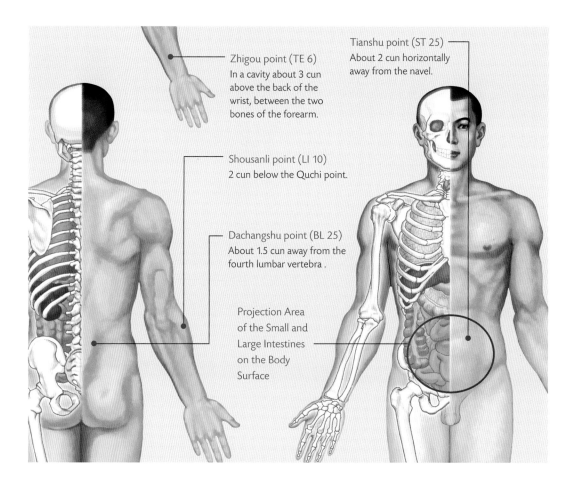

Zhigou point (TE 6)
In a cavity about 3 cun above the back of the wrist, between the two bones of the forearm.

Tianshu point (ST 25)
About 2 cun horizontally away from the navel.

Shousanli point (LI 10)
2 cun below the Quchi point.

Dachangshu point (BL 25)
About 1.5 cun away from the fourth lumbar vertebra .

Projection Area of the Small and Large Intestines on the Body Surface

Recommended Procedures

1. The Projection Area of the Small and Large Intestines on the Body Surface
Methods: Use the surface-scraping daily to scrape the area around the navel either from left to right or vice versa. Exert large pressure with slow speed until mild heat is felt on the abdomen as the best effect.

3. Dachangshu Point and Tianshu Point
Methods: Use the surface-scraping to scrape Dachangshu point on the back from up to down and use the surface-scraping to scrape Tianshu point on the abdomen from up to down.

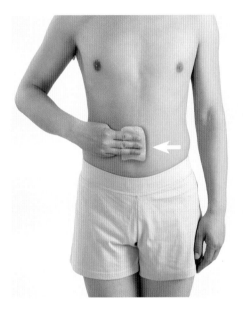

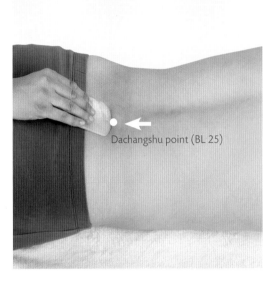

Dachangshu point (BL 25)

2. Shousanli Point and Zhigou Point
Methods: Use the surface-scraping to scrape Shousanli point and Zhigou point on the back of arm from up to down.

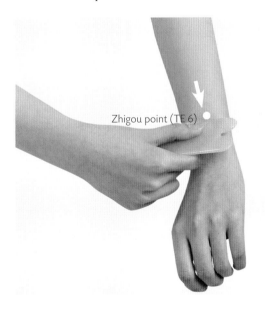

Zhigou point (TE 6)

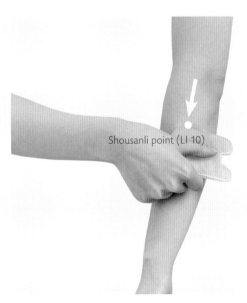

Shousanli point (LI 10)

Therapies to Increase the Curative Effect

• Nut porridge: 10 grams of walnut kernels, pine nuts, sesame, almonds and semen boitae respectively, plus 50 grams of rice. Hard nuts are pounded to pieces to be boiled into porridge with rice to be eaten for breakfast and supper each day. This porridge serves to replenish vital energy, nourish blood and strengthen intestinal movement.

• Knock at belt channel: As Belt Channel surrounds the waist, one can knock at the left side and the right side of the waist. Before going to bed every evening, lie in bed and quickly knock at these two parts 100 to 300 times with hollow fists until soreness and numbness are felt. Then, use overlapped hands to move around the navel clockwise 30 times. In this way, constipation will soon be improved.

Other Methods of Expelling Intestinal Toxin

• Reasonable diet and frequent exercise, i.e., adjustment of diet, increase of the intake of dietary fiber and reinforcement of exercise at the same time, can promote intestinal tract movement and help the bowel movement.

• Good habits make bowel movement smoother. Discharging excrement at set time every day serves to form conditioned reflex. The establishment of desirable regularity can relax and smooth each bowel movement.

• Drinking more water serves to discharge accumulated excrement. Drinking pure boiled water of at least 1500 ml daily can effectively soften excrement and push excrement to the far-end of the colon. Drinking a glass of water on an empty stomach after getting up in the morning is the most effective.

• Kneading the abdomen can speed up bowel movement. Often kneading the abdomen is conducive to reinforcing abdominal muscles, promoting intestinal movement and accelerating the discharge of excrement while keeping germ-groups within intestines in a balance to prevent intestinal aging.

• Timely treatment of related diseases such as anal fissure, perianal infection and adnexitis can prevent or ease constipation.

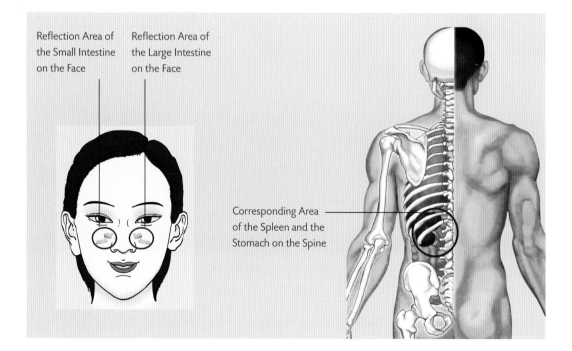

Reflection Area of the Small Intestine on the Face

Reflection Area of the Large Intestine on the Face

Corresponding Area of the Spleen and the Stomach on the Spine

Flabby Skin

According to Chinese medicine, spleen is in charge of muscles. People with nice functions of spleen and stomach can provide muscles with ample nutrition, making skin elastic and tight. These people can look younger than their peers. On the contrary, undesirable functions of spleen and stomach will lead to the reduction of skin elasticity and loosened skin at an early age. Scraping therapy should be concentrated on reinforcing the functions of spleen and stomach.

Recommended Procedures

1. Reflection Area of the Small and Large Intestines on the Face
Method: Use the flat-pressing and kneading to press and knead the area.

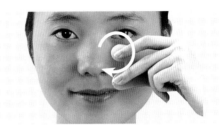

2. The Face
Method: With the face smeared evenly with the scraping cream for beautification, use the pulling method to scrape, i.e., place the scraping plate on the palm or use four fingers to clamp the scraping plate with fingers detached from skin, press while pushing the scraping plate down and up in slow and gentle whirling movements. The force of pressing should be greater than that of the pushing and moving. With one side of the cheek scraped, continue to scrape the other cheek.

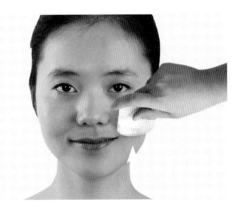

3. Corresponding Area of the Spleen and the Stomach on the Spine
Method: Use the surface-scraping and the dual-angle scraping to scrape the area from up to down.

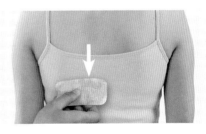

Expert Prompts
Excessive expelling of cutin will make skin thinner, resulting in the loss of natural protective screen of skin and making it more vulnerable to undesirable environment. At the same time, skin will become dry and sensitive, being apt to be loosened. Therefore, expelling the cutin once a week is enough. Oily and dusty face, or the face covered with cosmetics for a long time or cosmetics not fully done away with will lead to the blockage of pores, the imbalance of skin nutrition and even inflammation. If such a state remains for a long time, there will be the loss of skin tension and the phenomenon of loosened skin without elasticity. Therefore, it is very important to clean the face.

Fatigue

It is a subjective feeling of discomfort, resulting mainly from great pressure of life and work, over-exhaustion of energy and physique among people in modern times. Generally, fatigue is marked by a series of symptoms such as receding memory, dizziness, agitation, insomnia, soreness and pain of the waist and legs.

According to Chinese medicine, fatigue is associated with degeneration of inner organ functions and the imbalance of vital energy and blood. For instance, soreness and weakness of the waist and legs are mostly related to kidneys; short of breath and lacking strength are mostly concerned with lungs; spiritual fatigue is mostly linked with the heart while physical fatigue is mostly related to the spleen. Therefore, adjusting all inner organs is the key to easing fatigue.

Fatigue will occur whenever a disease develops into a certain stage, such as multiple sclerosis and cancer. Therefore, people of long-term fatigue failing to be relieved after rest should seek for timely check-up to see if it is caused by illness so as to receive timely treatment. Generally, pathological fatigue would arise without much physical power, which can cause a sense of inner weakness.

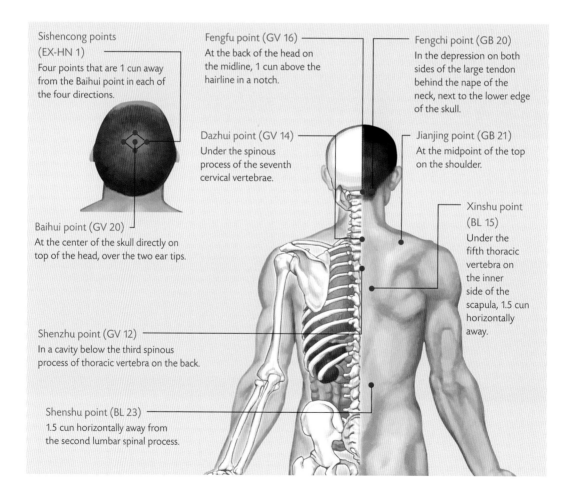

Sishencong points
(EX-HN 1)
Four points that are 1 cun away from the Baihui point in each of the four directions.

Fengfu point (GV 16)
At the back of the head on the midline, 1 cun above the hairline in a notch.

Fengchi point (GB 20)
In the depression on both sides of the large tendon behind the nape of the neck, next to the lower edge of the skull.

Dazhui point (GV 14)
Under the spinous process of the seventh cervical vertebrae.

Jianjing point (GB 21)
At the midpoint of the top on the shoulder.

Xinshu point
(BL 15)
Under the fifth thoracic vertebra on the inner side of the scapula, 1.5 cun horizontally away.

Baihui point (GV 20)
At the center of the skull directly on top of the head, over the two ear tips.

Shenzhu point (GV 12)
In a cavity below the third spinous process of thoracic vertebra on the back.

Shenshu point (BL 23)
1.5 cun horizontally away from the second lumbar spinal process.

Recommended Procedures

1. Baihui Point and Sishencong Points

Method: With Baihui point as the starting point, use the surface-scraping to scrape lightly toward Sishencong points, 10 to 20 times each time for one direction. The combing and scraping can also be used to scrape around with Baihui point as the center.

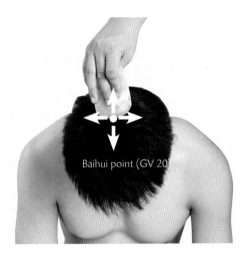

2. Fengfu Point, Dazhui Point and Shenzhu Point

Method: Use the surface-scraping to scrape 10 to 20 times from Fengfu point, Dazhui point to Shenzhu point, with stress on Dazhui point.

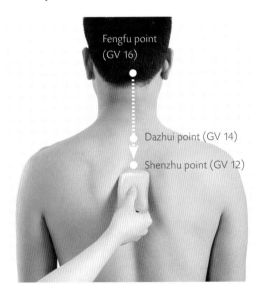

3. Fengchi Point and Jianjing Point

Method: Use the flat-scraping to scrape from Fengchi point to Jianjing point, 20 to 30 times on each side.

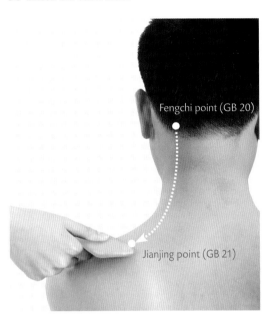

4. Xinshu Point and Shenshu Point

Method: Use the flat-scraping to scrape Xinshu point and Shenshu point of the Bladder Meridian on both sides of the spine, 10 to 20 times on each side.

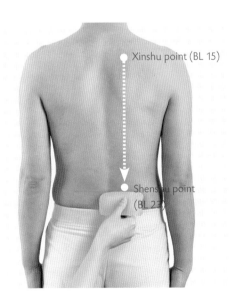

Forgetfulness

People enjoy the best memory around the age 20 and then cerebral functions would gradually decline. Memory would begin to go downhill around the age 25. The older the age, the worse the memory can be. Along with the acceleration of the rhythm in life, various kinds of pressure increase, so it is very common to see young and middle-aged people suffer from forgetfulness.

According to Chinese medicine, this is mostly due to weakness of the heart and spleen or the deficiency of essential vital energy, or the stasis of phlegm. Scraping therapy is conducive to improving forgetfulness.

Frequently using the brain is the most effective way of preventing and improving forgetfulness. Keeping a good mood and often taking part in physical exercise are also helpful to maintaining desirable memory and prolonging the aging of the brain.

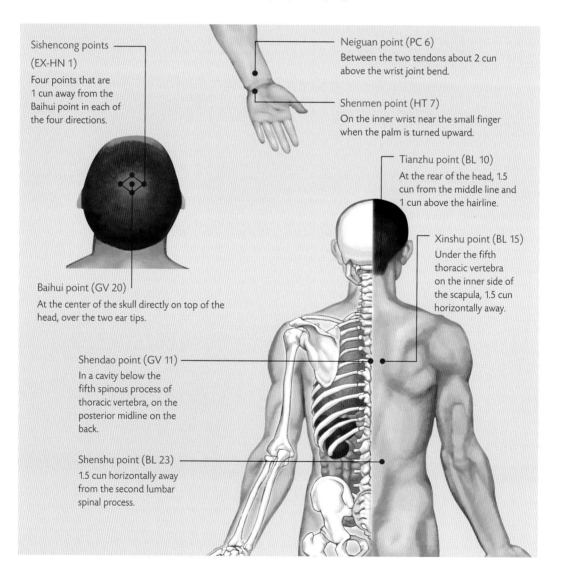

Sishencong points (EX-HN 1)
Four points that are 1 cun away from the Baihui point in each of the four directions.

Neiguan point (PC 6)
Between the two tendons about 2 cun above the wrist joint bend.

Shenmen point (HT 7)
On the inner wrist near the small finger when the palm is turned upward.

Tianzhu point (BL 10)
At the rear of the head, 1.5 cun from the middle line and 1 cun above the hairline.

Xinshu point (BL 15)
Under the fifth thoracic vertebra on the inner side of the scapula, 1.5 cun horizontally away.

Baihui point (GV 20)
At the center of the skull directly on top of the head, over the two ear tips.

Shendao point (GV 11)
In a cavity below the fifth spinous process of thoracic vertebra, on the posterior midline on the back.

Shenshu point (BL 23)
1.5 cun horizontally away from the second lumbar spinal process.

Recommended Procedures

1. Baihui Point and Sishenchong Points
Method: Use the flat-pressing and kneading to press and knead Baihui point and Sishenchong points on the head, until soreness and distention are felt. You can also use the multi-functional scraping comb to scrape and comb the top of the head and stimulate these acupoints at the same time.

3. Tianzhu Point, Shendao Point, Xinshu Point and Shenshu Point
Method: Use the surface-scraping to scrape Tianzhu point on the neck, Shendao point, Xinshu point and Shenshu point on the back from up to down.

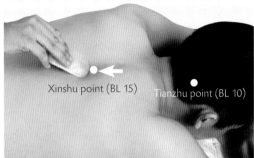

Xinshu point (BL 15)   Tianzhu point (BL 10)

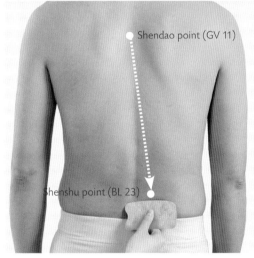

Shendao point (GV 11)

Shenshu point (BL 23)

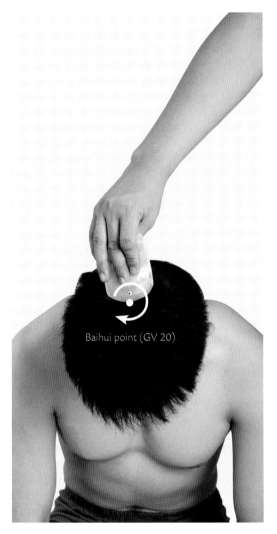

Baihui point (GV 20)

2. Neiguan Point and Shenmen Point
Method: Use the surface-scraping to scrape Neiguan point on the inside of the wrist from up to down, then use the angle-kneading to press and knead Shenmen point on the wrist.

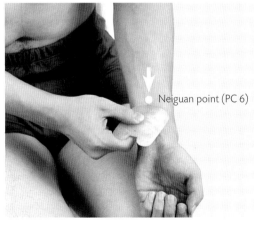

Neiguan point (PC 6)

Agitation

High pressure of work and life will set people in a state of high tension. Agitation, fidgety and depression will take place when people are under too much pressure for a long time beyond the tolerance of nerves, leading to the loss of emotional control. The state of undesirable moods for a long time without relief will result in the imbalance of endocrine and the nerve system as well as affect the physiological functions of other inner organs.

Agitation and fidgety will give rise to distending pain in lateral thorax, lack of appetite, the decline of immunity, sexual dysfunction among men, irregular menstruation, hyperplasia of mammary glands, aggravation of climacteric symptoms and chloasma on the face.

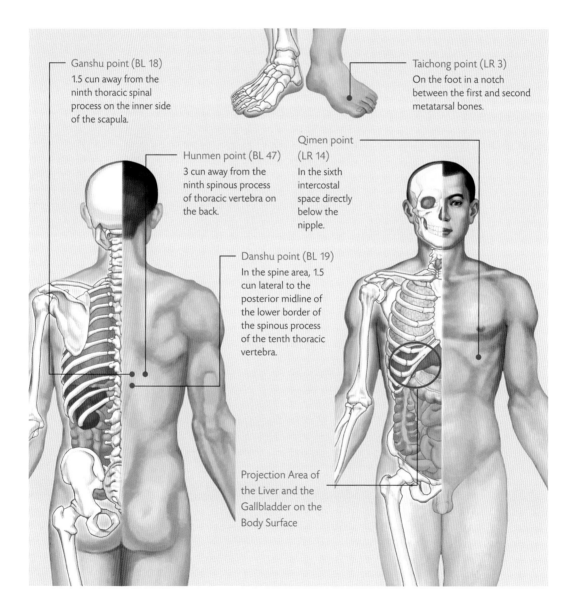

Ganshu point (BL 18)
1.5 cun away from the ninth thoracic spinal process on the inner side of the scapula.

Taichong point (LR 3)
On the foot in a notch between the first and second metatarsal bones.

Qimen point (LR 14)
In the sixth intercostal space directly below the nipple.

Hunmen point (BL 47)
3 cun away from the ninth spinous process of thoracic vertebra on the back.

Danshu point (BL 19)
In the spine area, 1.5 cun lateral to the posterior midline of the lower border of the spinous process of the tenth thoracic vertebra.

Projection Area of the Liver and the Gallbladder on the Body Surface

Recommended Procedures

1. Projection Area of the Liver and the Gallbladder on the Body Surface and Qimen Point

Method: Use the surface-scraping to slowly scrape the projection area of the liver and the gallbladder on the right side of the ribs from inside to outside, with stress on Qimen point. Heavy force and slow speed are needed when the projection area is scraped. Scraping is emphatically directed at areas of positive reactions such as pain and nodules.

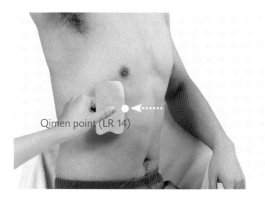

Qimen point (LR 14)

2. Taichong Point

Method: Use the vertical-pressing and kneading to press and knead Taichong point until soreness and distension are felt.

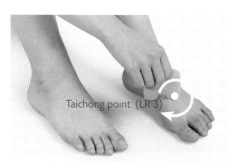

Taichong point (LR 3)

3. Ganshu Point, Hunmen Point and Danshu Point

Method: Use the surface-scraping and dual-angle scraping to scrape parts of Du Meridian, Jiaji points and Bladder Meridian paralleled with the liver and the gallbladder on the back, with emphasis on Ganshu point, Hunmen point and Danshu point.

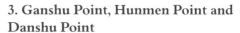

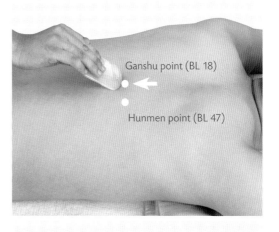

Ganshu point (BL 18)

Hunmen point (BL 47)

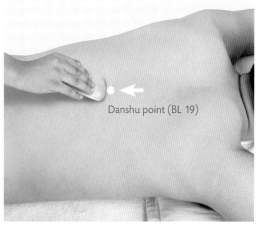

Danshu point (BL 19)

Therapies to Increase the Curative Effect

People with agitation are advised to eat more food that can disperse the liver and rectify vital energy, such as celery, tomatoes, turnips, oranges, grapefruits and tangerines, in addition to stopping smoking, setting a limit to alcoholic drinking and avoiding sweet, fatty or spicy food.

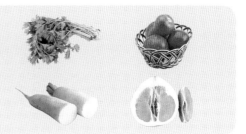

Stiff Neck

This is simple spasm of the neck muscle, mostly due to improper posture of sleep, fixed posture of the neck for a long time, sprain due to sudden turn, intrusion of the cold into the back of the neck, local damage or imbalance of vital energy regulation in related meridians. Scraping therapy can smooth related meridians and the circulation of blood and vital energy, so as to ease stiff muscles and relieve pain.

As for stiff neck, do not force to turn the neck around so as to avoid damage to the cervical vertebra. A hot-water bag, a hot towel or irradiation under the infrared ray bulb can all stop the pain, but attention must be paid to being scalded. Applying the pain-killing plaster to the painful area of the neck can also produce a quite ideal effect, but it is a taboo for pregnant women.

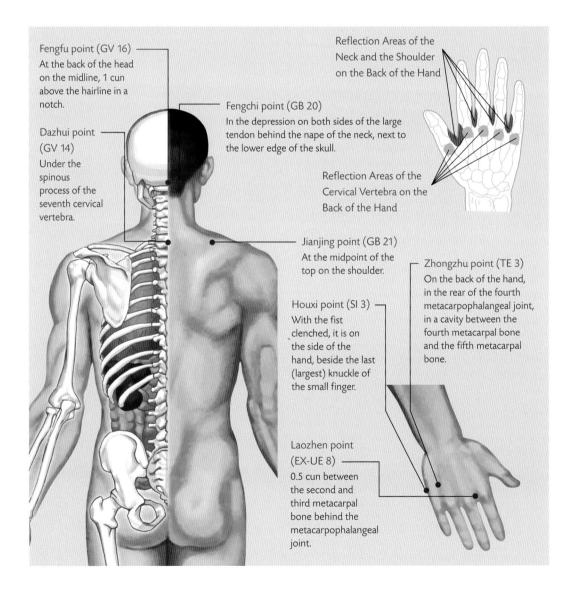

Fengfu point (GV 16)
At the back of the head on the midline, 1 cun above the hairline in a notch.

Dazhui point (GV 14)
Under the spinous process of the seventh cervical vertebra.

Reflection Areas of the Neck and the Shoulder on the Back of the Hand

Fengchi point (GB 20)
In the depression on both sides of the large tendon behind the nape of the neck, next to the lower edge of the skull.

Reflection Areas of the Cervical Vertebra on the Back of the Hand

Jianjing point (GB 21)
At the midpoint of the top on the shoulder.

Zhongzhu point (TE 3)
On the back of the hand, in the rear of the fourth metacarpophalangeal joint, in a cavity between the fourth metacarpal bone and the fifth metacarpal bone.

Houxi point (SI 3)
With the fist clenched, it is on the side of the hand, beside the last (largest) knuckle of the small finger.

Laozhen point (EX-UE 8)
0.5 cun between the second and third metacarpal bone behind the metacarpophalangeal joint.

Recommended Procedures

1. Reflection Areas of the Neck, the Shoulder and the Cervical Vertebra on the Back of the Hand

Method: Use the vertical-pressing and kneading to press and knead the areas. Try carefully to find the points of sensitivity to pain in the area of cervical vertebra, with emphasis on these points when kneading and pressing the areas.

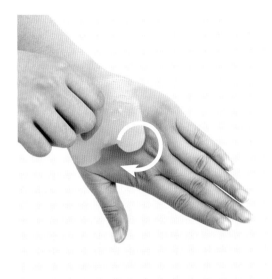

2. Fengfu Point, Dazhui Point, Fengchi Point and Jianjing Point

Method: Use the surface-scraping to scrape from Fengfu point to Dazhui point on Du Meridian from up to down. Then, use the single-angle scraping to scrape Fengchi point and use the surface-scraping to scrape from Fengchi point to Jianjing point.

3. Laozhen Point, Zhongzhu Point and Houxi Point

Method: Use the corner of the scraping plate to vertically press and knead Laozhen point and Zhongzhu point on the back of the hand of the affected side and then scrape Houxi point.

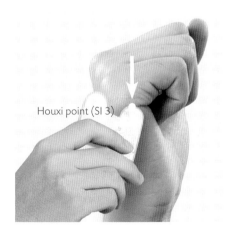

Houxi point (SI 3)

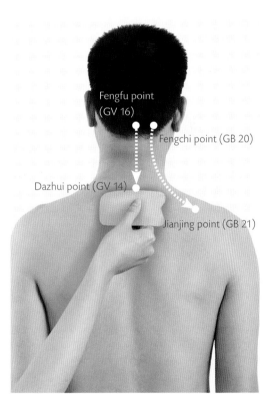

Fengfu point (GV 16)

Fengchi point (GB 20)

Dazhui point (GV 14)

Jianjing point (GB 21)

Insomnia

This refers to the illness caused by the disorder of the functions of inner organs, weakness of vital energy and blood and imbalance between yin and yang, leading to abnormal sleep. The patient of the minor case finds it difficult to fall asleep and easy to wake up. The patient of the serious case fails to sleep all night, coupled with headache, dizziness, palpitation, forgetfulness and lots of dreams, etc.

According to Chinese medicine, insomnia is caused by the seven human emotions, including anger, sorrow, fear, worry, hate and desire, resulting in the heart-kidney imbalance and the pathogenic fire generated by depression of the liver.

Regular routine of daily life is the most effective way for avoiding insomnia, i.e. going to bed and getting up at a designated time so as to establish an internal clock. Sometimes, it is unavoidable to sleep late, but one should get up on time as usual the next morning. On the weekend, try not to get up late, because more sleep is useless since the amount of sleep cannot be stored.

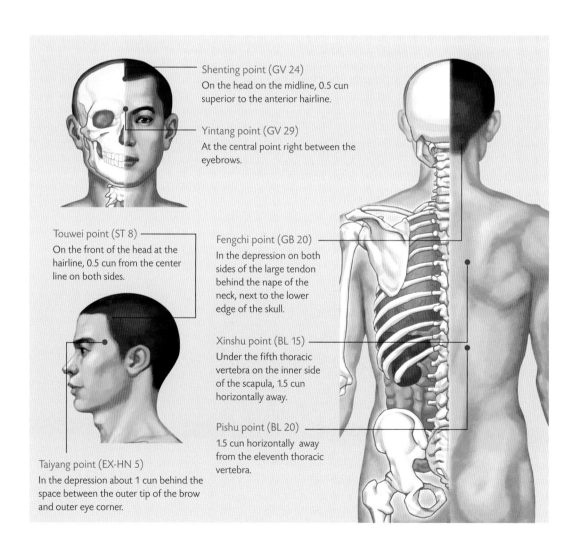

Shenting point (GV 24)
On the head on the midline, 0.5 cun superior to the anterior hairline.

Yintang point (GV 29)
At the central point right between the eyebrows.

Touwei point (ST 8)
On the front of the head at the hairline, 0.5 cun from the center line on both sides.

Fengchi point (GB 20)
In the depression on both sides of the large tendon behind the nape of the neck, next to the lower edge of the skull.

Xinshu point (BL 15)
Under the fifth thoracic vertebra on the inner side of the scapula, 1.5 cun horizontally away.

Pishu point (BL 20)
1.5 cun horizontally away from the eleventh thoracic vertebra.

Taiyang point (EX-HN 5)
In the depression about 1 cun behind the space between the outer tip of the brow and outer eye corner.

Recommended Procedures
1. Shenting Point, Yintang Point and Touwei Point

Method: Use the scraping plate to scrape gently from the middle of the forehead towards Touwei points on both sides of the hair line for 10 to 20 times. Then, use the corner of the scraping plate to press and knead Shenting point, Yintang point and Touwei point.

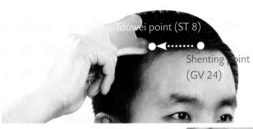

Touwei point (ST 8)
Shenting point (GV 24)

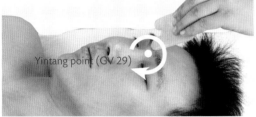

Yintang point (GV 29)

2. Taiyang Point and Fengchi Point

Method: Use the corner of the scraping plate to scrape from Taiyang point to the mastoid process and Fengchi point on the rear of the head via the upper part of the ear, 10 to 20 times on each side. And use the corner to press and knead Fengchi point.

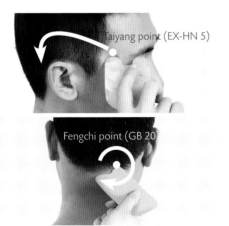

Taiyang point (EX-HN 5)
Fengchi point (GB 20)

3. Xinshu Point and Pishu Point

Method: Use the surface-scraping to scrape from Xinshu point to Pishu point on the back from up to down.

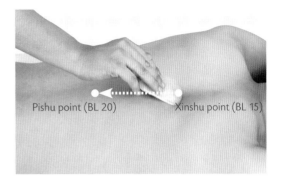

Pishu point (BL 20)
Xinshu point (BL 15)

4. The Sole and the Head

Method: Scrape the entire sole until the head and the sole feel heat before going to bed every evening. Use the surface-scraping to scrape the meridians of the entire head after getting up in the morning. Use the scraping comb made of buffalo horn to scrape in the order of the two sides, the top, and the rear of the head.

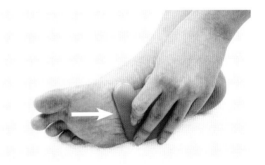

Therapies to Increase the Curative Effect
The diet-oriented prescription of helping sleep:
• 60-gram wheat without shells, 20-gram licorice and fifteen dates are boiled for oral use, once in the morning and once in the evening respectively.
• 15-gram lotus seeds with cores, 30-gram lily bulb and 12-gram lilyturf roots are boiled for oral use as drink.

Acute Conjunctivitis

It is also called "red-eye disease" marked by red and distended eyes, congestion, tears, secretion, the feeling of foreign bodies and heat. According to Chinese medicine, it is caused by pathogenic wind, heat and damp or internal heat in the liver and gallbladder. Therefore, scraping therapy chiefly serves to disperse pathogenic wind and expel heat.

Acute conjunctivitis is caused by germ-infection, being infectious to some extent. Therefore, the scraping plate should be used exclusively for a particular patient. With the scraping done each time, scraping instruments should be carefully washed and disinfected and that hands should also be washed, in order to avoid infection and cross infection.

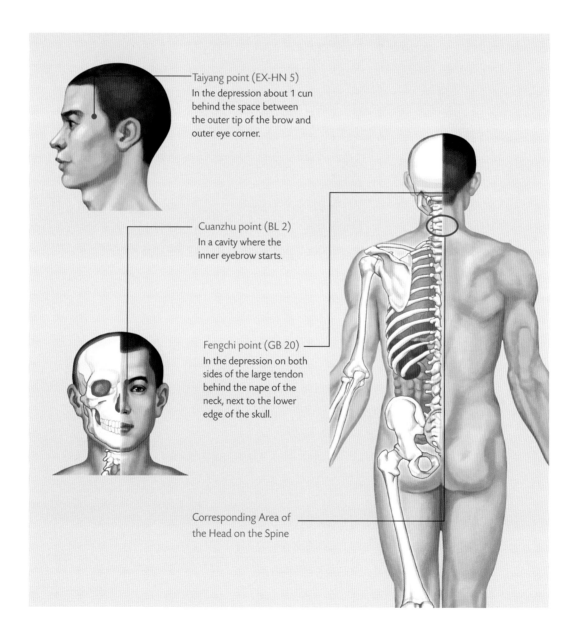

Taiyang point (EX-HN 5)
In the depression about 1 cun behind the space between the outer tip of the brow and outer eye corner.

Cuanzhu point (BL 2)
In a cavity where the inner eyebrow starts.

Fengchi point (GB 20)
In the depression on both sides of the large tendon behind the nape of the neck, next to the lower edge of the skull.

Corresponding Area of the Head on the Spine

Recommended Procedures
1. Corresponding Area of the Head on the Spine
Method: Use the surface-scraping and the dual-angle scraping to scrape the area from up to down.

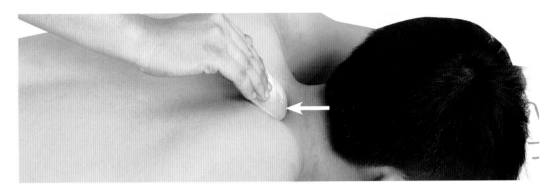

2. Taiyang Point, Cuanzhu Point and Fengchi Point
Method: Use the flat-pressing and kneading to press and knead Taiyang point on the affected side. Use the single-angle scraping to scrape Cuanzhu point on the affected side and Fengchi point on both sides of the head and neck.

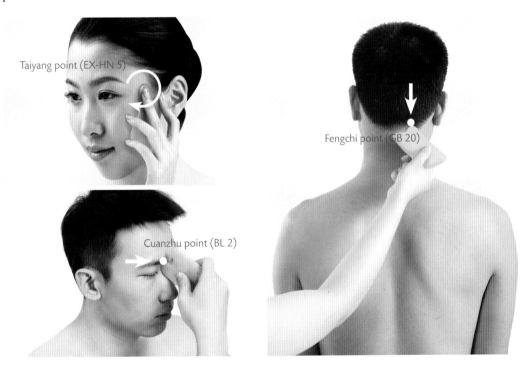

Taiyang point (EX-HN 5)

Cuanzhu point (BL 2)

Fengchi point (GB 20)

Therapy to Increase the Curative Effect
60-gram fresh chrysanthemum (or 15-gram dry chrysanthemum) is boiled for fumigating and washing the eyes before going to bed every evening, i.e., fumigating eyes from a distance and then washing the surrounding area of eyes with it.

Dry Eyes and Eye Strain

Reading and writing for a long time, watching the screen with great attention and blinking eyes less will all result in the reduction of the secretion of aqueous humor, dry eyes and eye fatigue. Inadequate illumination at the places of work and study can also lead to the muscle tension of eyes and excessive use of the eye's accommodation strength. Overloaded work of eyes is not only apt to result in eye fatigue, but also give rise to short-sightedness and other kinds of illness.

According to the Chinese medicine, the liver is closely associated with eyes. Therefore, dry eyes mostly reflects the lack of blood in the liver. Scraping the surrounding areas of eyes emphatically can smooth vital energy and blood, along with the scraping of Ganshu point and Danshu point, to tackle both symptoms and root causes of eye problems. The decline of eyesight can also be dealt with by this therapy.

So far, dry eyes cannot be fundamentally cured. In clinical practice, such a symptom is eased mostly by artificial tears and that the symptom will take place again once the application of artificial tears is stopped. An effective way to prevent dry eyes is to keep good habits of work and daily life. First of all, one should try to avoid watching TV and the mobile phone for a long time. Continuous watch for one hour requires a rest of 5 to 10 minutes. During the rest, one can look into the distance or do eye-exercise. It's better not to wear contact lens when using the computer for a long time, so as to reduce the degree of eye dryness. One who uses the computer very often should pay attention to their diet, i.e., eating more bean products, fish, milk, walnuts, rape, Chinese cabbage, water spinach, tomatoes, and fresh fruits.

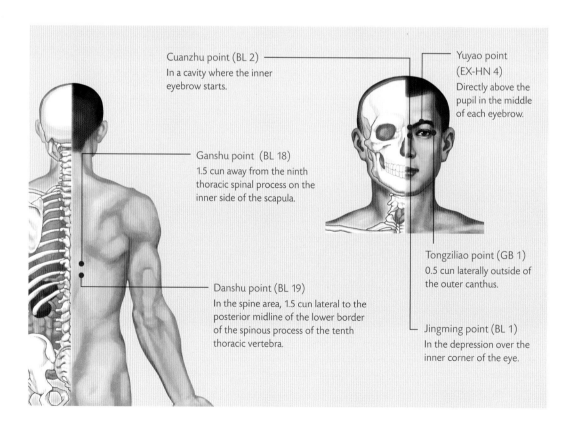

Cuanzhu point (BL 2)
In a cavity where the inner eyebrow starts.

Yuyao point (EX-HN 4)
Directly above the pupil in the middle of each eyebrow.

Ganshu point (BL 18)
1.5 cun away from the ninth thoracic spinal process on the inner side of the scapula.

Tongziliao point (GB 1)
0.5 cun laterally outside of the outer canthus.

Danshu point (BL 19)
In the spine area, 1.5 cun lateral to the posterior midline of the lower border of the spinous process of the tenth thoracic vertebra.

Jingming point (BL 1)
In the depression over the inner corner of the eye.

Recommended Procedures

1. Cuanzhu Point, Yuyao Point, Tongziliao Point and Jingming Point

Method: Use the corner of the scraping plate for beautification to press and knead Jingming point vertically. Then, use the flat-scraping to scrape from the inner eye-corner to Tongziliao point along the upper eye-rim, and then from the inner eye-corner to Tongziliao point along the lower eye-rim, with empahsis on pressing and kneading Cuanzhu point, Yuyao point and Tongziliao point. Gentle force is required for scraping the surrounding areas of eyes and that a little scraping cream can be applied to the scraping plate.

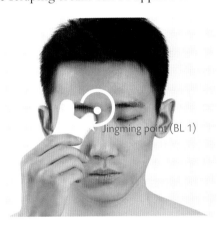
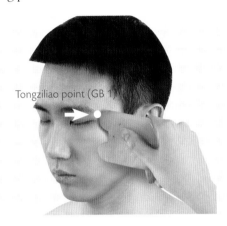

2. Ganshu Point and Danshu Point

Method: Use the surface-scraping to scrape from Ganshu point to Danshu point on the back from up to down repeatedly, until *sha* appears.

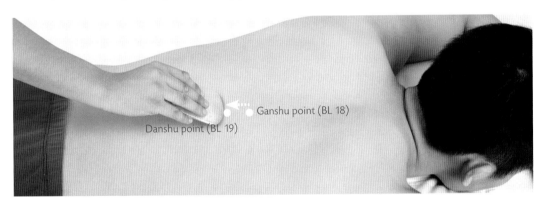

> **Therapy to Increase the Curative Effect**
>
> Porridge of Chinese wolfberries and mulberry fruit:
>
> Ingredients: Five grams of Chinese wolfberries, mulberry fruit and Chinese yam respectively plus five dates and 100-gram rice.
>
> The way of preparation: Washed rice is boiled together with other ingredients as porridge.
>
> The effect: Chinese wolfberries and mulberry fruit in it serve to tonify the liver and kidneys, while Chinese yam and dates are beneficial to the spleen and stomach. Eating this porridge in the morning and in the evening every day for a long time can either eliminate eye fatigue or reinforce physique.

Acne

They are commonly called "whelk." According to Chinese medicine, acne is caused by the accumulation of internal heat, stasis of liver energy and blood as well as imbalance between yin and yang. Too much psychological pressure will disturb the secretion of physiological hormones and lead to the imbalance of endocrine, making it possible for acne to appear. Therefore, people with acne should first learn to adjust work and life to eliminate tension.

Corresponding meridians and inner organs can be judged according to the area on which acne takes place. Instead of scraping the face, scraping therapy is only directed at adjusting the vital energy, blood, yin and yang of related meridians and organs so as to cure it fundamentally.

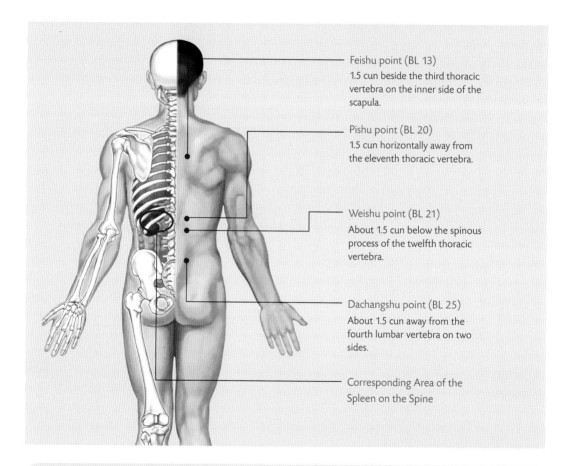

Feishu point (BL 13)
1.5 cun beside the third thoracic vertebra on the inner side of the scapula.

Pishu point (BL 20)
1.5 cun horizontally away from the eleventh thoracic vertebra.

Weishu point (BL 21)
About 1.5 cun below the spinous process of the twelfth thoracic vertebra.

Dachangshu point (BL 25)
About 1.5 cun away from the fourth lumbar vertebra on two sides.

Corresponding Area of the Spleen on the Spine

Expert Prompts
Acne is not supposed to be squeezed at random though they are annoying, because the squeeze is likely to result in such skin damage as the cavity, pigmentation and scars. Excessive force in squeezing the skin around acne will possibly damage related connective tissues and make inflammation worse, making it impossible to restore normal skin elasticity and forming acne-oriented cavities. Stasis of the tissues pressed will also be likely to form acne-oriented scars and pork marks.

Recommended Procedures
1. The Area of Left Ribs and the Corresponding Area of the Spleen on the Spine
Method: Use the flat-scraping to scrape the area of left ribs from inside to outside, and scrape the corresponding area of the spleen on the spine on the left of the back from up to down.

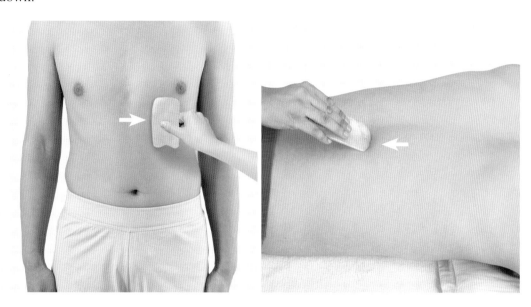

2. Feishu Point, Pishu Point, Weishu Point and Dachangshu Point
Method: Use the surface-scraping and the dual-angle scraping to scrape Feishu point, Pishu point, Weishu point and Dachangshu point of Bladder Meridian from up to down.

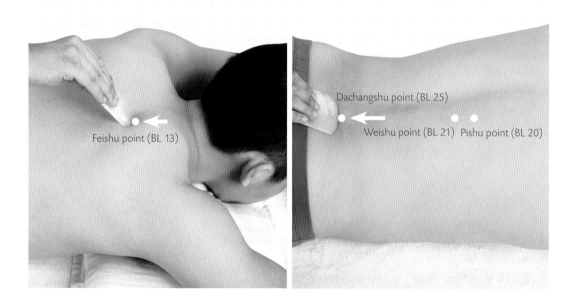

Feishu point (BL 13)

Dachangshu point (BL 25)

Weishu point (BL 21) Pishu point (BL 20)

Dark Circles

This is due to often staying up late, unstable mood, excessive slow blood flow in the eye veins, the lack of oxygen supply in eye cells, too much accumulation of carbon dioxide and metabolized waste in veins, leading to chromatosis around eyes as the under-eye dark circle.

Scraping the surrounding areas of eyes and related acupoints can smooth vital energy and blood in related areas, stimulate cells around eyes, expel edema, decompose pigments around eyes and lighten the under-eye dark circle.

Having enough sleep is very important for preventing the under-eye dark circles. The best time for fast asleep and tonifying the liver is between 22:00 at night and 2:00 in small hours. The under eye dark circle will be very serious if people fail to sleep during this period for long. Drinking more water can promote metabolism, expel waste in the body and reduce under-eye dark circles.

Recommended Procedures
Cuanzhu Point, Chengqi Point and Tongziliao Point
Method: Use the surface-scraping to scrape the face in order (refer to Page 45), with emphasis on acupoints around eyes. Use the single-angle scraping to scrape Cuanzhu point, Chengqi point and Tongziliao point, and try to find, press and knead the point of pain and nodules.

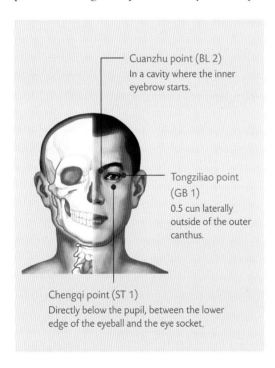

Cuanzhu point (BL 2)
In a cavity where the inner eyebrow starts.

Tongziliao point (GB 1)
0.5 cun laterally outside of the outer canthus.

Chengqi point (ST 1)
Directly below the pupil, between the lower edge of the eyeball and the eye socket.

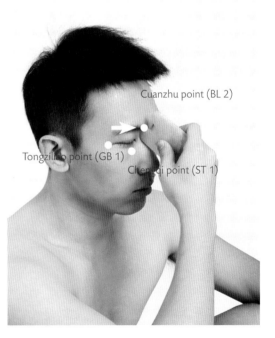

Cuanzhu point (BL 2)

Tongziliao point (GB 1)

Chengqi point (ST 1)

Therapy to Increase the Curative Effect
Use a towel to wrap a boiled egg without shells when it is still hot. The patient, with eyes closed, turn the egg around his/her eyes over ten times, since heat and massage can promote blood circulation of eyes, disperse blood stasis and ease the under-eye dark circles.

Puffiness of the Eye Socket

This is caused by undesirable blood circulation and stranded water. It can be easily caused by drinking lots of water before going to bed, often sitting unmoved for a long time, preferring to eat salty food, staying up late at night and undesirably slow metabolism. According to Chinese medicine, puffiness of the eye socket chiefly results from spleen weakness so that spleen should be adjusted emphatically.

Acute and chronic nephritis can lead to puffiness of the eye socket. It is suggested that the patient go to the hospital to receive check-up on kidney functions if the puffiness cannot be eliminated for a long time. Those with eye bags for a long time should be mindful of hyperlipemia, arteriosclerosis or coronary heart disease.

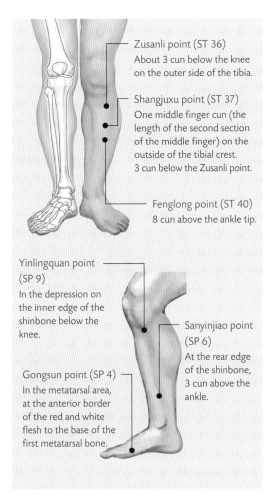

Zusanli point (ST 36)
About 3 cun below the knee on the outer side of the tibia.

Shangjuxu point (ST 37)
One middle finger cun (the length of the second section of the middle finger) on the outside of the tibial crest. 3 cun below the Zusanli point.

Fenglong point (ST 40)
8 cun above the ankle tip.

Yinlingquan point (SP 9)
In the depression on the inner edge of the shinbone below the knee.

Sanyinjiao point (SP 6)
At the rear edge of the shinbone, 3 cun above the ankle.

Gongsun point (SP 4)
In the metatarsal area, at the anterior border of the red and white flesh to the base of the first metatarsal bone.

Recommended Procedures
1. Zusanli Point, Shangjuxu Point and Fenglong Point
Method: Use the surface-scraping or the flat-pressing and kneading to scrape Zusanli point, Shangjuxu point and Fenglong point from up to down on the Stomach Meridian.

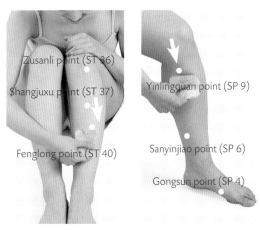

Zusanli point (ST 36)

Shangjuxu point (ST 37)

Yinlingquan point (SP 9)

Fenglong point (ST 40)

Sanyinjiao point (SP 6)

Gongsun point (SP 4)

2. Yinlingquan Point, Gongsun Point and Sanyinjiao Point
Method: Use the surface-scraping or the flat-pressing and kneading to scrape Yinlingquan point, Gongsun point and Sanyinjiao point on the Spleen Meridian.

Therapy to Increase the Curative Effect
With the face washed, use a hot and wet towel to be applied to eyes since the heat can promote blood circulation of eyes. Ten minutes later, use a cold and wet towel on the eyes for about one minute as it serves to contract blood vessels. With this done, smear eye-cream to keep moisture.

Chloasma

According to Chinese medicine, it is caused by the weakness of vital energy and blood, blockage of energy circulation and obstruction of micro-circulation due to stasis. Exhaustion, too much psychological pressure, and natural aging of the human body are all the elements leading to chloasma due to the weakness of vital energy and blood. Scraping therapy can smooth vital energy and blood stasis on the face and improve the functions of inner organs, curing chloasma fundamentally.

Those with chloasma should stop drinking alcohol, avoid eating spicy and irritating food, drink more water, eat more vegetables and fruit with vitamins, take in a variety of vitamins, particularly vitamin C, E and B. Keeping a pleasant mood is also very important in preventing and eliminating chloasma.

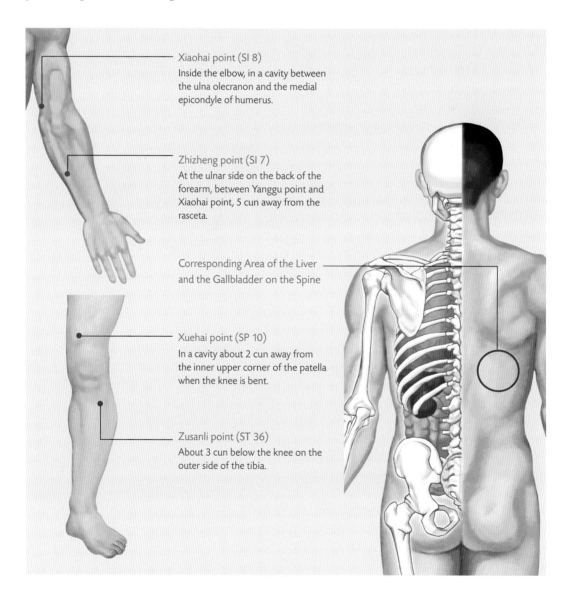

Xiaohai point (SI 8)
Inside the elbow, in a cavity between the ulna olecranon and the medial epicondyle of humerus.

Zhizheng point (SI 7)
At the ulnar side on the back of the forearm, between Yanggu point and Xiaohai point, 5 cun away from the rasceta.

Corresponding Area of the Liver and the Gallbladder on the Spine

Xuehai point (SP 10)
In a cavity about 2 cun away from the inner upper corner of the patella when the knee is bent.

Zusanli point (ST 36)
About 3 cun below the knee on the outer side of the tibia.

Recommended Procedures

1. The Areas with Chloasma

Method: With the face cleaned and the scraping cream smeared, push and scrape the forehead from inside to outside, with emphasis on scraping the areas with chloasma.

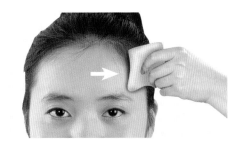

2. Corresponding Area of the Liver and the Gallbladder on the Spine

Method: Use the surface-scraping and the dual-angle scraping to scrape the area on the back.

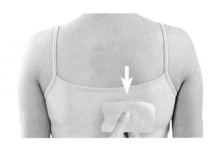

3. Xiaohai Point, Zhizheng Point, Zusanli Point and Xuehai Point

Method: Use the surface-scraping to scrape Xiaohai point and Zhizheng point of Small Intestine Meridian on upper limbs as well as Zusanli point of Stomach Meridian and Xuehai point of Spleen Meridian on lower limbs from up to down.

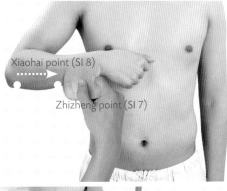

Xiaohai point (SI 8)

Zhizheng point (SI 7)

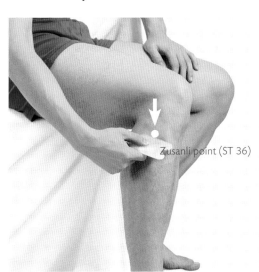

Zusanli point (ST 36)

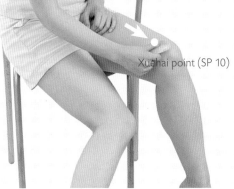

Xuehai point (SP 10)

Expert Prompts

In the market, there is a wide variety of freckle-curing creams. Mind that the stronger the effect of the cream is, the greater the harm it is to the skin due to its chemical elements. It is very likely to impair the pigment cells of skin. More freckles will appear after they are expelled for a short period of time, even to the extent of impairing the face.

Freckles

Freckles directly influence our facial beauty though they are not harmful to our health. According to Chinese medicine, freckles are associated with the weakness of kidneys and lungs. Kidneys are in charge of storing essential elements of the human body. Adequate essential elements and vigorous yang energy can speed up the decomposition of black pigment and obviously lighten freckles. Therefore, emphasis should be put on adjusting the functions of lungs and kidneys in the course of the scraping therapy.

The irradiation of ultraviolet will speed up the generation of lots of black pigment on the skin. Some stranded and precipitated black pigment in the skin lead to the formation and aggravation of freckles. Therefore, trying to avoid being exposed to the sunlight for a long time can effectively prevent and improve freckles.

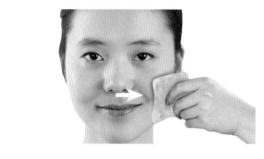

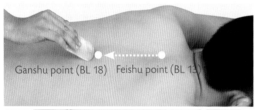

Ganshu point (BL 18)   Feishu point (BL 13)

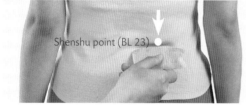

Shenshu point (BL 23)

Recommended Procedures

1. The Face

Method: With the face cleaned and the scraping cream smeared, use the flat-scraping to scrape the forehead, the surrounding areas of eyes, the cheeks, the surrounding areas of lips, the nose and the lower jaw from inside to outside in order (scraping on the nose should be done from up to down). Pressing and kneading should be emphatically done on the corresponding area of the lungs and the kidneys as well as areas with more freckles on the face, until the skin feels slightly hot and turns red.

2. Feishu Point, Ganshu Point and Shenshu Point

Method: Use the surface-scraping to scrape from Feishu point, Ganshu point to Shengshu point of Bladder Meridian on the back from up to down.

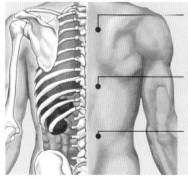

Feishu point (BL 13)
1.5 cun beside the third thoracic vertebra on the inner side of the scapula.

Ganshu point (BL 18)
1.5 cun away from the ninth thoracic spinal process on the inner side of the scapula.

Shenshu point (BL 23)
1.5 cun horizontally away from the second lumbar spinal process.

Holographic Area of the Lungs on the Face

Holographic Area of the Kidneys on the Face

Dry Skin

Women in modern times are generally marked by using cosmetics excessively, which will reduce the skin ability of secreting oil and lead to the lack of water in muscles. Climatic changes, insufficient sleep, fatigue, excessive reduction of weight and exclusive preference to a certain kind of food will also result in the imbalance of metabolism, the loss of skin vitality, being apt to result in dry and coarse skin.

Taking a bath in very hot water and using irritating soaps or cleaners can also give rise to dry skin. Dry skin is sometimes coupled with intolerable itching. Don't scratch it, in order to prevent the skin from being harmed or causing inflammation.

Since the flesh of the palm and the sole is quite thick, the scraping oil does not have to be applied. Scraping serves to promote the blood circulation of the palm and the sole. However, with the application of the scraping oil, the effect of beautification will be better. So, scraping with the scraping oil once a week can be adopted. After the scraping, pay attention to eating more juicy food.

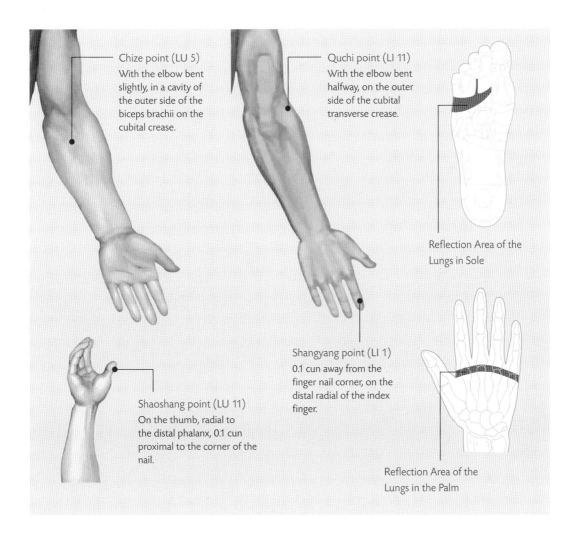

Chize point (LU 5)
With the elbow bent slightly, in a cavity of the outer side of the biceps brachii on the cubital crease.

Quchi point (LI 11)
With the elbow bent halfway, on the outer side of the cubital transverse crease.

Reflection Area of the Lungs in Sole

Shaoshang point (LU 11)
On the thumb, radial to the distal phalanx, 0.1 cun proximal to the corner of the nail.

Shangyang point (LI 1)
0.1 cun away from the finger nail corner, on the distal radial of the index finger.

Reflection Area of the Lungs in the Palm

Recommended Procedures

1. Chize Pioint, Shaoshang Point, Quchi Point and Shangyang Point

Method: With the method of smoothing the vital energy in the main and collateral channels, scrape the Lung Meridian and Large Intestine Meridian on the radial arm. Scrape from Chize point at the elbow joint downward to Shaoshang point at the thumb tip, and from Quchi point downward to Shangyang point at the index finger, once every day.

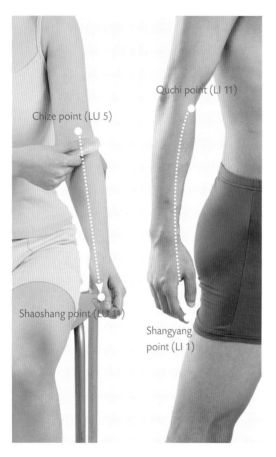

Quchi point (LI 11)

Chize point (LU 5)

Shaoshang point (LU 11)

Shangyang point (LI 1)

2. Reflection Area of the Lungs in the Palm

Method: Use the corner of the scraping plate to scrape the area until the skin in the area feels slightly hot. With one palm done, turn to the other palm.

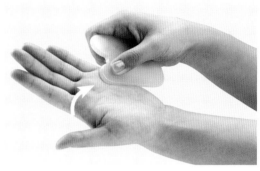

3. Reflection Area of the Lungs in Sole

Method: With feet cleaned, use the single-angle scraping to scrape the area until the skin feels slightly hot. With one foot done, turn to the other foot.

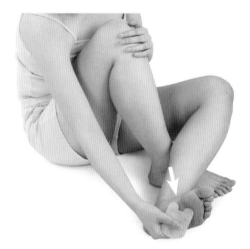

Therapy to Increase the Curative Effect

In dry season, eating some carrots can moisten skin. β-carotene rich in carrots can be converted into vitamin A in the human body, which can protect the skin surface and make the skin tender, moistened, glossy and elastic.

Points of attention: β-carotene is fat-soluble substance. It can be turned into vitamin A only when it is dissolved in oil. Therefore, carrots should be fried, or eaten together with other kinds of oily food.

Dull Complexion

The skin color is decided by liver functions. Liver is in charge of vital energy and blood all over the body. It is also an important organ of expelling toxin. Lots of metabolized substances in the inner environment of the human body are expelled and dealt with by the liver. Therefore, attention should be paid to expelling toxin in the liver when it comes to dull complexion. Scraping therapy focuses on soothing liver, benefiting gallbladder, eliminating stasis and expelling toxin.

Generally, scraping bladder meridian can bring about a little *sha* and that urine will be a bit more turbid than usual. These are manifestations of expelling accumulated toxin. With the scraping therapy done persistently for two months, skin will gradually become fair and light-complexioned. Thanks to smooth circulation of vital energy circulation, people will feel pleasant and that gray hair and the fall-off of hair can also be improved.

Recommended Procedures
1. Corresponding Area of the Liver and the Gallblader on the Spine on the Right Back
Method: Use the flat-scraping to scrape the area from up to down.

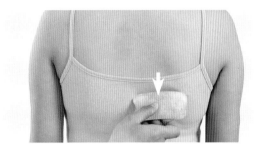

2. Ganshu Point, Hunmen Point, Danshu Point and Yanggang Point
Method: Use the flat-scraping to scrape Ganshu point, Hunmen point, Danshu point and Yanggang point of bladder meridian from up to down, i.e., from Ganshu point to Danshu point, and from Hunmen point to Yanggang point from up to down.

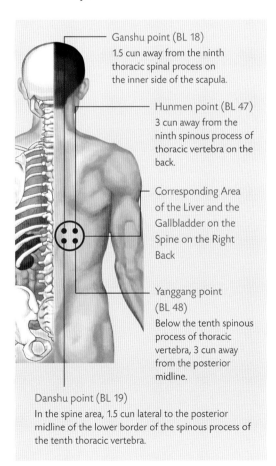

Ganshu point (BL 18)
1.5 cun away from the ninth thoracic spinal process on the inner side of the scapula.

Hunmen point (BL 47)
3 cun away from the ninth spinous process of thoracic vertebra on the back.

Corresponding Area of the Liver and the Gallbladder on the Spine on the Right Back

Yanggang point (BL 48)
Below the tenth spinous process of thoracic vertebra, 3 cun away from the posterior midline.

Danshu point (BL 19)
In the spine area, 1.5 cun lateral to the posterior midline of the lower border of the spinous process of the tenth thoracic vertebra.

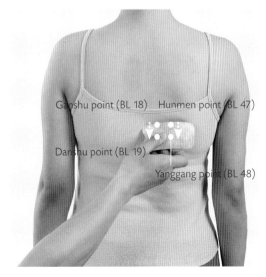

Skin Itch

According to Chinese medicine, it is caused by the intrusion of wind into the weak physique and the wind struggles with blood and vital energy. Together with the application of medicine on the affected area, scraping therapy can produce a desirable effect on stopping the itch. The wound on the skin, if any, should not be scraped and should be carefully avoided.

Recommended Procedures

1. Fengchi Point
Method: Use the single-angle scraping to scrape Fengchi points on both sides of the neck from up to down.

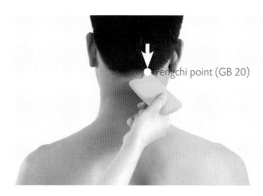

Fengchi point (GB 20)

2. Dazhui Point and Shenzhu Point
Method: Use the surface-scraping to scrape from Dazhui point to Shenzhu point on the back.

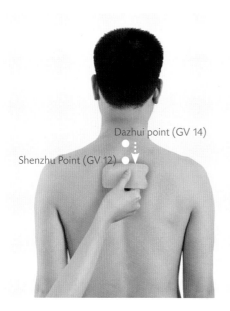

Dazhui point (GV 14)
Shenzhu Point (GV 12)

3. Quchi Point and Shousanli Point
Method: Use the single-angle scraping to scrape from Quchi point to Shousanli point of Large Intestine Meridian on both sides.

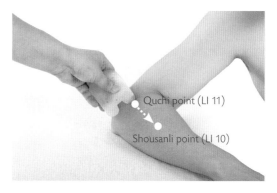

Quchi point (LI 11)
Shousanli point (LI 10)

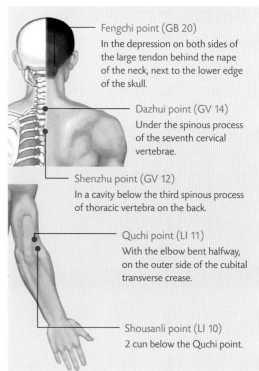

Fengchi point (GB 20)
In the depression on both sides of the large tendon behind the nape of the neck, next to the lower edge of the skull.

Dazhui point (GV 14)
Under the spinous process of the seventh cervical vertebrae.

Shenzhu point (GV 12)
In a cavity below the third spinous process of thoracic vertebra on the back.

Quchi point (LI 11)
With the elbow bent halfway, on the outer side of the cubital transverse crease.

Shousanli point (LI 10)
2 cun below the Quchi point.

Eczema

This is a kind of allergic disease. According to Chinese medicine, it is chiefly associated with the pathogenic damp which can contain heat in the form of damp-heat. Eczema is generally marked by erythema, blisters, erosion, itch and pimples. Generally, it attacks repeatedly due to pathogenic damp.

People with eczema must pay attention to the adjustment of diet, follow two points as below:

1. Eat light food of low sugar and low salt, avoid irritating and oily food.

2. Eat more food that can reduce internal heat and damp as well as more food rich in vitamins and minerals, more fruits and green vegetables.

Recommended Procedures

1. The Healthy Side

Method: Use the surface-scraping to scrape the healthy side corresponding to eczema.

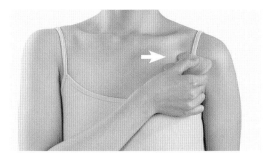

2. Yinlingquan Point and Sanyinjiao Point

Method: Use the surface-scraping to scrape from Yinlingquan point to Sanyinjiao point on both sides of lower limbs.

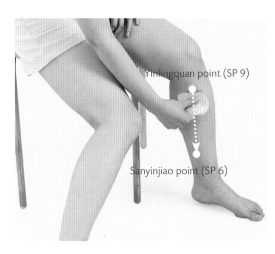

3. Quchi Point and Shousanli point

Method: Use the surface-scraping to scrape from Quchi point to Shousanli point on both sides of upper limbs.

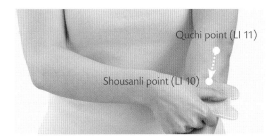

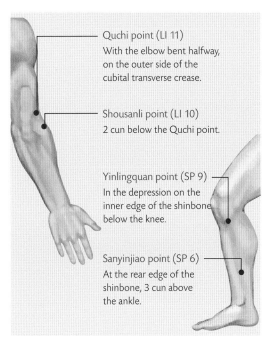

Quchi point (LI 11)
With the elbow bent halfway, on the outer side of the cubital transverse crease.

Shousanli point (LI 10)
2 cun below the Quchi point.

Yinlingquan point (SP 9)
In the depression on the inner edge of the shinbone below the knee.

Sanyinjiao point (SP 6)
At the rear edge of the shinbone, 3 cun above the ankle.

Chilblain

This is a kind of limited and inflammatory illness at the end area manifested by congestive distention on the chilled area and itch of skin when it turns warm. Erosion and ulcer will take place on the affected area for serious cases. The course of this illness is quite long with repeated attacks in winter, making it difficult to be cured fundamentally.

The affected area is generally at the end of hands and feet. Scraping therapy mainly serves to smooth the circulation of vital energy and blood in related areas. Therefore, scraping is generally done near the affected area without considering concrete acupoints.

It is normal to have pain at the place with deformed and distended nodules during scraping. The area being scraped will gradually go through a process from being ice-cold to being warm, driving the cold to the end of fingers. The symptom will be obviously eased if the scraping is done persistently once or twice every day. With the scraping done, do not touch the cold water within three hours to prevent the intrusion of pathogenic cold.

Recommended Procedures

1. Chilblain on Hands
Method: Use the surface-scraping to scrape from the wrist to fingers. The joints and both sides of each finger should be scraped. Scrape the palm before scraping the hand back for 20 times or so successively. Do not scrape the wound on the skin.

2. Chilblain on Feet
Method: Use the surface-scraping to scrape from the heel to the toes for 20 to 30 times and then from the ankle to the toes for 20 to 30 times until related skin feels warm. You should not scrape the wound on the skin.

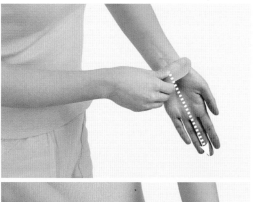

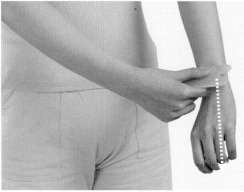

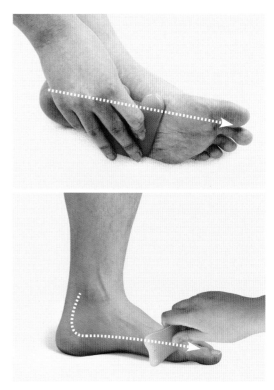

Cold Hands and Feet

According to Chinese medicine, ice-cold hands and feet are associated with the deficiency of yang energy in inner organs and slow blood flow. Hands and feet often in an ice-cold state, if not dealt with timely, will lead to depression and serious fear of the cold for a long time. Scraping therapy can restore and smooth the circulation of vital energy and blood, easing the symptom of ice-cold hands and feet.

Doing physical exercise frequently is the best way for preventing and controlling the symptom of ice-cold hands and feet. Walking fast for 30 minutes after getting up every morning can promote the circulation of vital energy and blood as well as keeping hands and feet warm for a whole day. People can also try to climb stairs or jump up and down to sweat a little to reinforce the body's ability of adjusting temperature. Walking around during the break of work and moving fingers and toes from time to time can all help to stimulate blood circulation.

Recommended Procedures

1. Hand
Method: Use the surface-scraping to scrape the palm from up to down, until the palm feels heat and turns red, or use the groove of the scraping plate to scrape from the finger roots to finger tips, until fingers feel heat and turn red.

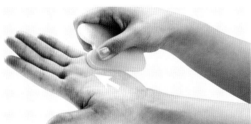

3. Sanyinjiao Point
Method: Use the flat-scraping to scrape Sanyinjiao point on both sides of lower limbs from up to down with light force, until the shins feel heat.

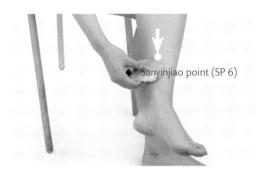

Sanyinjiao point (SP 6)

2. Sole
Method: Use the surface-scraping to scrape the sole, until the sole feels heat and turns red. Use the corner of the scraping plate to emphatically press and knead Yongquan point, until the sole feels heat.

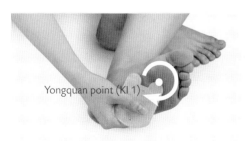

Yongquan point (KI 1)

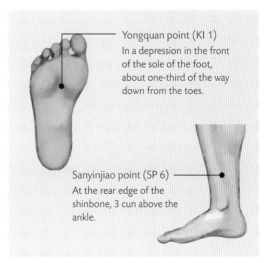

Yongquan point (KI 1)
In a depression in the front of the sole of the foot, about one-third of the way down from the toes.

Sanyinjiao point (SP 6)
At the rear edge of the shinbone, 3 cun above the ankle.

Neurodermitis

This is a kind of chronic skin inflammation manifested with paroxysmal itch and skin lichenification. It often takes place on the area subject to friction without a clear cause. However, according to general understanding, it is associated with long-time scraping, friction, mental factors and certain irritation from outside.

In principle, stopping itch is the main purpose for the patient with neurodermitis. The patient should avoid the irritation of thermal physics and mechanical contact such as sunlight, scraping and friction, in addition to avoiding over-tension and mental irritation plus the restriction over alcohol, coffee and spicy food.

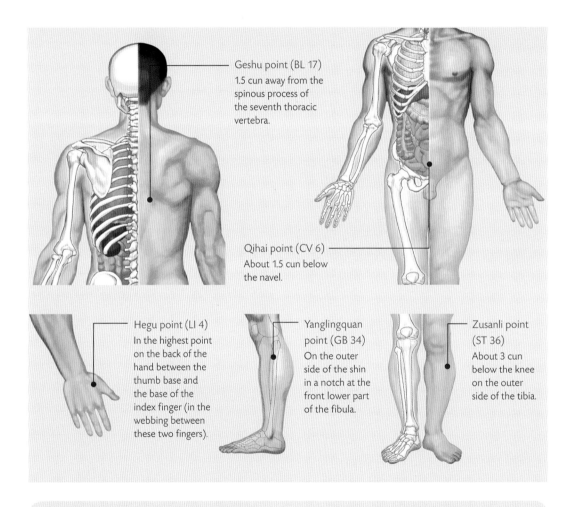

Geshu point (BL 17)
1.5 cun away from the spinous process of the seventh thoracic vertebra.

Qihai point (CV 6)
About 1.5 cun below the navel.

Hegu point (LI 4)
In the highest point on the back of the hand between the thumb base and the base of the index finger (in the webbing between these two fingers).

Yanglingquan point (GB 34)
On the outer side of the shin in a notch at the front lower part of the fibula.

Zusanli point (ST 36)
About 3 cun below the knee on the outer side of the tibia.

Therapy to Increase the Curative Effect
25-gram old tea leaves, 25-gram artemisia argyi, 50-gram old ginger and two pieces of purple garlic. The mashed garlic, sliced old ginger and tea leaves are boiled in water for five minutes with a little salt added. Such solution is used to wash the affected area (the up-mentioned dose is set for two days), which can expel inflammation and kill gems as an auxiliary method for curing neurodermitis.

Recommended Procedures

1. Qihai Point

Method: Use the single-angle scraping to scrape Qihai point 30 times from up to down, with the force gradually increased until a sense of strong soreness and distention is felt in the related area.

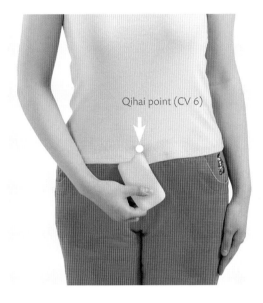

Qihai point (CV 6)

2. Yanglingquan Point and Zusanli Point

Method: Use the surface-scraping to scrape from Yanglingquan point to Zusanli point on both sides of lower limbs 30 times with a little heavy force, until *sha* appears.

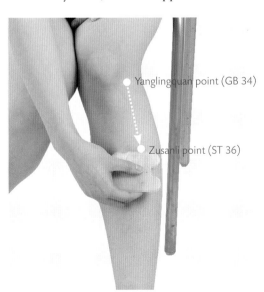

Yanglingquan point (GB 34)

Zusanli point (ST 36)

3. Hegu Point

Method: Use the corner of the scraping plate to scrape Hegu point 30 times from up to down, until the skin turns red.

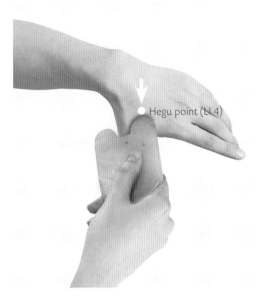

Hegu point (LI 4)

4. Geshu Point

Method: Use the surface-scraping to scrape Geshu point on the back 30 times from up to down with a little heavy force until purplish *sha* speckles appear.

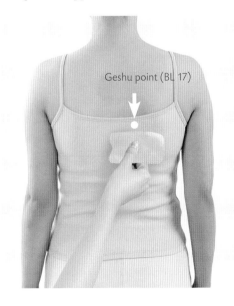

Geshu point (BL 17)

Urticaria

Also called "wind measles," it is marked by "wind patches" in different sizes and forms. The patient would feel burnt and extremely itching as well as abdominal pain and diarrhea, and even to the extent of laryngeal edema or shock. This disease attacks repeatedly and cannot be cured easily. According to Chinese medicine, it is mainly due to the imbalance of vital energy and blood. Scraping therapy can prevent and cure it through soothing the inner functions and expelling malignant elements.

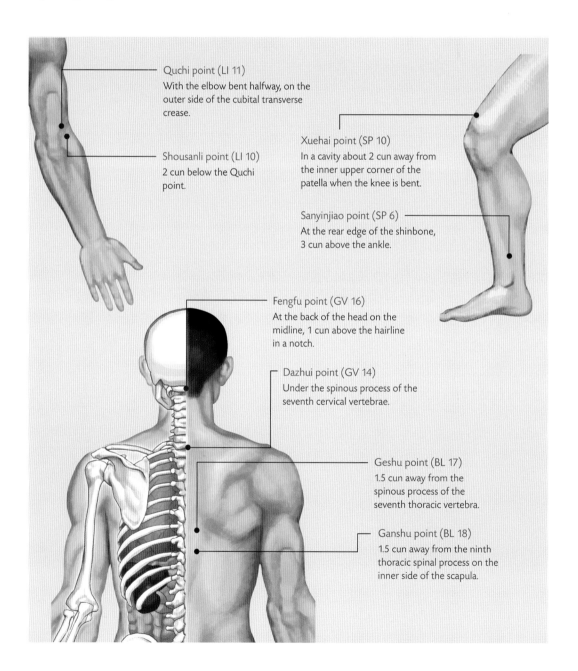

Quchi point (LI 11)
With the elbow bent halfway, on the outer side of the cubital transverse crease.

Shousanli point (LI 10)
2 cun below the Quchi point.

Xuehai point (SP 10)
In a cavity about 2 cun away from the inner upper corner of the patella when the knee is bent.

Sanyinjiao point (SP 6)
At the rear edge of the shinbone, 3 cun above the ankle.

Fengfu point (GV 16)
At the back of the head on the midline, 1 cun above the hairline in a notch.

Dazhui point (GV 14)
Under the spinous process of the seventh cervical vertebrae.

Geshu point (BL 17)
1.5 cun away from the spinous process of the seventh thoracic vertebra.

Ganshu point (BL 18)
1.5 cun away from the ninth thoracic spinal process on the inner side of the scapula.

Recommended Procedures

1. Fengfu Point and Dazhui Point

Method: Use the single-angle scraping to scrape from Fengfu point to Dazhui point on the rear of the neck.

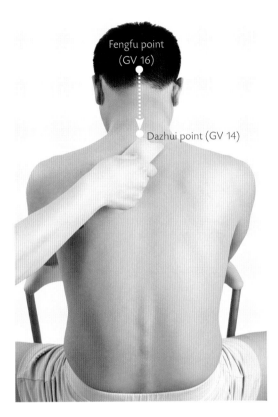

2. Quchi Point and Shousanli Point

Method: Use the single-angle scraping to scrape from Quchi point to Shousanli point of Large Intestine Meridian on both sides.

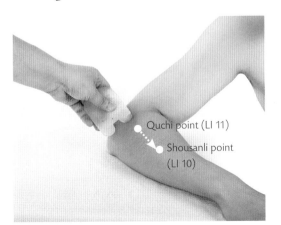

3. Geshu Point and Ganshu Point

Method: Use the surface-scraping to scrape from Geshu point to Ganshu point on the back.

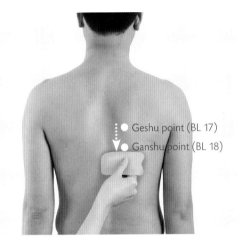

4. Xuehai Point and Sanyinjiao Point

Method: Use the surface-scraping to scrape from Xuehai point to Sanyinjiao point of Spleen Meridian on both sides.

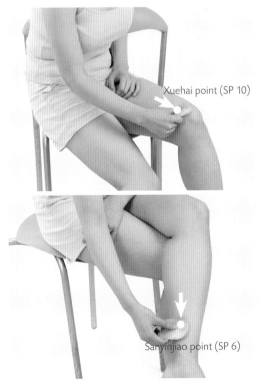

Shingles

This is a virus-oriented disease marked by belt-like blisters in groups as painful as being burnt. It mostly goes around the waist. The pain often continues until measles completely disappear, sometimes lasting for several months.

The area with blisters and measles must not be scraped directly. Scraping can be done around the affected area with a little force. Blisters must not be scraped.

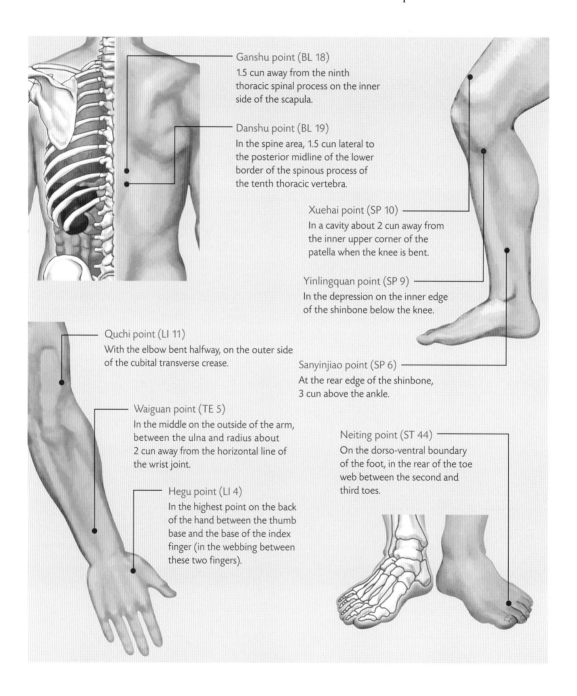

Ganshu point (BL 18)
1.5 cun away from the ninth thoracic spinal process on the inner side of the scapula.

Danshu point (BL 19)
In the spine area, 1.5 cun lateral to the posterior midline of the lower border of the spinous process of the tenth thoracic vertebra.

Xuehai point (SP 10)
In a cavity about 2 cun away from the inner upper corner of the patella when the knee is bent.

Yinlingquan point (SP 9)
In the depression on the inner edge of the shinbone below the knee.

Quchi point (LI 11)
With the elbow bent halfway, on the outer side of the cubital transverse crease.

Sanyinjiao point (SP 6)
At the rear edge of the shinbone, 3 cun above the ankle.

Waiguan point (TE 5)
In the middle on the outside of the arm, between the ulna and radius about 2 cun away from the horizontal line of the wrist joint.

Neiting point (ST 44)
On the dorso-ventral boundary of the foot, in the rear of the toe web between the second and third toes.

Hegu point (LI 4)
In the highest point on the back of the hand between the thumb base and the base of the index finger (in the webbing between these two fingers).

Recommended Procedures

1. Ganshu Point and Danshu Point

Method: Use the surface-scraping to scrape from Ganshu point to Danshu point on the back for about 30 times, until *sha* appears.

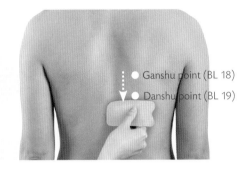

Ganshu point (BL 18)
Danshu point (BL 19)

2. Quchi Point, Waiguan Point and Hegu Point

Method: Use the single-angle scraping to scrape Quchi point, Waiguan point and Hegu point on both sides of lower limbs from up to down.

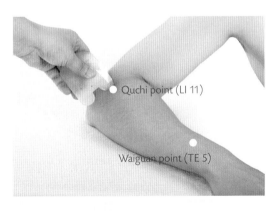

Quchi point (LI 11)
Waiguan point (TE 5)

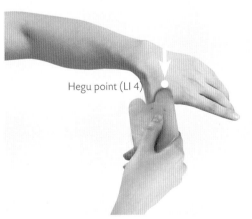

Hegu point (LI 4)

3. Xuehai Point, Yinlingquan Point, Sanyinjiao Point and Neiting point

Method: Use the surface-scraping to scrape from Xuehai point to Yinlingquan point and Sanyinjiao point inside lower limbs from up to down, then use the single-angle scraping to scrape Neiting point on the back of the foot.

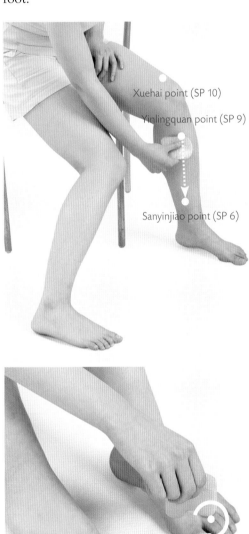

Xuehai point (SP 10)
Yinlingquan point (SP 9)
Sanyinjiao point (SP 6)
Neiting point (ST 44)

Flat Warts

As neoplasm on the skin-surface, they are caused by human papilloma virus. Appearing flat and smooth without causing any discomfort to people, they often take place on the face and hand back of youngsters. The patient generally does not feel about it, but suffers from itch before they disappear. It is often marked by a slow pathological change as benign illness without serious harm generally. It can last for 3 to 4 years and disappear automatically in one or two years. It is better not to scrape the itching area and timely treatement at the specialized hospital is required so as to prevent it from spreading to other parts of the body.

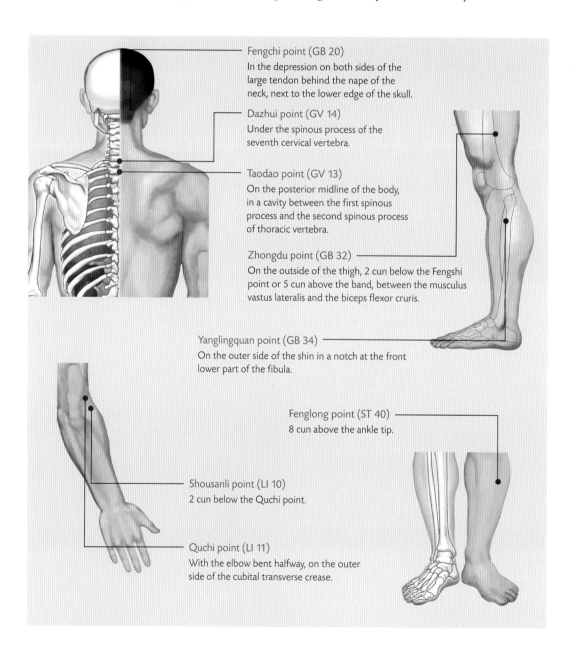

Fengchi point (GB 20)
In the depression on both sides of the large tendon behind the nape of the neck, next to the lower edge of the skull.

Dazhui point (GV 14)
Under the spinous process of the seventh cervical vertebra.

Taodao point (GV 13)
On the posterior midline of the body, in a cavity between the first spinous process and the second spinous process of thoracic vertebra.

Zhongdu point (GB 32)
On the outside of the thigh, 2 cun below the Fengshi point or 5 cun above the band, between the musculus vastus lateralis and the biceps flexor cruris.

Yanglingquan point (GB 34)
On the outer side of the shin in a notch at the front lower part of the fibula.

Fenglong point (ST 40)
8 cun above the ankle tip.

Shousanli point (LI 10)
2 cun below the Quchi point.

Quchi point (LI 11)
With the elbow bent halfway, on the outer side of the cubital transverse crease.

Recommended Procedures

1. Fengchi Point

Method: Use the single-angle scraping to scrape Fengchi point on both sides on the rear of the neck.

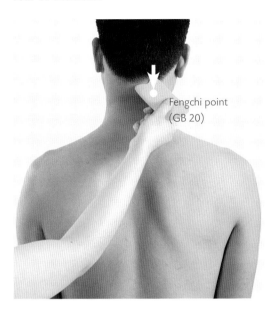

Fengchi point (GB 20)

3. Quchi Point and Shousanli Point

Method: Use the single-angle scraping to scrape from Quchi point to Shousanli point on both sides from up to down.

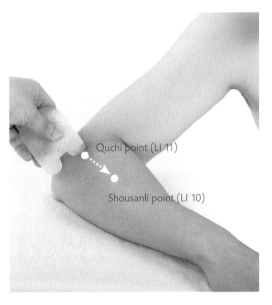

Quchi point (LI 11)

Shousanli point (LI 10)

2. Dazhui Point and Taodao Point

Method: Use the surface-scraping to scrape from Dazhui point to Taodao point on the back from up to down.

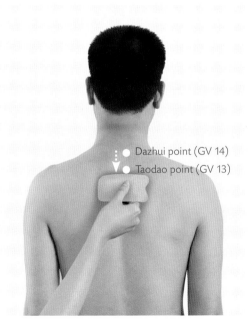

Dazhui point (GV 14)

Taodao point (GV 13)

4. Zhongdu Point, Yanglingquan Point and Fenglong Point

Method: Use the single-angle scraping to scrape Zhongdu point, Yanglingquan point and Fenglong point on both sides of the Gallbladder Meridian from up to down.

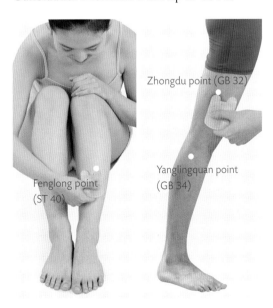

Zhongdu point (GB 32)

Yanglingquan point (GB 34)

Fenglong point (ST 40)

Facioplegia

....

Also called "facial paralysis," it attacks very quickly. Usually, it is marked by muscle paralysis on one side of the face and wry mouth and eyes. It occurs frequently in spring and autumn mostly with male patients aged from 20 to 40, and occasionally among children. Some patients will feel painful in the rear of and below the ears as well as on the face in the early stage. Sometimes, there will be the decline or disappearance of taste sense of tongue in the affected side. Scraping therapy can improve the illness to a certain extent. If it is central facioplegia (i.e., facial paralysis caused by the organic injury of cerebral nerves), scraping therapy can be coupled with the treatment of "sequela of apoplexy" mentioned in this chapter (Page 167).

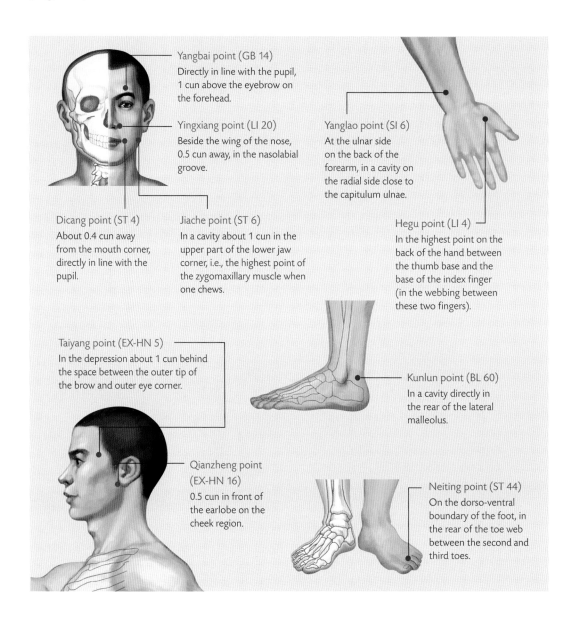

Yangbai point (GB 14)
Directly in line with the pupil, 1 cun above the eyebrow on the forehead.

Yingxiang point (LI 20)
Beside the wing of the nose, 0.5 cun away, in the nasolabial groove.

Yanglao point (SI 6)
At the ulnar side on the back of the forearm, in a cavity on the radial side close to the capitulum ulnae.

Dicang point (ST 4)
About 0.4 cun away from the mouth corner, directly in line with the pupil.

Jiache point (ST 6)
In a cavity about 1 cun in the upper part of the lower jaw corner, i.e., the highest point of the zygomaxillary muscle when one chews.

Hegu point (LI 4)
In the highest point on the back of the hand between the thumb base and the base of the index finger (in the webbing between these two fingers).

Taiyang point (EX-HN 5)
In the depression about 1 cun behind the space between the outer tip of the brow and outer eye corner.

Kunlun point (BL 60)
In a cavity directly in the rear of the lateral malleolus.

Qianzheng point (EX-HN 16)
0.5 cun in front of the earlobe on the cheek region.

Neiting point (ST 44)
On the dorso-ventral boundary of the foot, in the rear of the toe web between the second and third toes.

Recommended Procedures

1. Taiyang Point, Qianzheng Point, Yangbai Point, Yingxiang Point, Dicang Point and Jiache Point

Method: Use the corner of the scraping plate to press and knead Taiyang point and Qianzheng point on the affected side. Use the flat-pressing and kneading to press and knead Yangbai point, Yingxiang point and Dicang point on the affected side, and scrape from Dicang point to Jiache point.

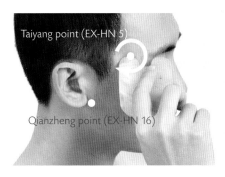

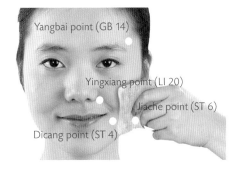

2. Yanglao Point and Hegu Point

Method: Use the corner of the scraping plate to scrape Yanglao point on the healthy side of the upper limbs from up to down and use the flat-pressing and kneading to scrape Hegu point of Large Intestine Meridian on the healthy side of upper limbs.

3. Kunlun Point and Neiting Point

Method: Use the flat-pressing and kneading to scrape Kunlun point on the healthy side of lower limbs, and vertically press and knead Neiting point of Stomach Meridian on the healthy side of lower limbs.

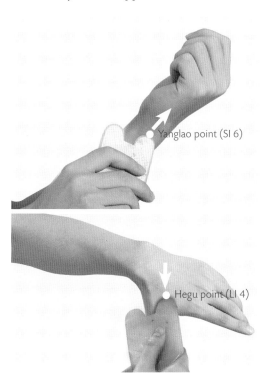

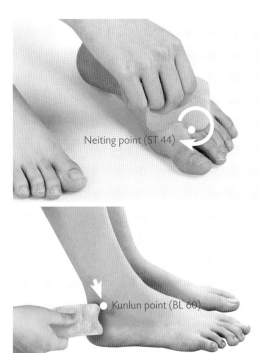

Along with the increase of age, vital energy and blood in the human body begin to weaken. Hair turning gray is a natural phenomenon. But if hair turns gray at an early age, it prompts problems with health. According to Chinese medicine, gray hair at an early age is mainly due to the deficiency of liver and kidney functions and the weakness of vital energy and blood, requiring the tonification of the liver and kidneys to benefit vital energy and blood circulation. Together with diet adjustment, scraping therapy serves to smooth the circulation of vital energy and blood with a curative effect to a certain extent.

Recommended Procedures

1. Head

Method: Use the multi-functional scraping comb to scrape the entire head from the front to the rear 30 times, twice every day.

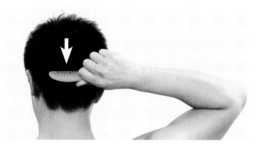

2. Xuehai Point

Method: Use the surface-scraping to scrape Xuehai point on both sides of lower limbs 30 times, and use the corner of the scraping plate to scrape the point with force, until soreness and distension are felt. The appearance of *sha* is not necessary.

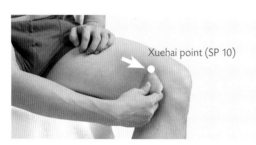

Xuehai point (SP 10)

3. Ganshu Point and Shenshu Point

Method: Use the surface-scraping to scrape Ganshu point and Shenshu point on both sides on the back for 30 times respectively with a little heavy force. The appearance of *sha* is not necessary.

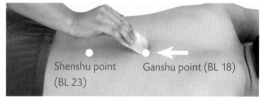

Shenshu point (BL 23)   Ganshu point (BL 18)

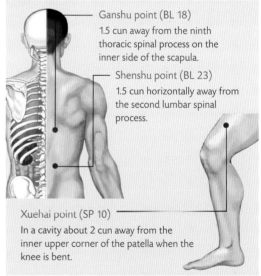

Ganshu point (BL 18)
1.5 cun away from the ninth thoracic spinal process on the inner side of the scapula.

Shenshu point (BL 23)
1.5 cun horizontally away from the second lumbar spinal process.

Xuehai point (SP 10)
In a cavity about 2 cun away from the inner upper corner of the patella when the knee is bent.

Therapy to Increase the Curative Effect

10-gram polygonum multiflorum, 20-gram Chinese wolfberry, 30-gram wild chrysanthemum, two dates,10-gram dried rehmannia roots and an appropriate amount of rock candy are boiled or brewed in boiling water for drink. Long-term drinking can moisten hair.

Hair Loss

A healthy adult will see the fall-off of 50 to 100 hairs every day. If the number of hairs falling off increases obviously and the hair line changes obviously or the hair becomes obviously finer and softer, one should be mindful of the hair loss problem. The fall-off of hair can be caused by quick rhythm of life, great pressure of work and undesirable habits of diet.

Perming or dyeing hair are both detrimental to the hair quality, being apt to result in the fall-off of hair. Hair is not supposed to be washed every day. Washing hair once every two days is enough. With hair washed, it is better to let hair dry itself. Electric hair dryer should not be too hot. According to Chinese medicine, the inadequacy of vital energy and blood is the main reason for the loss of hair. Scraping related acupoints can help to smooth vital energy and blood circulation and tonify hair, so as to prevent and cure the loss of the hair. The hair root can be further firmed and hair will look healthy and glossy by often eating those food that can tonify kidneys and hair, such as black sesame, walnuts, bean products, kelp or laver.

Recommended Procedures

1. Head
Method: Use the multi-functional scraping comb to scrape the entire head from the front to the rear 30 times, twice every day.

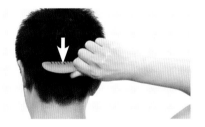

2. Fengchi Point
Method: Use the corner of the scraping plate to forcefully scrape Fengchi point on both sides on the neck, until soreness and distension are felt.

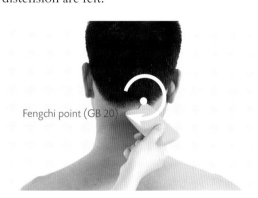

Fengchi point (GB 20)

3. Ganshu Point and Shenshu Point
Method: Use the surface-scraping to scrape Ganshu point and Shenshu point on both sides on the back from up to down, until *sha* appears.

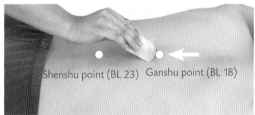

Shenshu point (BL 23) Ganshu point (BL 18)

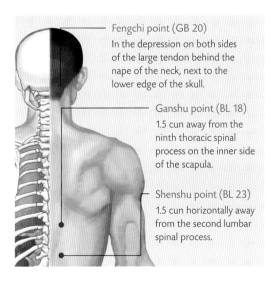

Fengchi point (GB 20)
In the depression on both sides of the large tendon behind the nape of the neck, next to the lower edge of the skull.

Ganshu point (BL 18)
1.5 cun away from the ninth thoracic spinal process on the inner side of the scapula.

Shenshu point (BL 23)
1.5 cun horizontally away from the second lumbar spinal process.

Aching and Stiff Shoulders and Neck

This happens frequently to white-collar workers. Many people believe that neck-shoulder soreness and pain are equivalent to cervical spondylosis. In fact, most of the neck-shoulder soreness, pain and stiffness are caused by siting for a long time, great pressure on shoulders, muscle trauma and stasis of vital energy and blood. Scraping the neck can smooth tendons, invigorate blood and quickly reduce or eliminate soreness and pain.

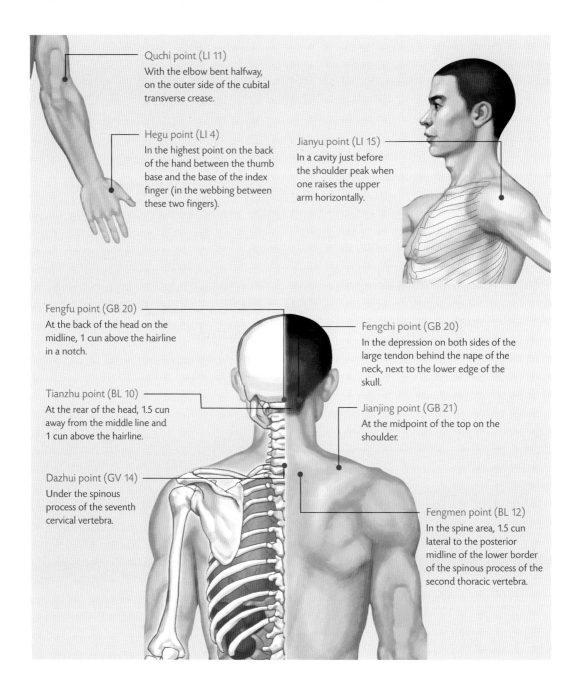

Quchi point (LI 11)
With the elbow bent halfway, on the outer side of the cubital transverse crease.

Hegu point (LI 4)
In the highest point on the back of the hand between the thumb base and the base of the index finger (in the webbing between these two fingers).

Jianyu point (LI 15)
In a cavity just before the shoulder peak when one raises the upper arm horizontally.

Fengfu point (GB 20)
At the back of the head on the midline, 1 cun above the hairline in a notch.

Fengchi point (GB 20)
In the depression on both sides of the large tendon behind the nape of the neck, next to the lower edge of the skull.

Tianzhu point (BL 10)
At the rear of the head, 1.5 cun away from the middle line and 1 cun above the hairline.

Jianjing point (GB 21)
At the midpoint of the top on the shoulder.

Dazhui point (GV 14)
Under the spinous process of the seventh cervical vertebra.

Fengmen point (BL 12)
In the spine area, 1.5 cun lateral to the posterior midline of the lower border of the spinous process of the second thoracic vertebra.

Recommended Procedures

1. Fengfu Point and Dazhui Point

Method: Use the surface-scraping to scrape from Fengfu point to Dazhui point of Du Meridian from up to down, until *sha* appears.

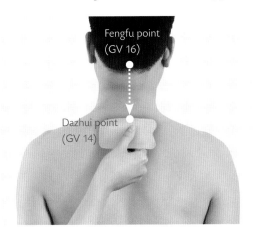

2. Tianzhu Point and Fengmen Point

Method: Use the surface-scraping to scrape Tianzhu point and Fengmen point of Bladder Meridian from up to down, 15 to 20 times on each side, until *sha* appears. With one side done, scrape the other side.

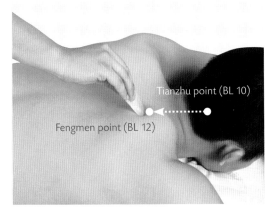

3. Fengchi Point and Jianjing Point

Method: Use the surface-scraping to scrape from Fengchi point to Jianjing point toward the shoulder-end, 15 to 20 times on each side, until *sha* appears. With one side done, scrape the other side.

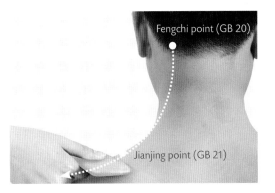

4. Jianyu Point, Quchi Point and Hegu Point

Method: Use the surface-scraping to scrape Jianyu point, Quchi point and Hegu point along Large Intestine Meridian for 15 to 20 times while pressing and kneading Hegu point several times, until soreness and distension are felt. With one side done, scrape the other.

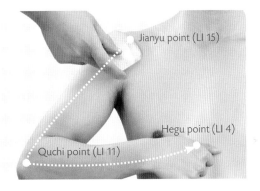

Therapy to Increase the Curative Effect

Stand or sit, chest out and looking up. Raise one shoulder to the highest level and circle with the shoulder top. Both shoulders can circle at the same time clockwise or counter clockwise, 15 times in one direction respectively. However, make sure to move slowly and gently. Often doing neck-shoulder exercise can effectively ease neck-shoulder soreness and pain. The above-mentioned movements can be done at any time and any place, since it is both convenient and effective.

Back Waist Pain

This often happens to many people, particularly to middle-aged and old people, due to irregular life, lack of rest or physical exercise as well as intrusion of the cold. It can also be caused by the insufficiency of yang energy in kidneys resulting in the intrusion of the wind-cold and stasis of vital energy and blood. Scraping can smooth meridians and the circulation of vital energy and blood, expel wind and disperse the cold, invigorate blood, expel stasis, and stop pain.

The speed-up of the loss of calcium among middle-aged and old people will lead to osteoporosis as well as waist-back pain. Scraping therapy can only ease such symptom for the time-being, but cannot cure it, patients require timely medical check-up for treatment.

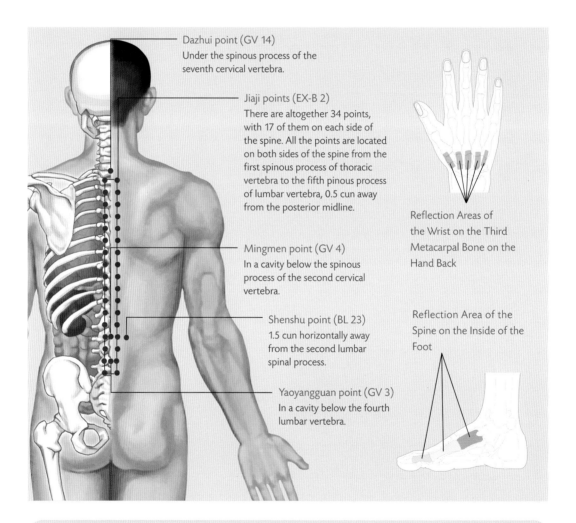

Dazhui point (GV 14)
Under the spinous process of the seventh cervical vertebra.

Jiaji points (EX-B 2)
There are altogether 34 points, with 17 of them on each side of the spine. All the points are located on both sides of the spine from the first spinous process of thoracic vertebra to the fifth pinous process of lumbar vertebra, 0.5 cun away from the posterior midline.

Mingmen point (GV 4)
In a cavity below the spinous process of the second cervical vertebra.

Shenshu point (BL 23)
1.5 cun horizontally away from the second lumbar spinal process.

Yaoyangguan point (GV 3)
In a cavity below the fourth lumbar vertebra.

Reflection Areas of the Wrist on the Third Metacarpal Bone on the Hand Back

Reflection Area of the Spine on the Inside of the Foot

Therapy to Increase the Curative Effect
Sit with the arms clasped round knees and stretch the spine naturally to relax the spine joints and muscular ligaments. Before going to bed in the evening or getting up in the morning, keeping this position for 2 to 3 minutes can ease waist-back pain.

Recommended Procedures

1. The Waist and the Back
Method: Use the surface-scraping to scrape the painful area of the waist and the back from up to down, until *sha* appears.

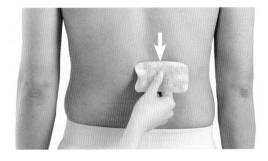

2. The Reflection Area of the Wrist on the Third Metacarpal Bone on the Hand Back and the Reflection Area of the Spine on the Inside of the Foot
Method: Use the pushing and scraping to gently scrape the reflection area of the wrist on the third metacarpal bone on hand back with possible points of pain. Use the single-angle scraping to scrape from back to front the reflection area of the spine on the inside of the foot.

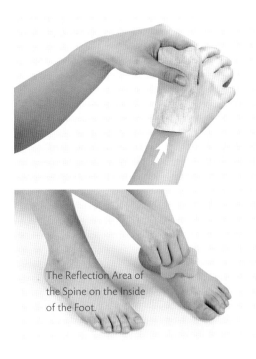

The Reflection Area of the Spine on the Inside of the Foot.

3. Dazhui Point, Yaoyangguan Point and Jiaji Points
Method: Use the surface-scraping to scrape from Dazhui point to Yaoyangguan point on both sides on the back from up to down. Then, use the dual-angle scraping to scrape Jiaji points on both sides.

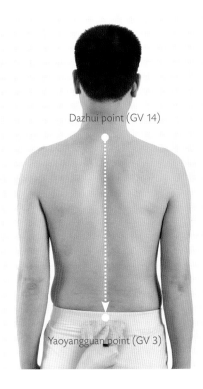

Dazhui point (GV 14)

Yaoyangguan point (GV 3)

4. Mingmen Point and Shenshu Point
Method: Use the surface-scraping to scrape Mingmen point and Shenshu point on the back from up to down.

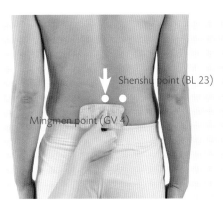

Shenshu point (BL 23)

Mingmen point (GV 4)

Lower Limb Ache

Due to busy work, many people in modern times always take a bus or drive a car instead of taking a walk, lacking physical exercise. Consequently, they often feel sore, painful and weak in lower limbs. Middle-aged and old people often feel sore, painful and heavy in lower limbs due to weakened body functions, insufficient supply or blockage of vital energy and blood in addition to the lack of physical exercise. Scraping can smooth meridians, vital energy and blood, and promote blood circulation and fluid metabolism, producing a very good effect on easing soreness and pain in lower limbs.

Varicose veins will also lead to soreness and pain in lower limbs, which is not suitable for the scraping. If the symptom of varicose veins is not serious, it is acceptable if the patient pays attention to the rest and does not stand for a long time. If it is serious, surgical operation can be adopted. However, after the operation, attention should be paid to protection, and standing and sitting for a long time are not allowed.

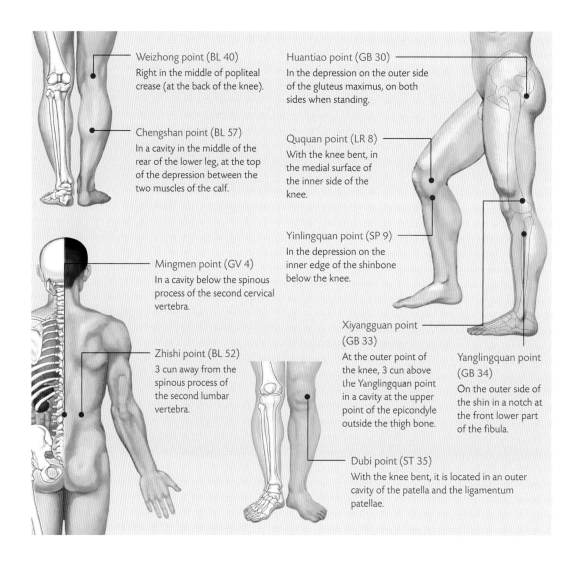

Weizhong point (BL 40)
Right in the middle of popliteal crease (at the back of the knee).

Chengshan point (BL 57)
In a cavity in the middle of the rear of the lower leg, at the top of the depression between the two muscles of the calf.

Mingmen point (GV 4)
In a cavity below the spinous process of the second cervical vertebra.

Zhishi point (BL 52)
3 cun away from the spinous process of the second lumbar vertebra.

Huantiao point (GB 30)
In the depression on the outer side of the gluteus maximus, on both sides when standing.

Ququan point (LR 8)
With the knee bent, in the medial surface of the inner side of the knee.

Yinlingquan point (SP 9)
In the depression on the inner edge of the shinbone below the knee.

Xiyangguan point (GB 33)
At the outer point of the knee, 3 cun above the Yanglingquan point in a cavity at the upper point of the epicondyle outside the thigh bone.

Yanglingquan point (GB 34)
On the outer side of the shin in a notch at the front lower part of the fibula.

Dubi point (ST 35)
With the knee bent, it is located in an outer cavity of the patella and the ligamentum patellae.

Recommended Procedures

1. Weizhong Point and Chengshan Point

Method: Use the surface-scraping to scrape Weizhong point on the rear of the knee and Chengshan point on the rear of the shin from up to down, or use the single-angle pressing and kneading to press and knead these two acupoints 15 to 20 times respectively, until soreness and distension are felt.

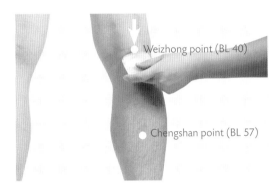

Weizhong point (BL 40)

Chengshan point (BL 57)

2. Mingmen Point and Zhishi Point

Method: Use the surface-scraping to scrape Mingmen point and Zhishi point on the waist from up to down respectively, until the skin turns red or *sha* appears.

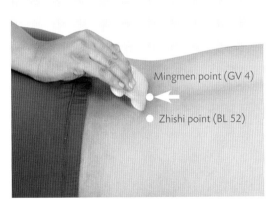

Mingmen point (GV 4)

Zhishi point (BL 52)

3. Huantiao Point and Dubi Point

Method: Use the single-angle pressing and kneading to press and knead Huantiao point 15 to 20 times with a little heavy force until soreness and distension are felt. Then, press Dubi point on the knee gently.

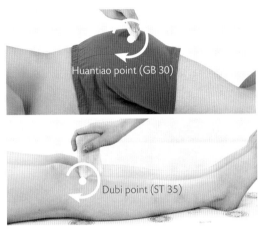

Huantiao point (GB 30)

Dubi point (ST 35)

4. Xiyangguan Point, Yanglingquan Point, Ququan Point and Yinlingquan Point

Method: Use the surface-scraping to scrape from Xiyangguan poin to Yanglingquan point on the lateral knee as well as Ququan point and Yinlingquan point on the medial knee.

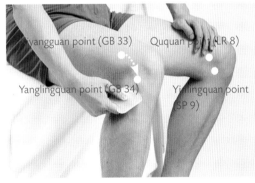

Xiyangguan point (GB 33)   Ququan point (LR 8)

Yanglingquan point (GB 34)   Yinlingquan point (SP 9)

Therapy to Increase the Curative Effect

Try to stand on the tiptoe to ease the soreness and pain in lower limbs when one stands, walks or sits down for a long time. Stand with two legs closed and two feet stand on the tiptoe to limit, drop down and then stand on the tiptoe again, do this for 12 times and 2 to 3 groups each time. This can effectively relax muscles of lower limbs, particularly the shin muscle, while producing an effect on preventing varicose veins or edema.

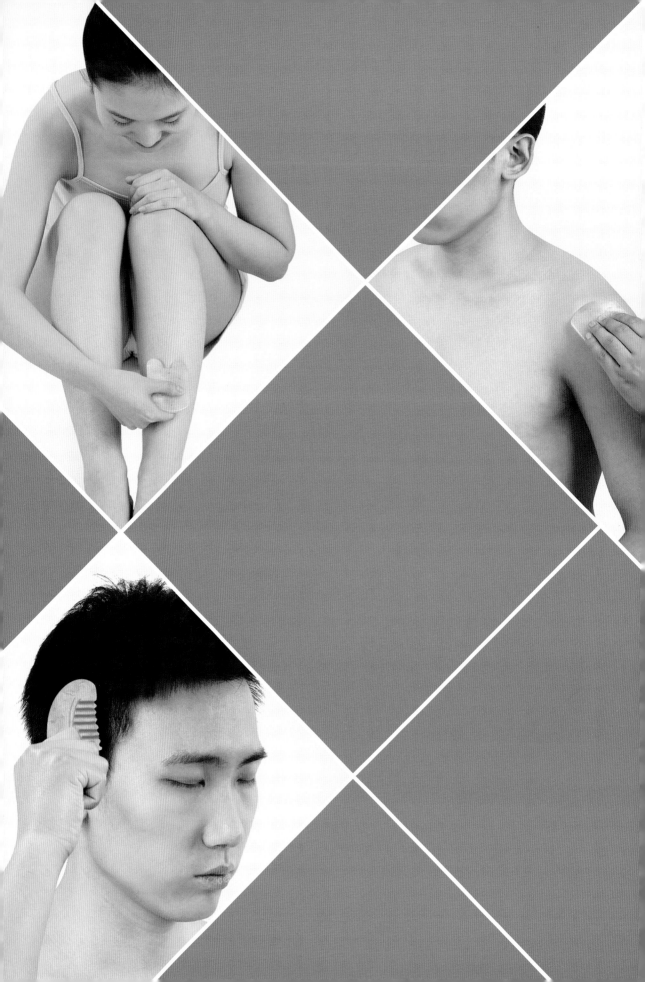

CHAPTER FOUR
Use *Gua Sha* to Detoxify Internal Organs to Prevent and Treat Chronic Diseases

Attention should be paid both to medical treatment and regulation in dealing with chronic diseases. Scraping therapy is a simple and effective way to regulate chronic diseases, as it can stimulate and smooth meridians, the circulation of vital energy and blood as well as expel toxin in all inner organs. With toxin in the body expelled, and the ability of resistance to diseases reinforced, recuperation of health will get twice the result with half of the efforts.

Hypertension

It is often coupled with headache, dizziness, tinnitus, insomnia, palpitation, chest distress and agitation, etc. Long-term high blood pressure will lead to pathological changes in such organs as the heart, brain, kidneys and retina. Scraping therapy can adjust the functions of the heart, brain and kidneys, producing a certain auxiliary effect of dealing with this illness.

High blood pressure is also likely to be a complexion caused by a certain kind or several kinds of other diseases. Under such circumstance, reducing the blood pressure can only relieve the symptom. Only by targeting at the primary cause of high blood pressure can it be cured fundamentally.

The intake of the amount of salt must be brought under control on the part of the patient. In particular, those who are fond of eating salty food should gradually make a change. As recommended by China Public Union of Nutrition, the intake of salt for a healthy adult should not exceed 5 grams per day, and 3 to 4 grams for the patient of high blood pressure.

Recommended Procedures
1. Projection Area of the Heart on the Chest, Corresponding Area of the Heart and the Kidneys on the Back
Method: Use the flat-scraping to scrape from inside to outside the projection area of the heart on the chest and the corresponding area of the heart on the back. Use the surface-scraping to scrape the corresponding area of the kidneys on the back.

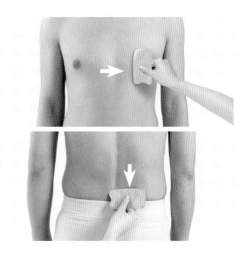

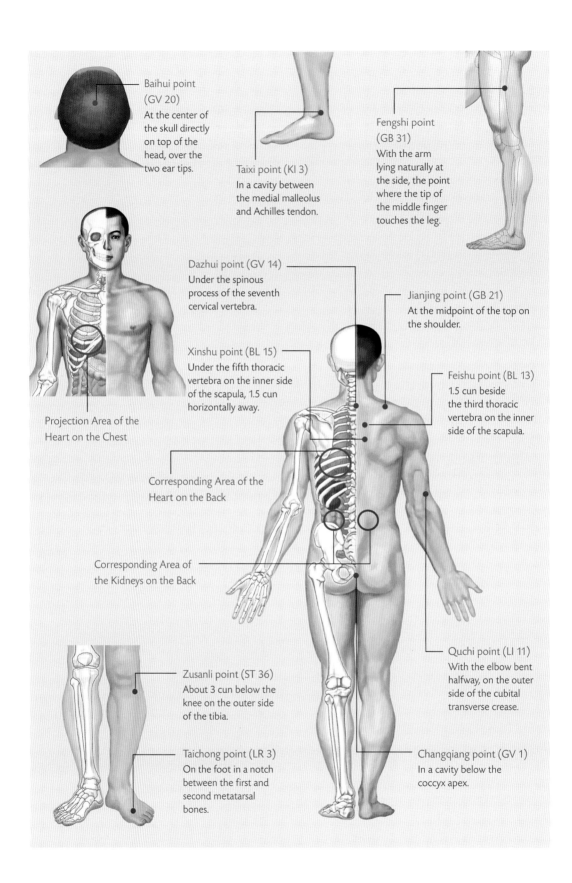

Baihui point (GV 20)
At the center of the skull directly on top of the head, over the two ear tips.

Taixi point (KI 3)
In a cavity between the medial malleolus and Achilles tendon.

Fengshi point (GB 31)
With the arm lying naturally at the side, the point where the tip of the middle finger touches the leg.

Dazhui point (GV 14)
Under the spinous process of the seventh cervical vertebra.

Jianjing point (GB 21)
At the midpoint of the top on the shoulder.

Xinshu point (BL 15)
Under the fifth thoracic vertebra on the inner side of the scapula, 1.5 cun horizontally away.

Feishu point (BL 13)
1.5 cun beside the third thoracic vertebra on the inner side of the scapula.

Projection Area of the Heart on the Chest

Corresponding Area of the Heart on the Back

Corresponding Area of the Kidneys on the Back

Zusanli point (ST 36)
About 3 cun below the knee on the outer side of the tibia.

Taichong point (LR 3)
On the foot in a notch between the first and second metatarsal bones.

Quchi point (LI 11)
With the elbow bent halfway, on the outer side of the cubital transverse crease.

Changqiang point (GV 1)
In a cavity below the coccyx apex.

2. Baihui Point and Jianjing Point

Method: Use the surface-scraping to scrape from the head top to the rear hairline, including Baihui point on the top of the head. Then, use the surface-scraping to scrape Jianjing point from inside to outside.

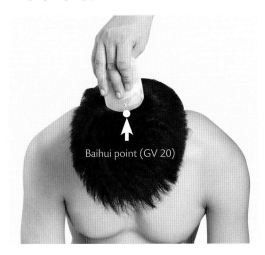

Baihui point (GV 20)

3. Dazhui Point, Changqiang Point, Feishu Point and Xinshu Point

Method: Use the surface-scraping to scrape from Dazhui point to Changqiang point of Du Meridian on the back in sections from up to down. Then, scrape from Feishu point to Xinshu point of Bladder Meridian on both sides from up to down.

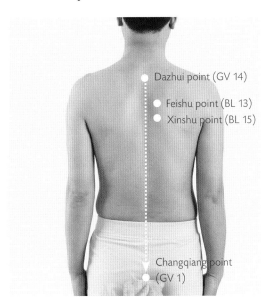

Dazhui point (GV 14)
Feishu point (BL 13)
Xinshu point (BL 15)
Changqiang point (GV 1)

4. Quchi Point, Fengshi Point, Zusanli Point, Taixi Point and Taichong Point

Method: Use the single-angle scraping to scrape Quchi points on both sides, Fengshi point, Zusanli point and Taixi point of lower limbs. Then, use the vertical-pressing and kneading to press and knead Taixi point on the foot.

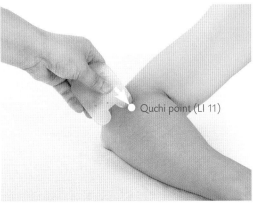

Quchi point (LI 11)

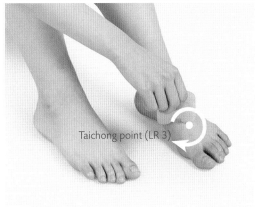

Taichong point (LR 3)

Therapy to Increase the Curative Effect

Corn stigma tea: 500 grams of fresh corn stigma, washed and sliced, is boiled in the casserole with water of 600 ml under soft fire until 300 ml is left behind. Then, it is filtered through the gauze to be in a state of juice added with an appropriate amount of white sugar for oral use as tea, one dose each day to be drunk in several times. Corn stigma serves to reduce heat, expel dampness, smooth urine discharge and lower down blood pressure, suitable for treating all kinds of high blood pressure.

Obesity

This refers to obvious overweight and thicker fat layer in the body to a considerable extent. Or rather, it is a state of too much accumulation of triglyceride. Obesity can be caused by hereditary factors, imbalance of metabolism, the ways of diet and daily life as well as mental factors. Obesity can lead to various pathological changes as well as a sense of inferiority, agitation and depression as psychological illness. Persisting in receiving scraping therapy can produce considerable effects on adjusting body fat, fluid metabolism, and the prevention and treatment of obesity.

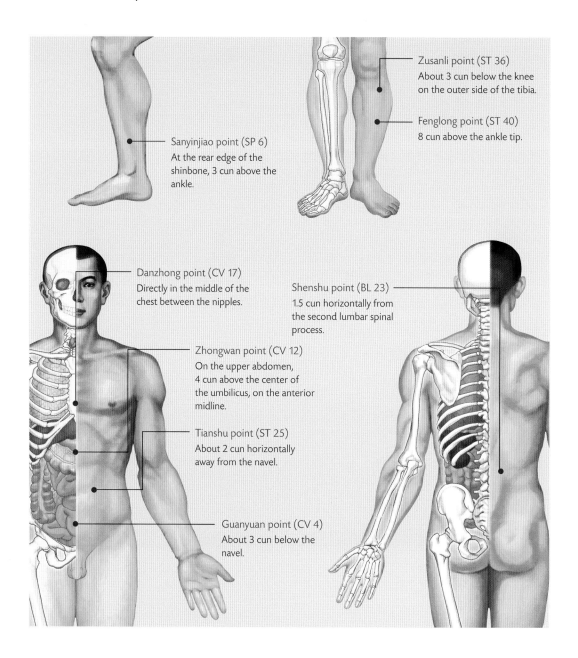

Zusanli point (ST 36)
About 3 cun below the knee on the outer side of the tibia.

Fenglong point (ST 40)
8 cun above the ankle tip.

Sanyinjiao point (SP 6)
At the rear edge of the shinbone, 3 cun above the ankle.

Danzhong point (CV 17)
Directly in the middle of the chest between the nipples.

Shenshu point (BL 23)
1.5 cun horizontally from the second lumbar spinal process.

Zhongwan point (CV 12)
On the upper abdomen, 4 cun above the center of the umbilicus, on the anterior midline.

Tianshu point (ST 25)
About 2 cun horizontally away from the navel.

Guanyuan point (CV 4)
About 3 cun below the navel.

Recommended Procedures

1. Shenshu Point

Method: Use the surface-scraping to scrape Shenshu point on the back from up to down, until the skin turns red or *sha* speckles take form.

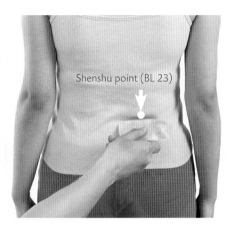

Shenshu point (BL 23)

3. Sanyinjiao Point, Zusanli Point and Fenglong Point

Method: Use the surface-scraping to scrape Sanyinjiao point on the inside of the lower limbs and Zusanli point on the outside of the shin from up to down respectively 30 times, with a little heavy force. The appearance of *sha* is not necessary.

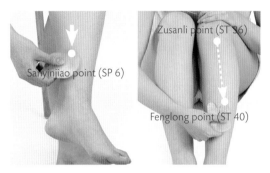

Zusanli point (ST 36)
Sanyinjiao point (SP 6)
Fenglong point (ST 40)

2. Danzhong Point, Zhongwan Point, Tianshu Point and Guanyuan Point

Method: Use the angle-scraping to gently scrape Danzhong point from up to down, until the skin turns red. Then use the surface-scraping to gently scrape Zhongwan point on the abdomen from up to down, as well as the surrounding areas of the navel and Tianshu point for 30 times respectively. Finally, scrape Guanyuan point from up to down, until the skin turns red.

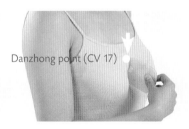

Danzhong point (CV 17)

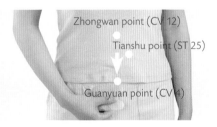

Zhongwan point (CV 12)
Tianshu point (ST 25)
Guanyuan point (CV 4)

Expert Prompts

The key of preventing and curing obesity lies in formulating and adhering to correct principles of diet as follows:

• The arrangement of diet should be based on the situation of different individuals, marked by appropriateness, balance, reasonable structure and persistence in healthy diet.

• The time and amount of three meals should be set and that the speed of eating should be brought under control. Eat less for the supper and don't eat late at night.

• Exert control over the intake of total energy, particularly the intake of the amount of fat. The reduction of energy must be based on the principle of ensuring the normal activities of human body. Generally, the intake of energy for an adult should be around 4184 kilojoules every day.

• Eat light food, be sure to take enough protein, eat more assorted grains rich in dietary fibers as well as fresh vegetables and fruits rich in vitamins and mineral substances.

Diabetes

It is a common disease caused by interaction between hereditary factors and environmental factors. According to Chinese medicine, it is called "drinking and urine," mainly marked by hyperglycaemia in clinical practice. There are such common symptoms as drinking more, urinating more, eating more and becoming thin. Long-term diabetes will lead to chronic harm and functional obstruction to various tissues, particularly to eyes, kidneys, heart, blood vessels and nerves.

The increase of glycogen content in the skin of diabetes patient will create a nice environment for the infection by moulds and germs. Therefore, the scraping oil must be applied to protect the skin when the scraping is done. It should be done gently to prevent the wounds on the skin from being infected. The far-end of limbs is not sensitive, requiring more care.

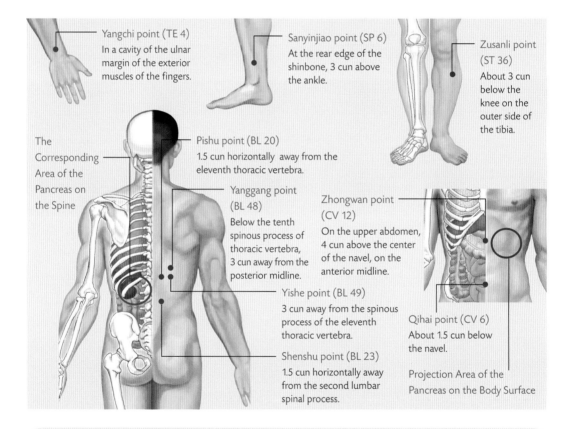

Yangchi point (TE 4)
In a cavity of the ulnar margin of the exterior muscles of the fingers.

Sanyinjiao point (SP 6)
At the rear edge of the shinbone, 3 cun above the ankle.

Zusanli point (ST 36)
About 3 cun below the knee on the outer side of the tibia.

The Corresponding Area of the Pancreas on the Spine

Pishu point (BL 20)
1.5 cun horizontally away from the eleventh thoracic vertebra.

Yanggang point (BL 48)
Below the tenth spinous process of thoracic vertebra, 3 cun away from the posterior midline.

Zhongwan point (CV 12)
On the upper abdomen, 4 cun above the center of the navel, on the anterior midline.

Yishe point (BL 49)
3 cun away from the spinous process of the eleventh thoracic vertebra.

Qihai point (CV 6)
About 1.5 cun below the navel.

Shenshu point (BL 23)
1.5 cun horizontally away from the second lumbar spinal process.

Projection Area of the Pancreas on the Body Surface

Therapies to Increase the Curative Effect
Use the surface-scraping to scrape Shaofu point and Taiyuan point from up to down for the patients who drink more.

Use the vertical-pressing and kneading to scrape Neiting point and use the surface-scraping to scrape Lougu point on both sides of the Spleen Meridian from up to down for the patients who eat more.

Use the flat-pressing and kneading to scrape Taixi point and the surface-scraping to scrape Sanyinjiao point for the patients who urinate more.

Recommended Procedures

1. The Corresponding Area of Pancreas on the Spine

Method: Use the surface-scraping and the dual-angle scraping to scrape the area from up to down.

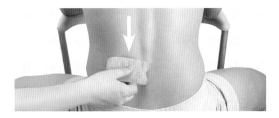

2. The Projection Area of Pancreas on the Body Surface

Method: Use the flat-scraping to scrape the area on the ribs from inside to outside.

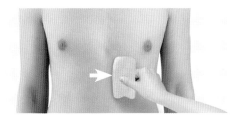

3. Pishu Point, Shenshu Point, Yanggang Point and Yishe Point

Method: Use the surface-scraping to scrape from Pishu point to Shenshu point and from Yanggang point to Yishe point of Bladder Meridian on both sides on the back.

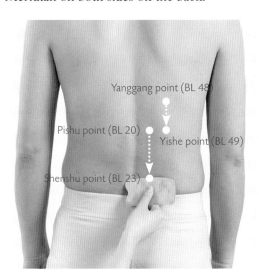

Yanggang point (BL 48)
Pishu point (BL 20)
Yishe point (BL 49)
Shenshu point (BL 23)

4. Zhongwan Point and Qihai Point

Method: Use the surface-scraping to scrape from Zhongwan point to Qihai point of Ren Meridian from up to down on the abdomen (scraping is done respectively on the upper part and the lower part, with Shenque point as the border).

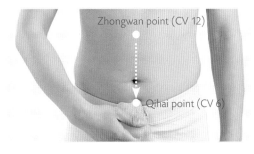

Zhongwan point (CV 12)
Qihai point (CV 6)

5. Yangchi Point, Zusanli Point and Sanyinjiao Point

Method: Use the flat-pressing and kneading to press and knead Yangchi point on the wrist. Use the corner of the scraping plate to scrape Zusanli point and Sanyinjiao point on lower limbs from up to down.

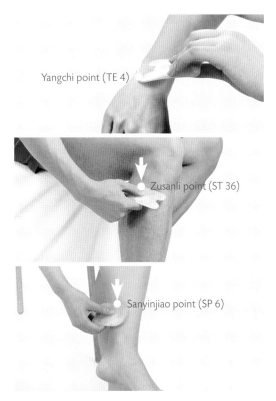

Yangchi point (TE 4)
Zusanli point (ST 36)
Sanyinjiao point (SP 6)

Coronary Heart Disease

It is also called coronary atherosclerosis cardiopathy caused by abnormal fat metabolism and stenosis of the artery because of fat precipitation in the blood, resulting in the obstruction of blood-flow, the lack of blood in the heart and angina. Patients of this kind mostly suffer from hypercholesteremia and high blood pressure as well as have the habit of smoking, often accompanied by diabetes and obesity. Scraping therapy is conducive to smoothing the heart vessel and producing certain effects on easing and reducing the attack of angina.

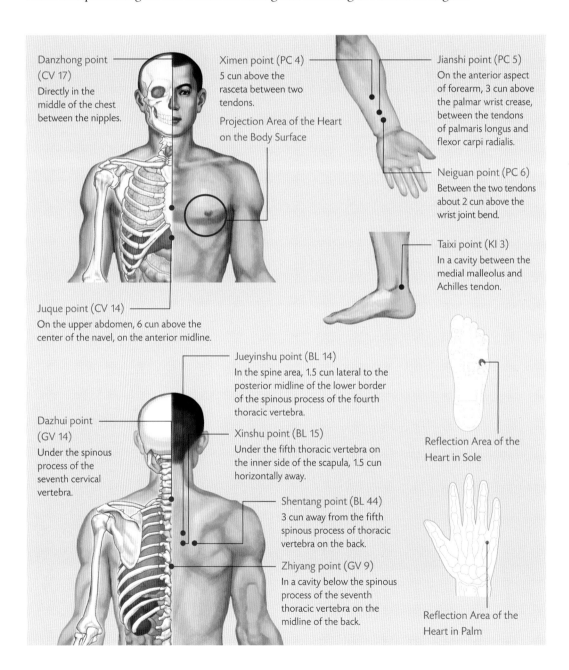

Danzhong point (CV 17)
Directly in the middle of the chest between the nipples.

Ximen point (PC 4)
5 cun above the rasceta between two tendons.

Projection Area of the Heart on the Body Surface

Jianshi point (PC 5)
On the anterior aspect of forearm, 3 cun above the palmar wrist crease, between the tendons of palmaris longus and flexor carpi radialis.

Neiguan point (PC 6)
Between the two tendons about 2 cun above the wrist joint bend.

Taixi point (KI 3)
In a cavity between the medial malleolus and Achilles tendon.

Juque point (CV 14)
On the upper abdomen, 6 cun above the center of the navel, on the anterior midline.

Jueyinshu point (BL 14)
In the spine area, 1.5 cun lateral to the posterior midline of the lower border of the spinous process of the fourth thoracic vertebra.

Dazhui point (GV 14)
Under the spinous process of the seventh cervical vertebra.

Xinshu point (BL 15)
Under the fifth thoracic vertebra on the inner side of the scapula, 1.5 cun horizontally away.

Shentang point (BL 44)
3 cun away from the fifth spinous process of thoracic vertebra on the back.

Zhiyang point (GV 9)
In a cavity below the spinous process of the seventh thoracic vertebra on the midline of the back.

Reflection Area of the Heart in Sole

Reflection Area of the Heart in Palm

Recommended Procedures

1. Projection Area of the Heart on the Body Surface, Danzhong Point and Juque Point

Method: Use the flat-scraping to scrape the projection area from inside to outside. Use the single-angle scraping to scrape Danzhong point and Juque point of Ren Meridian from up to down.

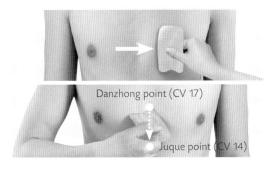

Danzhong point (CV 17)

Juque point (CV 14)

2. Jianshi Point, Neiguan Point, Taixi Point and Ximen Point

Method: Use the surface-scraping to scrape from Ximen point to Jianshi point and Neiguan point of Pericardium Meridian on both sides of upper limbs from up to down. Use the flat-pressing and kneading to press and knead Taixi point of Kidney Meridian on lower limbs.

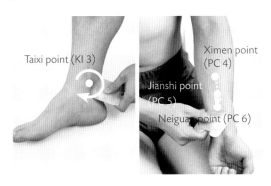

Taixi point (KI 3)

Ximen point (PC 4)

Jianshi point (PC 5)

Neiguan point (PC 6)

3. Reflection Areas of the Heart on Palm and the Sole

Method: Use the single-angle pressing and kneading to scrape the areas.

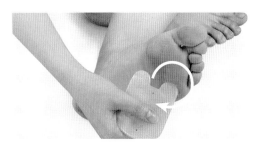

4. Dazhui Point, Zhiyang Point, Jueyinshu Point, Xinshu Point and Shentang Point

Method: Use the surface-scraping to scrape from Dazhui point to Zhiyang point on Du Meridian on the back from up to down, and scrape Jueyinshu point, Xinshu point and Shentang point of Bladder Meridian.

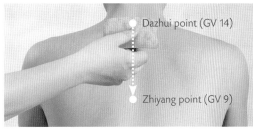

Dazhui point (GV 14)

Zhiyang point (GV 9)

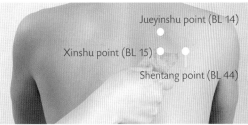

Jueyinshu point (BL 14)

Xinshu point (BL 15)

Shentang point (BL 44)

Emergency Measures for Rescuing Patients with Coronary Heart Disease and Angina

• Once angina attacks, rest is needed at once along with taking medicine. Generally, a rest and in-take of medicine can ease angina in just one or two minutes.

• If medicine is not available when it attacks, one can forcefully press and knead Ximen point and Neiguan point mentioned above. Another person can also help to press and knead the patient's Zhiyang point, which can quickly ease angina.

• After a short rest with the pain eased, go to the hospital quickly for treatment.

Rheumatic Heart Disease

It is marked by repeated attacks of rheumatism, leading to chronic harm to cardiac valves, the narrow-down of the valve-opening or valvular insufficiency, which causes the change of hemodynamics, incompensation of cardiac functions and congestive heart-failure. According to Chinese medicine, this disease is associated with insufficiency of vital energy and blood, failure of heart yang and intrusion of wind-damp. Scraping therapy can improve the symptom of this disease.

Patients of rheumatic heart disease are strictly forbidden to take part in heavy physical labor in order to avoid the burden on the heart. Patients coupled with insufficiency of cardiac functions or in rheumatism should absolutely lie in bed for rest. Pay attention to rheumatic symptoms caused by the infection of the respiratory tract which will make it worse.

Patients with insufficiency of cardiac functions should control the in-take of water and the sodium salt. Eating food preserved with salt is a taboo.

Scraping therapy can promote the breakage of blood capillaries and stimulate new circulation in the wake of it. Although it can improve the symptom, it can also add burden to the heart. Therefore, it is not suitable for patients of serious heart diseases to receive scraping therapy.

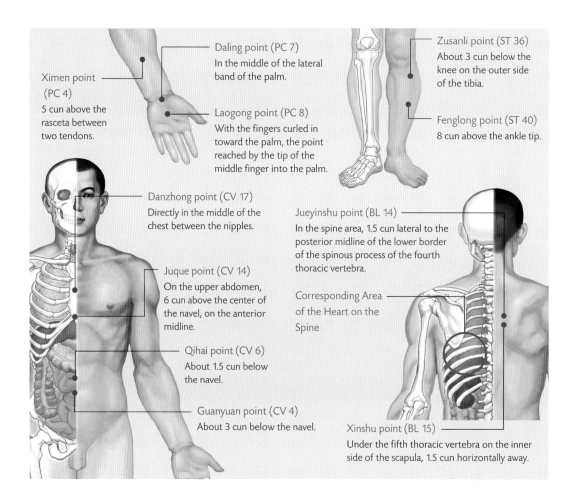

Daling point (PC 7)
In the middle of the lateral band of the palm.

Ximen point (PC 4)
5 cun above the rasceta between two tendons.

Laogong point (PC 8)
With the fingers curled in toward the palm, the point reached by the tip of the middle finger into the palm.

Zusanli point (ST 36)
About 3 cun below the knee on the outer side of the tibia.

Fenglong point (ST 40)
8 cun above the ankle tip.

Danzhong point (CV 17)
Directly in the middle of the chest between the nipples.

Jueyinshu point (BL 14)
In the spine area, 1.5 cun lateral to the posterior midline of the lower border of the spinous process of the fourth thoracic vertebra.

Juque point (CV 14)
On the upper abdomen, 6 cun above the center of the navel, on the anterior midline.

Corresponding Area of the Heart on the Spine

Qihai point (CV 6)
About 1.5 cun below the navel.

Guanyuan point (CV 4)
About 3 cun below the navel.

Xinshu point (BL 15)
Under the fifth thoracic vertebra on the inner side of the scapula, 1.5 cun horizontally away.

Recommended Procedures

1. Corresponding Area of the Heart on the Spine, Jueyinshu Point and Xinshu Point

Method: Use the flat-scraping to scrape the coresponding area from up to down. Use the corner of the scraping plate to scrape Jueyinshu point and Xinshu point on both sides.

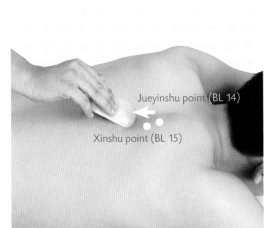

Jueyinshu point (BL 14)

Xinshu point (BL 15)

2. Ximen Point, Daling Point and Laogong Point

Method: Use the corner of the scraping plate to scrape from Ximen point to Daling point on the inside of the upper limbs from up to down. Use the corner of the scraping plate to press and knead Laogong point of the palm.

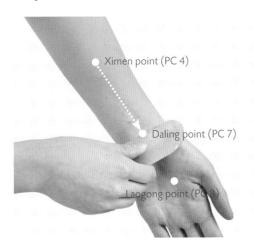

Ximen point (PC 4)

Daling point (PC 7)

Laogong point (PC 8)

3. Danzhong Point, Juque Point, Qihai Pointand Guanyuan Point

Method: Use the corner of the scraping plate to scrape from Danzhong point to Juque point on the chest, and from Qihai point to Guanyuan point on the abdomen from up to down.

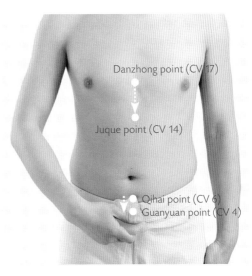

Danzhong point (CV 17)

Juque point (CV 14)

Qihai point (CV 6)
Guanyuan point (CV 4)

4. Zusanli Point and Fenglong Point

Method: Use the surface-scraping to scrape from Zusanli point to Fenglong point of Stomach Meridian on the outside of he lower limbs from up to down.

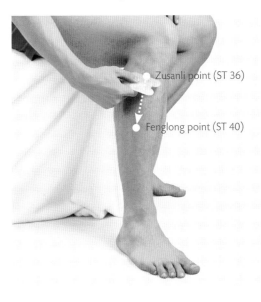

Zusanli point (ST 36)

Fenglong point (ST 40)

Hyperlipemia

Caused by the disorder of lipid metabolism, it is closely linked with unreasonable diet and the lack of physical exercise, which will give rise to such cardiovascular diseases as fat liver, high blood pressure, arteriosclerosis and coronary heart disease. Timely adjustment must be made if the blood lipid is found too high. Scraping therapy can promote blood circulation and speed up fluid metabolism, which can play an active role in preventing and curing hyperlipemia.

Patients of hyperlipemia should eat light food, drink more water and often do physical exercise while reducing the in-take of food with high cholesterol, such as pork, beef or mutton, so as to reduce the burden of fat metabolism in the system of digestion. Also, eat less spicy, oily and sweet food. Eat fish once every week, since there is a low content of fat and a high content of protein. Eat more fruits, vegetables, cereals and beans of various kinds. Drink water frequently can help to expel toxin, and drink an appropriate amount of green tea, which is not supposed to be too strong. Physical exercise can consume redundant fat in blood. Patients of hyperlipemia had better persist in walking and slow-running every day. Patients of hyperlipemia without other complications should maintain a medium degree of exercise, such as slow-running 3 to 5 kilometers every day. Those with minor high blood pressure, obesity, and diabetes should follow the principle of feeling no obvious physical discomfort in their exercise.

Recommended Procedures

1. Ximen Point, Neiguan Point, Quchi Point, Xuehai Point, Zusanli Point, Gongsun Point, and Fenglong Point
Method: Use the surface-scraping to scrape from Ximen point to Neiguan point on the wrist and Quchi point on the elbow and Xuehai point on lower limbs. Use the surface-scraping or the flat-pressing and kneading to press and knead Zusanli point, Gongsun point, and Fenglong point.

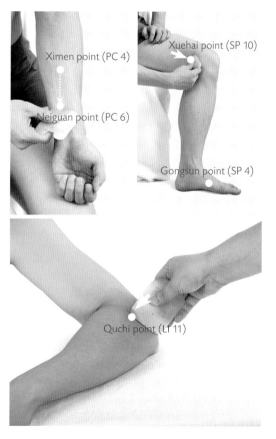

Ximen point (PC 4)

Neiguan point (PC 6)

Xuehai point (SP 10)

Gongsun point (SP 4)

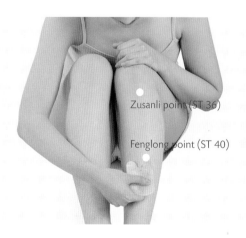

Zusanli point (ST 36)

Fenglong point (ST 40)

Quchi point (LI 11)

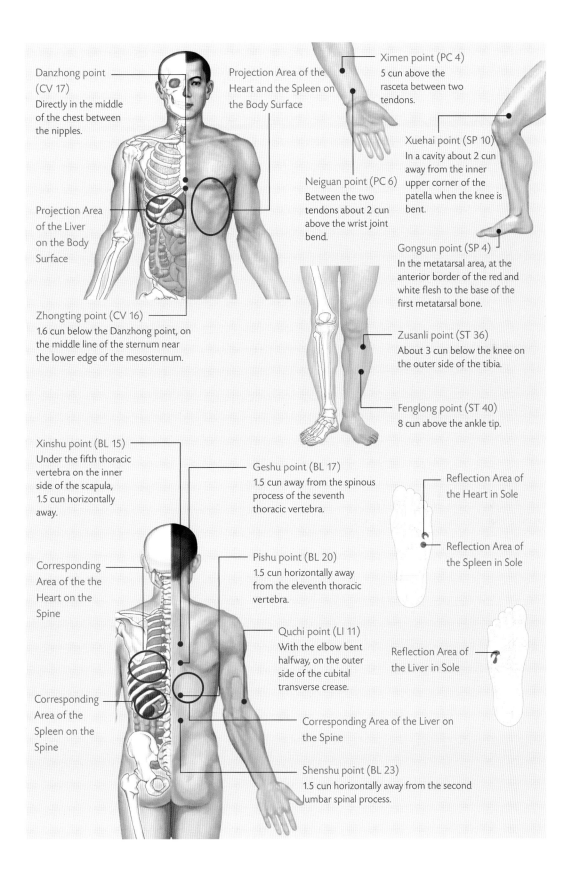

Danzhong point
(CV 17)
Directly in the middle
of the chest between
the nipples.

Projection Area of the
Heart and the Spleen on
the Body Surface

Ximen point (PC 4)
5 cun above the
rasceta between two
tendons.

Xuehai point (SP 10)
In a cavity about 2 cun
away from the inner
upper corner of the
patella when the knee is
bent.

Neiguan point (PC 6)
Between the two
tendons about 2 cun
above the wrist joint
bend.

Projection Area
of the Liver
on the Body
Surface

Gongsun point (SP 4)
In the metatarsal area, at the
anterior border of the red and
white flesh to the base of the
first metatarsal bone.

Zhongting point (CV 16)
1.6 cun below the Danzhong point, on
the middle line of the sternum near
the lower edge of the mesosternum.

Zusanli point (ST 36)
About 3 cun below the knee on
the outer side of the tibia.

Fenglong point (ST 40)
8 cun above the ankle tip.

Xinshu point (BL 15)
Under the fifth thoracic
vertebra on the inner
side of the scapula,
1.5 cun horizontally
away.

Geshu point (BL 17)
1.5 cun away from the spinous
process of the seventh
thoracic vertebra.

Reflection Area of
the Heart in Sole

Reflection Area of
the Spleen in Sole

Corresponding
Area of the the
Heart on the
Spine

Pishu point (BL 20)
1.5 cun horizontally away
from the eleventh thoracic
vertebra.

Quchi point (LI 11)
With the elbow bent
halfway, on the outer
side of the cubital
transverse crease.

Reflection Area of
the Liver in Sole

Corresponding
Area of the
Spleen on the
Spine

Corresponding Area of the Liver on
the Spine

Shenshu point (BL 23)
1.5 cun horizontally away from the second
lumbar spinal process.

2. Corresponding Areas of the Heart, the Liver and the Spleen on the Spine, Xinshu Point, Geshu Point, Pishu Point and Shenshu Point

Method: Use the surface-scraping and the dual-angle scraping to scrape corresponding areas of the heart, the liver and the spleen on the spine from up to down. Use the surface-scraping to scrape from Xinshu point, Geshu point, Pishu point to Shenshu point.

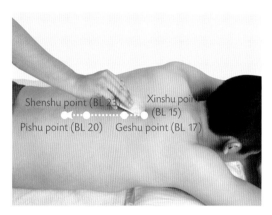

Shenshu point (BL 23)
Xinshu point (BL 15)
Pishu point (BL 20)
Geshu point (BL 17)

3. Reflection Areas of the Heart, the Liver and the Spleen in Palm and Sole

Method: Use the surface-scraping to scrape these areas.

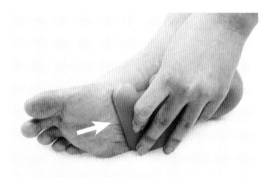

4. Projection Areas of the Heart, the Spleen and the Liver on Body Surface, Danzhong Point and Zhongting Point

Method: Use the flat-scraping to scrape the projection areas from inside to outside. Use the single-angle scraping to scrape Danzhong point and Zhongting point.

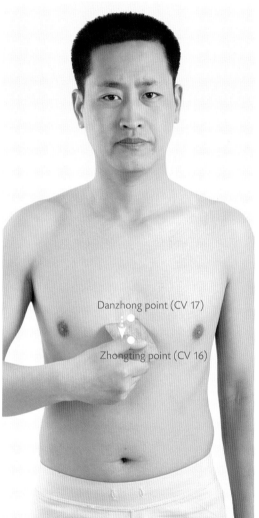

Danzhong point (CV 17)

Zhongting point (CV 16)

Therapy to Increase the Curative Effect

Onions immersed in red wine: Take three onions and one bottle of red grape wine (750 ml). Peeled onions are cut into eight equal parts and put into a glass bottle with red grape wine, covered tightly and put aside at a cool place for seven days. Then, the liquid is filtered, put into another bottle and stored in the refrigerator. Twenty to fifty millimeters every day. Long-term oral use can produce a considerable effect on softening blood vessels and reducing blood fat.

Sequela of Apoplexy

Old people with high blood pressure, diabetes, and hyperlipemia are apt to suffer from apoplexy which can damage cerebral nerve cells or cause death in a few minutes due to the lack of oxygen. The functions of this part of cerebral nerve cells will lose, leading to the sequela of apoplexy.

The sequela of apoplexy is often marked by paralysis and numbness of one side of the body, facial paralysis and difficulty in verbal expression, etc. According to Chinese medicine, it is mainly due to the channel blockage because of blood stasis, obstruction of collateral paths because of wind phlegm, the deficiency of kidney yin, the rise of liver yang, inadequacy of essentials and blood as well as the neglect of nurturing tendons. Scraping therapy can produce a quite good effect to restore some physiological functions.

The rehabilitation treatment of the sequela of apoplexy in the early stage is very important. The best time for ideal recovery is within three months after the occurrence of the illness. The time for recovery will be slow if such a disease lasts for over two years. Gentle scraping therapy is required for patients of this kind and heavy force is forbidden.

Basic Scraping Therapy

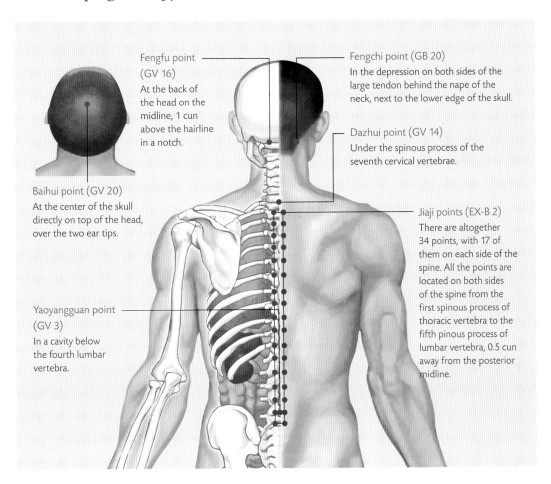

Fengfu point (GV 16)
At the back of the head on the midline, 1 cun above the hairline in a notch.

Fengchi point (GB 20)
In the depression on both sides of the large tendon behind the nape of the neck, next to the lower edge of the skull.

Dazhui point (GV 14)
Under the spinous process of the seventh cervical vertebrae.

Baihui point (GV 20)
At the center of the skull directly on top of the head, over the two ear tips.

Jiaji points (EX-B 2)
There are altogether 34 points, with 17 of them on each side of the spine. All the points are located on both sides of the spine from the first spinous process of thoracic vertebra to the fifth pinous process of lumbar vertebra, 0.5 cun away from the posterior midline.

Yaoyangguan point (GV 3)
In a cavity below the fourth lumbar vertebra.

Recommended Procedures

1. The Head

Method: Use the multifunctional scraping comb to scrape the entire head, look for the point of pain, which should be emphatically scraped.

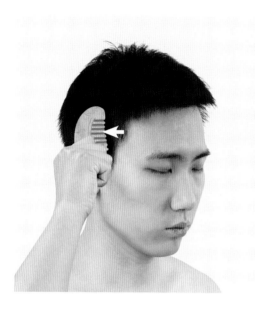

3. Baihui Point, Fengchi Point and Fengfu Point

Method: Use the single-angle scraping to scrape from the top of the head to Baihui point and scrape Fengchi point on the rear of the head from up to down. Use the surface-scraping to scrape Fengchi point on the rear of the neck from up to down.

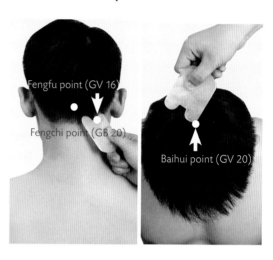

2. Dazhui Point, Yaoyangguan Point and Jiaji Points

Method: Use the surface-scraping to scrape from Dazhui point to Yaoyangguan point from up to down. Then, use the dual-angle scraping to scrape Jiaji points on both sides from up to down.

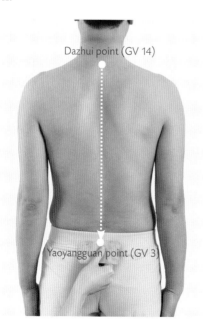

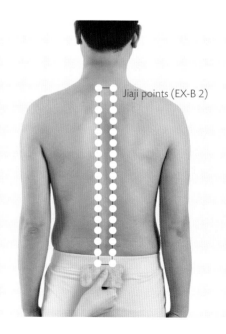

Scraping Therapy According to the Symptoms

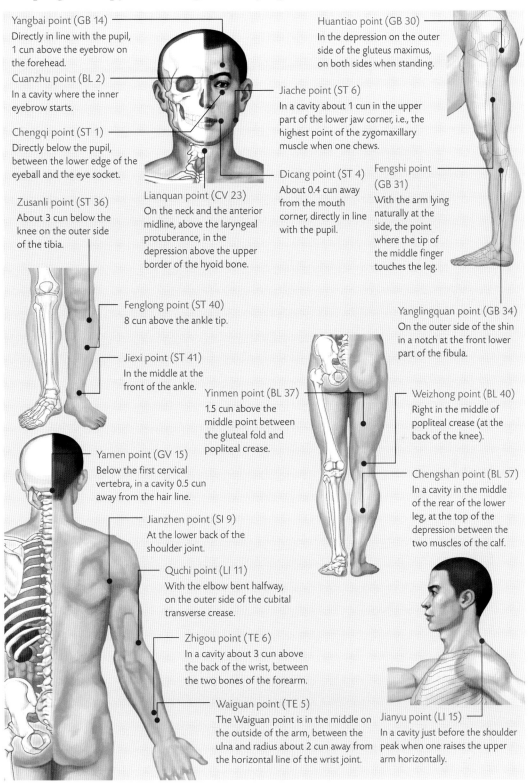

Yangbai point (GB 14)
Directly in line with the pupil, 1 cun above the eyebrow on the forehead.

Cuanzhu point (BL 2)
In a cavity where the inner eyebrow starts.

Chengqi point (ST 1)
Directly below the pupil, between the lower edge of the eyeball and the eye socket.

Zusanli point (ST 36)
About 3 cun below the knee on the outer side of the tibia.

Lianquan point (CV 23)
On the neck and the anterior midline, above the laryngeal protuberance, in the depression above the upper border of the hyoid bone.

Fenglong point (ST 40)
8 cun above the ankle tip.

Jiexi point (ST 41)
In the middle at the front of the ankle.

Huantiao point (GB 30)
In the depression on the outer side of the gluteus maximus, on both sides when standing.

Jiache point (ST 6)
In a cavity about 1 cun in the upper part of the lower jaw corner, i.e., the highest point of the zygomaxillary muscle when one chews.

Dicang point (ST 4)
About 0.4 cun away from the mouth corner, directly in line with the pupil.

Fengshi point (GB 31)
With the arm lying naturally at the side, the point where the tip of the middle finger touches the leg.

Yanglingquan point (GB 34)
On the outer side of the shin in a notch at the front lower part of the fibula.

Yinmen point (BL 37)
1.5 cun above the middle point between the gluteal fold and popliteal crease.

Yamen point (GV 15)
Below the first cervical vertebra, in a cavity 0.5 cun away from the hair line.

Jianzhen point (SI 9)
At the lower back of the shoulder joint.

Quchi point (LI 11)
With the elbow bent halfway, on the outer side of the cubital transverse crease.

Zhigou point (TE 6)
In a cavity about 3 cun above the back of the wrist, between the two bones of the forearm.

Waiguan point (TE 5)
The Waiguan point is in the middle on the outside of the arm, between the ulna and radius about 2 cun away from the horizontal line of the wrist joint.

Weizhong point (BL 40)
Right in the middle of popliteal crease (at the back of the knee).

Chengshan point (BL 57)
In a cavity in the middle of the rear of the lower leg, at the top of the depression between the two muscles of the calf.

Jianyu point (LI 15)
In a cavity just before the shoulder peak when one raises the upper arm horizontally.

Recommended Procedures

1. For Patients with Difficulty in Verbal Expression: Yamen Point and Lianquan Point

Method: With the basic scraping therapy done, use the surface-scraping to scrape Yamen point on the rear of the head and Lianquan point on the front of the neck.

3. For Patients with Facial Paralysis: Dicang Point, Jiache Point, Chengqi Point, Yangbai Point and Cuanzhu Point

Method: With the basic scraping therapy done, use the flat-pressing and kneading to press and knead Dicang point, Jiache point, Chengqi point, and Yangbai point on the face. Then, use the corner of the scraping plate to press Cuanzhu point.

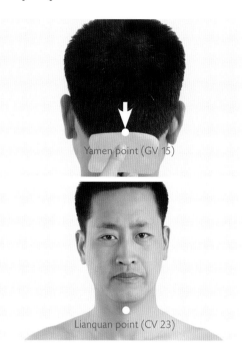

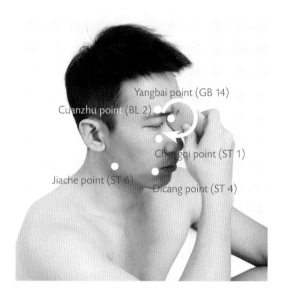

2. For Patients with Upper-Limb Paralysis: Jianyu Point, Jianzhen Point, Quchi Point, Zhigou Point, and Waiguan Point

Method: With the basic scraping therapy done, use the surface-scraping to scrape Jianyu point, Jianzhen point, Quchi point, Zhigou point, and Waiguan point on upper limbs from up to down.

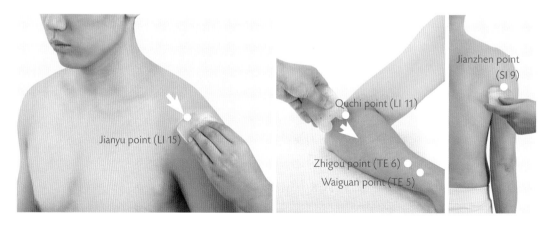

4. For Patients with Lower-Limb Paralysis: Huantiao Point, Fengshi Point, Yanglingquan Point, Zusanli Point, Fenglong Point, Jiexi Point, Yinmen Point, Weizhong Point, and Chengshan Point

Method: With the basic scraping therapy done, use the surface-scraping to scrape from Huantiao point to Fengshi point and Yanglingquan point of Gallbladder Maridian on lower limbs from up to down, from Zusanli point to Fenglong point and Jiexi point of Stomach Meridian, and from Yingmen point to Weizhong point and Chengshan point of Bladder Meridian on lower limbs.

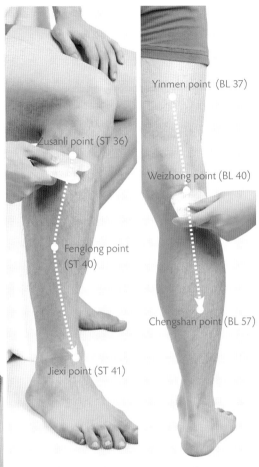

Yinmen point (BL 37)

Zusanli point (ST 36)

Weizhong point (BL 40)

Fenglong point (ST 40)

Chengshan point (BL 57)

Jiexi point (ST 41)

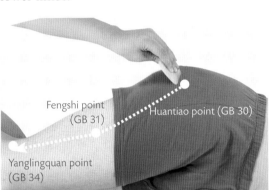

Fengshi point (GB 31)

Huantiao point (GB 30)

Yanglingquan point (GB 34)

Chronic Bronchitis

Commonly seen among old people, it is not obvious in the early stage. Chronic bronchitis mostly occurs in winter and subsides after warm spring. It is mainly marked by chronic cough or cough with sputa which is white and sticky, or with minor cough and light sputa, but attacks once the patient catches a cold. Failure to cure it in the early stage will make it worse in the late stage and stay every year. The course of this disease often repeats itself, to the extent of causing complications like emphysema and pulmonary heart disease. Scraping particular acupoints can play the role of dispersing lung energy, stopping cough, resolving sputum and relieving asthma, very helpful to ease and cure this disease.

Smoking is the most important reason for chronic bronchitis. Though giving up smoking cannot completely cure chronic bronchitis, it can obviously delay the development of its course, partially recovering lung functions. Reasonable nutrition, physical exercise, reinforcement of the physique, and prevention of the cold are all beneficial to the prevention of chronic bronchitis among old people.

Recommended Procedures

1. Dazhui Point, Dingchuan Point, Dazhu Point, Fengmen Point and Feishu Point

Method: Use the surface-scraping to scrape from Dazhui point, Dingchuan point, Dashu point, Fengmen point to Feishu point until *sha* appears.

2. Tiantu Point and Zhongfu Point

Method: Use the corner of the scraping plate to scrape Tiantu point and Zhongfu point from up to down respectively. Then, press and knead each acupoint respectively for 30 times in whirls, until *sha* appears.

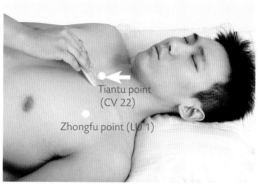

Tiantu point (CV 22)

Zhongfu point (LU 1)

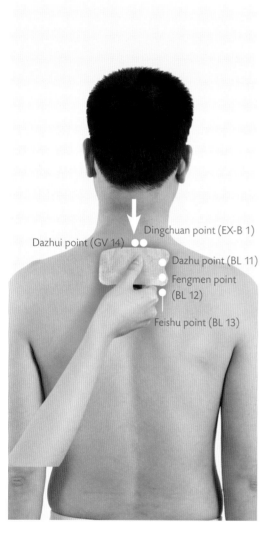

Dazhui point (GV 14)

Dingchuan point (EX-B 1)

Dazhu point (BL 11)

Fengmen point (BL 12)

Feishu point (BL 13)

3. Chize Point and Taiyuan Point

Method: Use the surface-scraping to scrape Chize point and Taiyuan point on upper limbs from up to down respectively, with the extent of force increasing gradually, until *sha* appears.

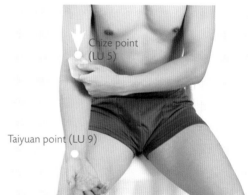

Chize point (LU 5)

Taiyuan point (LU 9)

Therapies to Increase the Curative Effect

• 15-gram sweet apricot kernels are mashed repeatedly with water added to be filtered into juice, added with one spoon of honey to be drunk with boiled water. Twice or three times a day.

• 500-gram pumpkins peeled off and cut into small pieces are boiled together with 15 dates and an appropriate amount of brown sugar to be drunk once or twice a day.

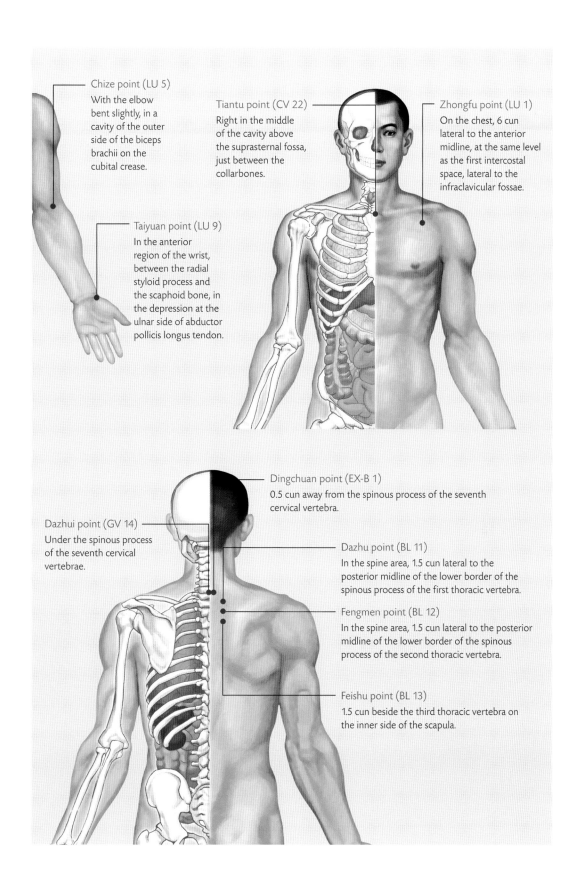

Chize point (LU 5)
With the elbow bent slightly, in a cavity of the outer side of the biceps brachii on the cubital crease.

Taiyuan point (LU 9)
In the anterior region of the wrist, between the radial styloid process and the scaphoid bone, in the depression at the ulnar side of abductor pollicis longus tendon.

Tiantu point (CV 22)
Right in the middle of the cavity above the suprasternal fossa, just between the collarbones.

Zhongfu point (LU 1)
On the chest, 6 cun lateral to the anterior midline, at the same level as the first intercostal space, lateral to the infraclavicular fossae.

Dingchuan point (EX-B 1)
0.5 cun away from the spinous process of the seventh cervical vertebra.

Dazhui point (GV 14)
Under the spinous process of the seventh cervical vertebrae.

Dazhu point (BL 11)
In the spine area, 1.5 cun lateral to the posterior midline of the lower border of the spinous process of the first thoracic vertebra.

Fengmen point (BL 12)
In the spine area, 1.5 cun lateral to the posterior midline of the lower border of the spinous process of the second thoracic vertebra.

Feishu point (BL 13)
1.5 cun beside the third thoracic vertebra on the inner side of the scapula.

Chronic Rhinitis

There are many reasons for the disease. Acute rhinitis can be turned into a chronic one if it fails to be cured with repeated attacks. Excessive smoking and alcoholic drinks can also lead to chronic rhinitis. Environmental factors, such as smogs and coal-dust, flour or chemical substances as well as sharp changes of the temperature and humidity are also extremely apt to result in chronic rhinitis. Chronic rhinitis is mainly marked by the increase of nasal discharge as well as intermittent and alternate nasal obstruction. Scraping therapy can function as smoothing the nose, inducing mild diaphoresis and opening the inhibited lung-energy, which are conducive to easing the congestion and swelling of nasal mucosa.

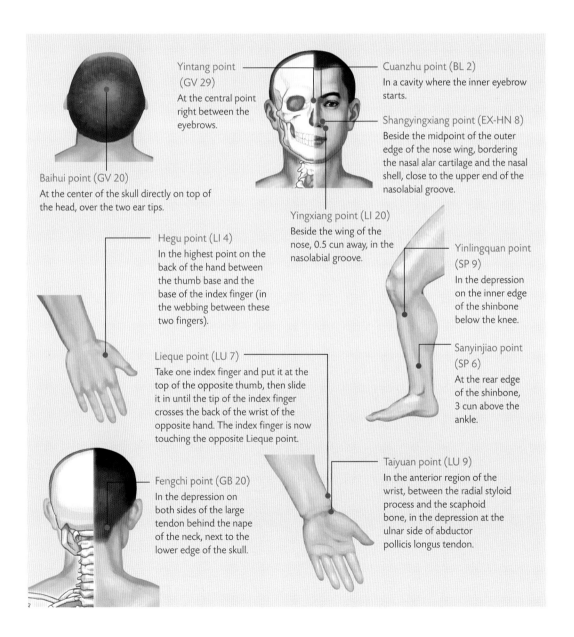

Yintang point (GV 29)
At the central point right between the eyebrows.

Cuanzhu point (BL 2)
In a cavity where the inner eyebrow starts.

Shangyingxiang point (EX-HN 8)
Beside the midpoint of the outer edge of the nose wing, bordering the nasal alar cartilage and the nasal shell, close to the upper end of the nasolabial groove.

Baihui point (GV 20)
At the center of the skull directly on top of the head, over the two ear tips.

Yingxiang point (LI 20)
Beside the wing of the nose, 0.5 cun away, in the nasolabial groove.

Hegu point (LI 4)
In the highest point on the back of the hand between the thumb base and the base of the index finger (in the webbing between these two fingers).

Yinlingquan point (SP 9)
In the depression on the inner edge of the shinbone below the knee.

Lieque point (LU 7)
Take one index finger and put it at the top of the opposite thumb, then slide it in until the tip of the index finger crosses the back of the wrist of the opposite hand. The index finger is now touching the opposite Lieque point.

Sanyinjiao point (SP 6)
At the rear edge of the shinbone, 3 cun above the ankle.

Fengchi point (GB 20)
In the depression on both sides of the large tendon behind the nape of the neck, next to the lower edge of the skull.

Taiyuan point (LU 9)
In the anterior region of the wrist, between the radial styloid process and the scaphoid bone, in the depression at the ulnar side of abductor pollicis longus tendon.

Recommended Procedures

1. Yintang Point, Cuanzhu Point, Shangyingxiang Point and Yingxiang Point

Method: Use the corner of the scraping plate to press and knead Yintang point, Cuanzhu point, Shangyingxiang point and Yingxiang point on the face.

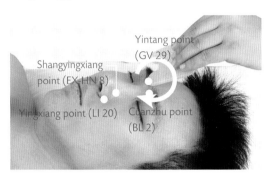

3. Baihui Point and Fengchi Point

Method: Use the single-angle scraping to scrape Baihui point on the top of the head and Fengchi point on both sides at the rear of the neck.

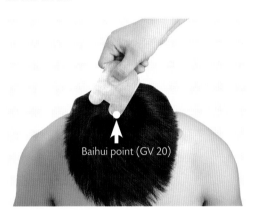

2. Lieque Point, Taiyuan Point and Hegu Point

Method: Use the surface-scraping to scrape from Lieque point to Taiyuan point on upper limbs. Use the flat-pressing and kneading to press and knead Hegu point on the hand back.

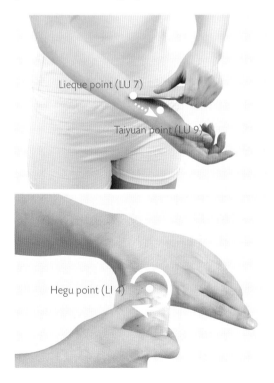

4. Yinlingquan Point and Sanyinjiao Point

Method: Use the surface-scraping to scrape from Yinlingquan point to Sanyinjiao point on lower limbs.

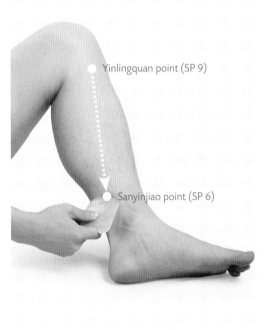

Allergic Rhinitis

It is chronic inflammation of nasal mucosa caused by atopic individual contact allergen. Allergic rhinitis is mainly featured by nasal itch, sneeze, too much nasal discharge and distention of nasal mucosa, which can induce simultaneous occurrence of bronchial asthma, nasosinusitis, nasal polyps, otitis media, or allergic conjunctivitis, etc.

Allergrc rhinitis is typical of paroxysmal and continuous sneezes, along with lots of watery snots, nasal congestion and itch. The sense of smell among some patients declines, but temporarily. Generally, the symptoms will be reduced or controlled after proper treatment.

Avoiding allergen is the most effective way for preventing and curing allergic rhinitis. Try to avoid all doubtful or confirmed allergens as much as possible, including all kinds of allergen-oriented inhalations, food and substances in contact so as to reduce the incidence. Air-conditioning is also an important element for resulting in allergic rhinitis. People of allergic physique should try to avoid it.

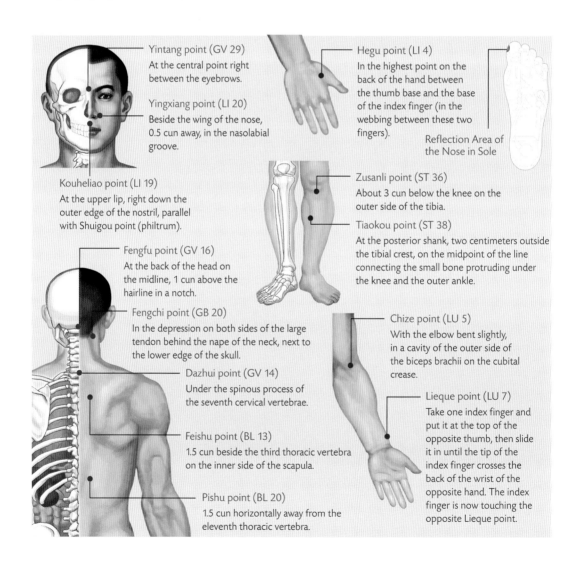

Yintang point (GV 29)
At the central point right between the eyebrows.

Yingxiang point (LI 20)
Beside the wing of the nose, 0.5 cun away, in the nasolabial groove.

Kouheliao point (LI 19)
At the upper lip, right down the outer edge of the nostril, parallel with Shuigou point (philtrum).

Fengfu point (GV 16)
At the back of the head on the midline, 1 cun above the hairline in a notch.

Fengchi point (GB 20)
In the depression on both sides of the large tendon behind the nape of the neck, next to the lower edge of the skull.

Dazhui point (GV 14)
Under the spinous process of the seventh cervical vertebrae.

Feishu point (BL 13)
1.5 cun beside the third thoracic vertebra on the inner side of the scapula.

Pishu point (BL 20)
1.5 cun horizontally away from the eleventh thoracic vertebra.

Hegu point (LI 4)
In the highest point on the back of the hand between the thumb base and the base of the index finger (in the webbing between these two fingers).

Reflection Area of the Nose in Sole

Zusanli point (ST 36)
About 3 cun below the knee on the outer side of the tibia.

Tiaokou point (ST 38)
At the posterior shank, two centimeters outside the tibial crest, on the midpoint of the line connecting the small bone protruding under the knee and the outer ankle.

Chize point (LU 5)
With the elbow bent slightly, in a cavity of the outer side of the biceps brachii on the cubital crease.

Lieque point (LU 7)
Take one index finger and put it at the top of the opposite thumb, then slide it in until the tip of the index finger crosses the back of the wrist of the opposite hand. The index finger is now touching the opposite Lieque point.

Recommended Procedures

1. Reflection Area of the Nose in Sole
Method: Use the corner of the scraping plate to press and knead the area until soreness and distension are felt.

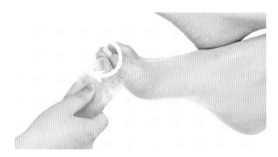

2. Fengchi Point, Fengfu Point, Dazhui Point, Feishu Point and Pishu Point
Method: Use the corner of the scraping plate to press and knead Fengchi point of Gallbladder Meridian on both sides. Use the surface-scraping to scrape from Fengfu point to Dazhui point of Du Meridian from up to down, and from Feishu point to Pishu point of Bladder Meridian.

3. Kouheliao Point, Yingxiang Point and Yintang Point
Method: Use the single corner of the scraping plate to press and knead Kouheliao point, Yingxiang point and Yintang point.

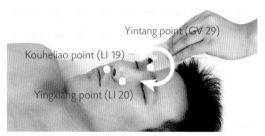

4. Hegu Point, Chize Point, Lieque Point, Zusanli Point and Tiaokou Point
Method: Use the surface-scraping to scrape Hegu point of Large Intestine Meridian on upper limbs from up to down, from Chize point to Lieque point of Lung Meridian and from Zusanli point to Tiaokou point of Stomach Meridian of lower limbs.

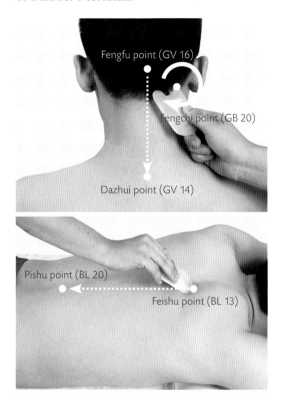

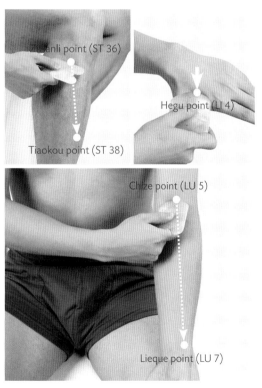

Presbyopia

This refers to old people who are gradually finding it difficult to read in short distance. It demonstrates the aging of human functions, but not a pathological state. Reading or watching too much is also a factor that cannot be overlooked. In order to prevent and cure presbyopia, pay attention to the hygiene of using eyes and reduce their tension on the one hand, use massage and scraping therapy to mobilize the vital energy and blood around eyes to nourish eyes on the other.

Recommended Procedures

1. Yanglao Point and Yanglaodian Point
Method: Use the vertical-pressing and kneading to press and knead Yanglao point on the back of the forearm and Yanglaodian point on the root of the small finger, until soreness and numbness are felt.

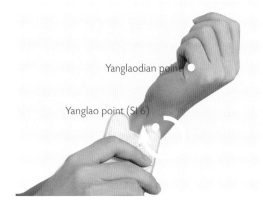

2. Ganshu Point and Shenshu Point
Method: Use the surface-scraping to scrape from Ganshu point to Shenshu point on the back from up to down, until the skin turns red.

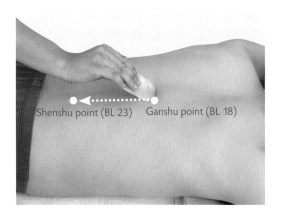

3. Jingming Point, Cuanzhu Point, and Tongziliao Point
Method: Use the vertical-pressing and kneading to press and knead Jingming point on the face. Use the flat-pressing and kneading to press and knead Cuanzhu point and Tongziliao point.

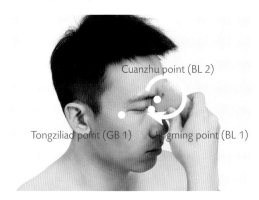

4. Guangming Point and Yangfu Point
Method: Use the surface-scraping to scrape from Guangming point to Yangfu point on the outside of the lower limbs from up to down.

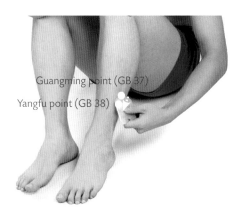

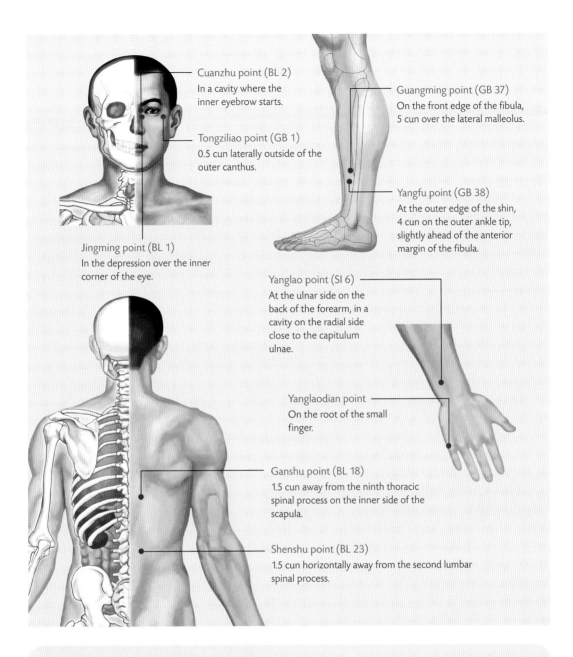

Cuanzhu point (BL 2)
In a cavity where the inner eyebrow starts.

Tongziliao point (GB 1)
0.5 cun laterally outside of the outer canthus.

Jingming point (BL 1)
In the depression over the inner corner of the eye.

Guangming point (GB 37)
On the front edge of the fibula, 5 cun over the lateral malleolus.

Yangfu point (GB 38)
At the outer edge of the shin, 4 cun on the outer ankle tip, slightly ahead of the anterior margin of the fibula.

Yanglao point (SI 6)
At the ulnar side on the back of the forearm, in a cavity on the radial side close to the capitulum ulnae.

Yanglaodian point
On the root of the small finger.

Ganshu point (BL 18)
1.5 cun away from the ninth thoracic spinal process on the inner side of the scapula.

Shenshu point (BL 23)
1.5 cun horizontally away from the second lumbar spinal process.

Therapies to Increase the Curative Effect

• Protecting eyes via hot compress: Apply the towel to eyes for several times when you wash face with warm water, which can smooth the circulation of the blood vessels of eyes and supply eye muscles with oxygen and nutrients. In free time, you can close eyes, rub your palms to make them warm and gently cover eyes with them for one minute.

• Looking into far distance at a designated time: Look into distance as far as possible to see green plants once or twice every day and then gradually move the eyesight closer from afar, which is conducive to improving eyesight and adjusting eye muscles.

Chronic Pharyngitis

The throat can experience different feelings when chronic pharyngitis attacks, such as the feeling of a foreign body, dryness, burning and slight pain as well as more and sticky secretions. Therefore, the patient often clears the throat and spits white sticky sputa. Scraping therapy can ease it to a certain extent.

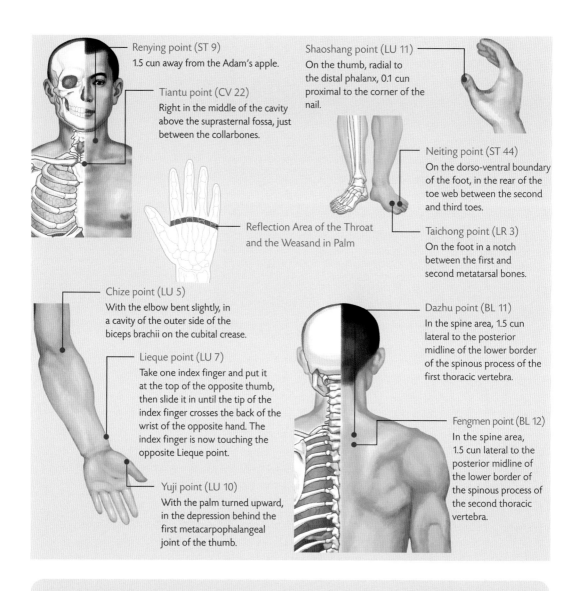

Renying point (ST 9)
1.5 cun away from the Adam's apple.

Tiantu point (CV 22)
Right in the middle of the cavity above the suprasternal fossa, just between the collarbones.

Shaoshang point (LU 11)
On the thumb, radial to the distal phalanx, 0.1 cun proximal to the corner of the nail.

Neiting point (ST 44)
On the dorso-ventral boundary of the foot, in the rear of the toe web between the second and third toes.

Reflection Area of the Throat and the Weasand in Palm

Taichong point (LR 3)
On the foot in a notch between the first and second metatarsal bones.

Chize point (LU 5)
With the elbow bent slightly, in a cavity of the outer side of the biceps brachii on the cubital crease.

Lieque point (LU 7)
Take one index finger and put it at the top of the opposite thumb, then slide it in until the tip of the index finger crosses the back of the wrist of the opposite hand. The index finger is now touching the opposite Lieque point.

Yuji point (LU 10)
With the palm turned upward, in the depression behind the first metacarpophalangeal joint of the thumb.

Dazhu point (BL 11)
In the spine area, 1.5 cun lateral to the posterior midline of the lower border of the spinous process of the first thoracic vertebra.

Fengmen point (BL 12)
In the spine area, 1.5 cun lateral to the posterior midline of the lower border of the spinous process of the second thoracic vertebra.

Therapy to Increase the Curative Effect
If pharyngitis attacks in spring, apart from scraping therapy, you can also press and knead Liver Meridian on the inside of the thigh, with stress on several points of pain above and below the knee and use the corner of the scraping plate to press and knead Taichong point between the big toe and the second toe.

Recommended Procedures

1. Reflection Area of the Throat and the Weasand in Palm

Method: Use the flat-pressing and kneading to scrape the area 30 to 50 times.

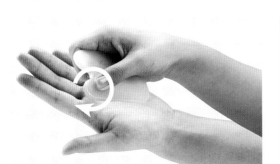

2. Chize Point, Lieque Point, Yuji Point and Shaoshang Point

Method: Use the flat-scraping to scrape from Chize point to Lieque point, and from Yuji point to Shaoshang point, until the skin turns red or *sha* appears.

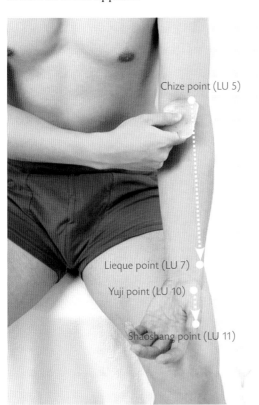

Chize point (LU 5)

Lieque point (LU 7)

Yuji point (LU 10)

Shaoshang point (LU 11)

3. Renying Point and Tiantu Point

Method: Use the flat scraping to gently scrape Renying point 15 to 30 times and then use the single-angle scraping to gently scrape Tiantu point, until *sha* appears.

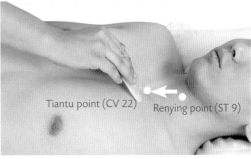

Tiantu point (CV 22)   Renying point (ST 9)

4. Taichong Point and Neiting Point

Method: Use the corner of the scraping plate to press and knead Taichong point and Neiting point on the foot back, until storng sorness and distention are felt or *sha* appears.

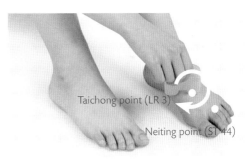

Taichong point (LR 3)

Neiting point (ST 44)

5. Dazhu Point and Fengmen Point

Method: Use the dual-angle scraping to scrape from Dazhu point to Fengmen point on the back, until *sha* appears.

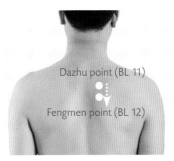

Dazhu point (BL 11)

Fengmen point (BL 12)

Chronic Pneumonia

If the course of pneumonia exceeds three months, it is regarded as chronic pneumonia marked by repeated attacks periodically and aggravation. There is no obvious symptom in the resting stage almost without cough, but the patient is apt to suffer from shortness of breath while running or climbing stairs. Scraping therapy is conducive to easing cough and fever in the course of pneumonia attack, enhancing physical resistance and preventing the recurrence of inflammation.

Active prevention of infection of the respiratory tract is an important measure for preventing and curing chronic pneumonia. The patient of chronic pneumonia should pay attention to the rest, avoid fatigue or places of lots of people with poor ventilation. He should eat food that can be easily digested, drink more water, eat more fruits, and avoid spicy and oily food, so as to prevent sputa due to internal heat which will trigger off or aggravate the symptom.

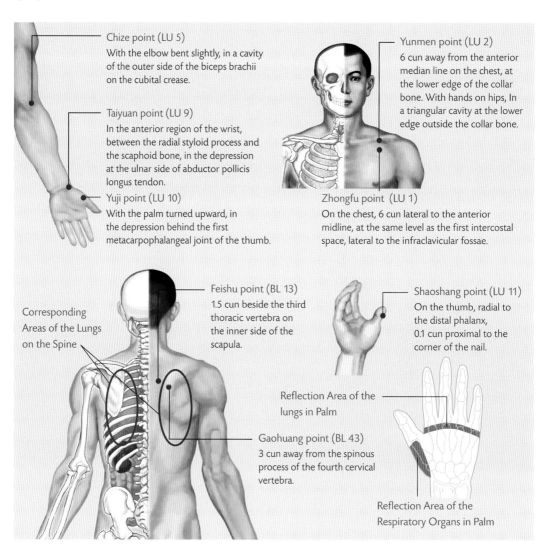

Chize point (LU 5)
With the elbow bent slightly, in a cavity of the outer side of the biceps brachii on the cubital crease.

Taiyuan point (LU 9)
In the anterior region of the wrist, between the radial styloid process and the scaphoid bone, in the depression at the ulnar side of abductor pollicis longus tendon.

Yuji point (LU 10)
With the palm turned upward, in the depression behind the first metacarpophalangeal joint of the thumb.

Yunmen point (LU 2)
6 cun away from the anterior median line on the chest, at the lower edge of the collar bone. With hands on hips, In a triangular cavity at the lower edge outside the collar bone.

Zhongfu point (LU 1)
On the chest, 6 cun lateral to the anterior midline, at the same level as the first intercostal space, lateral to the infraclavicular fossae.

Corresponding Areas of the Lungs on the Spine

Feishu point (BL 13)
1.5 cun beside the third thoracic vertebra on the inner side of the scapula.

Shaoshang point (LU 11)
On the thumb, radial to the distal phalanx, 0.1 cun proximal to the corner of the nail.

Reflection Area of the lungs in Palm

Gaohuang point (BL 43)
3 cun away from the spinous process of the fourth cervical vertebra.

Reflection Area of the Respiratory Organs in Palm

Recommended Procedures

1. Corresponding Areas of the Lungs on the Spine, Feishu Point and Gaohuang Point

Method: Use the surface-scraping to scrape the corresponding areas of the lungs, with stress on Feishu point and Gaohuang point.

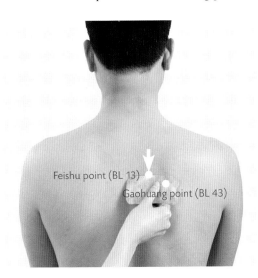

Feishu point (BL 13)
Gaohuang point (BL 43)

2. Chize Point, Taiyuan Point, Reflection Areas of the Lungs and the Respiratory Organs in Palm

Method: Use the flat-scraping to scrape from Chize point to Taiyuan point and the reflection areas in palm.

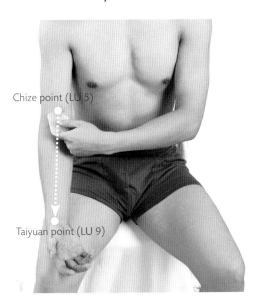

Chize point (LU 5)

Taiyuan point (LU 9)

3. Yunmen Point and Zhongfu Point

Method: Use the angle-scraping to scrape from Yunmen point to Zhongfu point of Lung Meridian from up to down.

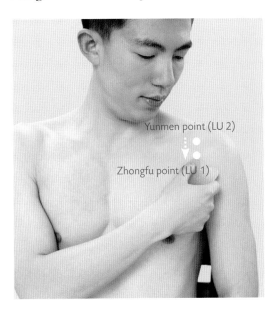

Yunmen point (LU 2)

Zhongfu point (LU 1)

4. Yuji point and Shaoshang point

Method: Use the angle-kneading to press and knead Yuji point and then use the flat-scraping to scrape from Yuji point to Shaoshang point.

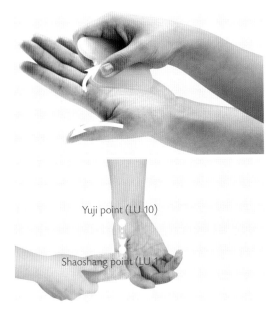

Yuji point (LU 10)

Shaoshang point (LU 11)

Asthma

This is a common disease of the respiratory system marked by repeated attacks. Generally, it is featured by paroxysmal short breath, chest distress, difficulty in breathing, wheezing, cough and cough with phlegm. Asthma can be induced by smog, dust, pollens, cold air, oily smoke, chemical smell and diet, etc. Scraping therapy in this section is applicable to bronchial asthma, asthmatic chronic bronchitis and obstructive emphysema as well as the difficulty in breathing caused by other kinds of diseases.

Patients of asthma should pay attention to avoiding factors of induction, such as dust, pollens, cold air or oily smoke. They should eat light food, avoid irritation, eat less, and avoid very salty, sweet, spicy, cold food, or alcoholic drinks. Try to avoid eating any kind of food which can induce the attack of bronchial asthma.

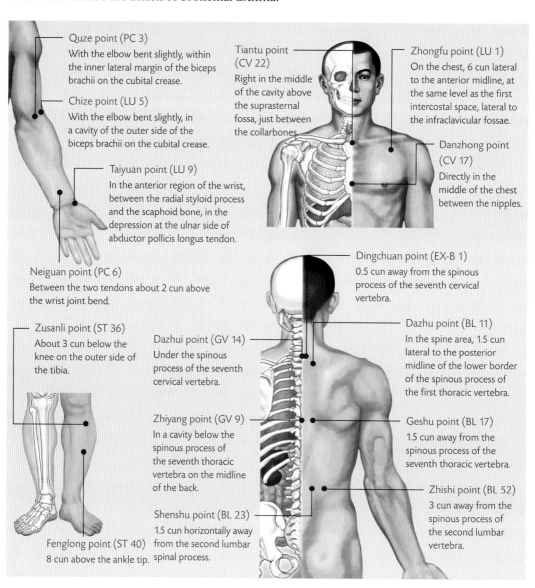

Quze point (PC 3)
With the elbow bent slightly, within the inner lateral margin of the biceps brachii on the cubital crease.

Chize point (LU 5)
With the elbow bent slightly, in a cavity of the outer side of the biceps brachii on the cubital crease.

Taiyuan point (LU 9)
In the anterior region of the wrist, between the radial styloid process and the scaphoid bone, in the depression at the ulnar side of abductor pollicis longus tendon.

Neiguan point (PC 6)
Between the two tendons about 2 cun above the wrist joint bend.

Zusanli point (ST 36)
About 3 cun below the knee on the outer side of the tibia.

Fenglong point (ST 40)
8 cun above the ankle tip.

Tiantu point (CV 22)
Right in the middle of the cavity above the suprasternal fossa, just between the collarbones.

Dazhui point (GV 14)
Under the spinous process of the seventh cervical vertebra.

Zhiyang point (GV 9)
In a cavity below the spinous process of the seventh thoracic vertebra on the midline of the back.

Shenshu point (BL 23)
1.5 cun horizontally away from the second lumbar spinal process.

Zhongfu point (LU 1)
On the chest, 6 cun lateral to the anterior midline, at the same level as the first intercostal space, lateral to the infraclavicular fossae.

Danzhong point (CV 17)
Directly in the middle of the chest between the nipples.

Dingchuan point (EX-B 1)
0.5 cun away from the spinous process of the seventh cervical vertebra.

Dazhu point (BL 11)
In the spine area, 1.5 cun lateral to the posterior midline of the lower border of the spinous process of the first thoracic vertebra.

Geshu point (BL 17)
1.5 cun away from the spinous process of the seventh thoracic vertebra.

Zhishi point (BL 52)
3 cun away from the spinous process of the second lumbar vertebra.

Recommended Procedures

1. Tiantu Point, Danzhong Point and Zhongfu Point

Method: Use the angle-scraping to scrape from Tiantu point to Danzhong point of Ren Meridian on the chest from up to down. Then, scrape the frontal chest from inside to outside, with stress on Zhongfu point of Lung Meridian on both sides.

3. Quze Point, Neiguan Point, Chize Point, Taiyuan Point, Zusanli Point and Fenglong Point

Method: Use the surface-scraping to scrape from Quze point, Neiguan point to the tip of the middle finger on both sides of upper limbs from up to down. In case of cough, add Chize point and Taiyuan point on both sides. In case of cough with phlegm, add Zusanli point and Fenglong point on both sides.

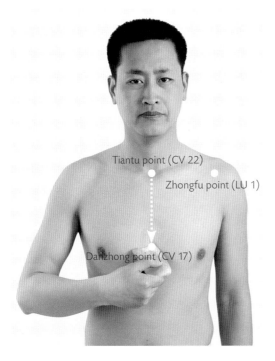

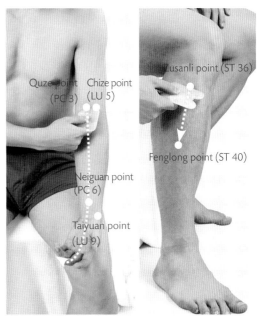

2. Dazhui Point, Zhiyang Point, Dazhu Point, Geshu Point, Zhishi Point, Shenshu Point and Dingchuan Point

Method: Use the surface-scraping to Scrape from Dazhui point to Zhiyang point of Du Meridian on the back. Scrape from Dazhu point to Geshu point, Zhishi point, Shenshu point ang Dingchuan point on both sides from up to down.

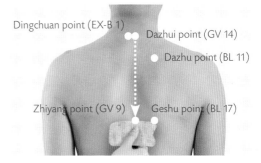

Therapy to Increase the Curative Effect

15-gram shelled-off ginkgo and an appropriate amount of white sugar are boiled. With this done, ginkgo, with its peel and core removed, is steamed for oral use. This prescription serves to contract lung energy and stops asthma, applicable to asthma marked by cough of a long time, lung weakness and reversed flow of vital energy.

Chronic Hepatitis

This is mostly caused by mistaken diagnosis or treatment of acute hepatitis, virus infection, disorder of immune system or the toxic effect of some medicine, resulting in the failure to cure hepatitis for a long time. It is mainly featured by exhaustion all over the body, declining appetite, abdominal distention, liver distention or dull pain.

Scraping therapy serves to smooth liver energy, benefit spleen, and reduce internal heat and dampness, exerting an active effect on the rehabilitation of chronic hepatitis.

Since alcoholics and medicine are metabolized by liver, patients of chronic hepatitis should give up alcoholic drinks and take medicine cautiously. They should follow the principle of eating food which is light, easily digestive and very nutritious, instead of eating lots of irritating food such as spring onions, ginger or garlic as well as fried and baked food. Mental factors have a quite big influence on chronic hepatitis. Therefore, patients should be optimistic and avoid fatigue.

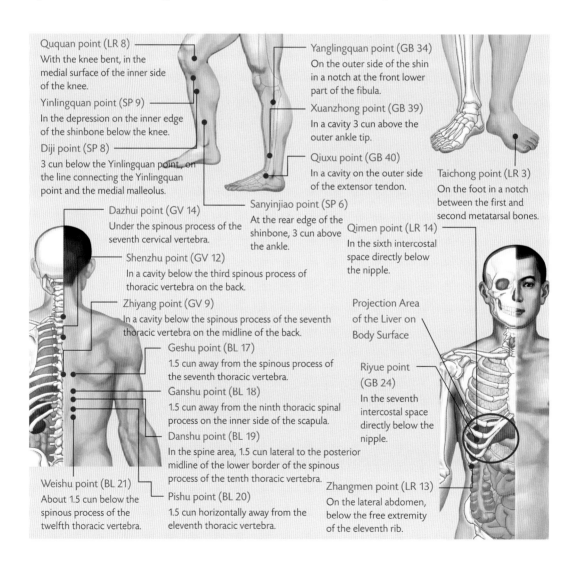

Ququan point (LR 8)
With the knee bent, in the medial surface of the inner side of the knee.

Yinlingquan point (SP 9)
In the depression on the inner edge of the shinbone below the knee.

Diji point (SP 8)
3 cun below the Yinlingquan point, on the line connecting the Yinlingquan point and the medial malleolus.

Yanglingquan point (GB 34)
On the outer side of the shin in a notch at the front lower part of the fibula.

Xuanzhong point (GB 39)
In a cavity 3 cun above the outer ankle tip.

Qiuxu point (GB 40)
In a cavity on the outer side of the extensor tendon.

Taichong point (LR 3)
On the foot in a notch between the first and second metatarsal bones.

Dazhui point (GV 14)
Under the spinous process of the seventh cervical vertebra.

Shenzhu point (GV 12)
In a cavity below the third spinous process of thoracic vertebra on the back.

Zhiyang point (GV 9)
In a cavity below the spinous process of the seventh thoracic vertebra on the midline of the back.

Geshu point (BL 17)
1.5 cun away from the spinous process of the seventh thoracic vertebra.

Ganshu point (BL 18)
1.5 cun away from the ninth thoracic spinal process on the inner side of the scapula.

Danshu point (BL 19)
In the spine area, 1.5 cun lateral to the posterior midline of the lower border of the spinous process of the tenth thoracic vertebra.

Weishu point (BL 21)
About 1.5 cun below the spinous process of the twelfth thoracic vertebra.

Pishu point (BL 20)
1.5 cun horizontally away from the eleventh thoracic vertebra.

Sanyinjiao point (SP 6)
At the rear edge of the shinbone, 3 cun above the ankle.

Qimen point (LR 14)
In the sixth intercostal space directly below the nipple.

Projection Area of the Liver on Body Surface

Riyue point (GB 24)
In the seventh intercostal space directly below the nipple.

Zhangmen point (LR 13)
On the lateral abdomen, below the free extremity of the eleventh rib.

Recommended Procedures

1. Projection Area of the Liver on the Body Surface, Qimen Point, Riyue Point and Zhangmen Point

Method: Use the surface-scraping to scrape the projection area from inside to outside, with stress on Qimen point, Riyue point and Zhangmen point on the right side.

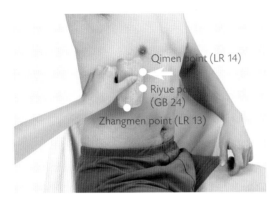

Qimen point (LR 14)

Riyue point (GB 24)

Zhangmen point (LR 13)

2. Dazhui Point, Shenzhu Point, Zhiyang Point, Geshu Point, Weishu Point, Ganshu Point, Danshu Point and Pishu Point

Method: Use the surface-scraping to scrape from Dazhui point along the posterior median line, via Shenzhu point to Zhiyang point from up to down. Then, use the surface-scraping to scrape from Geshu point on the back to Weishu point, with stress on Ganshu point, Danshu point and Pishu point.

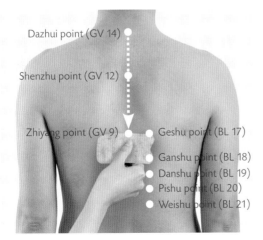

Dazhui point (GV 14)

Shenzhu point (GV 12)

Zhiyang point (GV 9)   Geshu point (BL 17)

Ganshu point (BL 18)

Danshu point (BL 19)

Pishu point (BL 20)

Weishu point (BL 21)

3. Ququan Point, Yinlingquan Point, Diji Point, Sanyinjiao Point, Taichong Point, Yanglingquan Point, Xuanzhong Point and Qiuxu Point

Method: Use the surface-scraping to scrape from Ququan point to Yinlingquan point, Diji point, Sanyinjiao point and Taichong point of Liver Meridian on lower limbs. Then, scrape from Yanglingquan point on the outside of the shin to Xuanzhong point and Qiuxu point of Gallbladder Meridian on lower limbs.

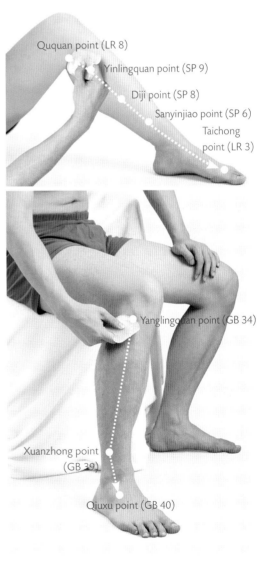

Ququan point (LR 8)

Yinlingquan point (SP 9)

Diji point (SP 8)

Sanyinjiao point (SP 6)

Taichong point (LR 3)

Yanglingquan point (GB 34)

Xuanzhong point (GB 39)

Qiuxu point (GB 40)

Fatty Liver

This is a pathological change caused by too much accumulation of fat within liver cells due to various reasons. It has many manifestations. People with minor symptom of fat liver only feel tired. People with medium or heavy symptoms of fat liver are marked by lack of appetite, exhaustion, nausea, vomit, loss of weight, dull pain in the liver or in the upper right abdomen.

Fat liver mostly results from eating too much sweet and oily food, or drinking too much alcoholics, or suffering from pathogenic damp-heat, or experiencing emotional disorder. Scraping therapy can expel fat and toxin, helpful to improve the symptom.

The most important for the patient of fat liver is to take control of the diet while persisting in doing physical exercise. Generally speaking, no medicine is needed if there is no inflammation.

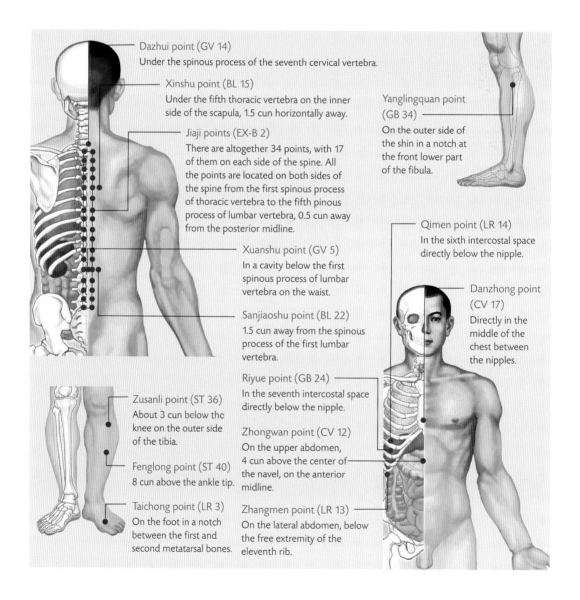

Dazhui point (GV 14)
Under the spinous process of the seventh cervical vertebra.

Xinshu point (BL 15)
Under the fifth thoracic vertebra on the inner side of the scapula, 1.5 cun horizontally away.

Jiaji points (EX-B 2)
There are altogether 34 points, with 17 of them on each side of the spine. All the points are located on both sides of the spine from the first spinous process of thoracic vertebra to the fifth pinous process of lumbar vertebra, 0.5 cun away from the posterior midline.

Xuanshu point (GV 5)
In a cavity below the first spinous process of lumbar vertebra on the waist.

Sanjiaoshu point (BL 22)
1.5 cun away from the spinous process of the first lumbar vertebra.

Yanglingquan point (GB 34)
On the outer side of the shin in a notch at the front lower part of the fibula.

Qimen point (LR 14)
In the sixth intercostal space directly below the nipple.

Danzhong point (CV 17)
Directly in the middle of the chest between the nipples.

Riyue point (GB 24)
In the seventh intercostal space directly below the nipple.

Zusanli point (ST 36)
About 3 cun below the knee on the outer side of the tibia.

Zhongwan point (CV 12)
On the upper abdomen, 4 cun above the center of the navel, on the anterior midline.

Fenglong point (ST 40)
8 cun above the ankle tip.

Taichong point (LR 3)
On the foot in a notch between the first and second metatarsal bones.

Zhangmen point (LR 13)
On the lateral abdomen, below the free extremity of the eleventh rib.

Recommended Procedures

1. Danzhong Point and Zhongwan Point

Method: Use the flat-scraping to scrape from Danzhong point to Zhongwan point from up to down. Then, use the flat-pressing and kneading to press and knead Zhongwan point 20 to 30 times.

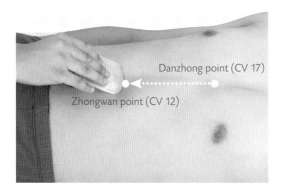

Danzhong point (CV 17)

Zhongwan point (CV 12)

2. Dazhui Point, Xuanshu Point, Xinshu Point, Sanjiaoshu Point and Jiaji Points

Method: Use the surface-scraping to scrape from Dazhui point to Xuanshu point of Du Meridian on the back from up to down, from Xinshu point to Sanjiaoshu point of Bladder Meridian. Use the dual-angle scraping to scrape Jiaji points on both sides.

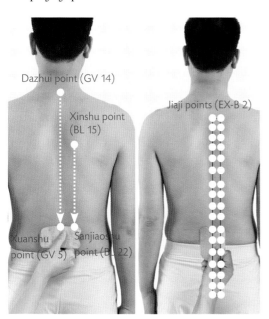

Dazhui point (GV 14)

Xinshu point (BL 15)

Jiaji points (EX-B 2)

Xuanshu point (GV 5)

Sanjiaoshu point (BL 22)

3. Qimen Point, Zhangmen Point, Riyue Point and Taichong Point

Method: Use the angle-scraping to scrape Qimen point, Zhangmen point and Riyue point on the chest and ribs from inside to outside. Use the angle-kneading to press and knead Taichong point on the foot 20 to 30 times, until soreness and distention are felt.

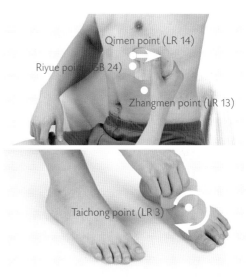

Qimen point (LR 14)

Riyue point (GB 24)

Zhangmen point (LR 13)

Taichong point (LR 3)

4. Yanglingquan Point, Zusanli Point and Fenglong Point

Method: Use the surface-scraping to scrape Yanglingquan point of Gallbladder Meridian on the outside of the lower limbs from up to down, and from Zusanli point to Fenglong point on the Stomach Meridian from up to down.

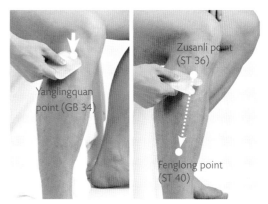

Yanglingquan point (GB 34)

Zusanli point (ST 36)

Fenglong point (ST 40)

Chronic Cholecystitis and Cholelithiasis

Chronic cholecystitis mostly goes together with gall-stones. A few cases of chronic cholecystitis are free from gall-stones. This disease is mostly chronic, and it can also be caused by repeated attacks of acute cholecystitis.

Chronic cholecystitis or cholelithiasis is mostly marked by gall-oriented indigestion, disgust at oily food, distention of upper abdomen, belching and burning in stomach. It is similar to ulcers or chronic appendicitis. When it attacks all of a sudden, there will be continuous sharp pain on the right ribs and upper abdomen. Sometimes, the pain will radiate to the right shoulder, often coupled with nausea and fever, etc.

Scraping therapy is only applicable to chronic cholecystitis as auxiliary treatment. The patient must go to the hospital if he/she is in the period of acute attack or at a time of sharp pain in the gallbladder, in order to receive timely treatment.

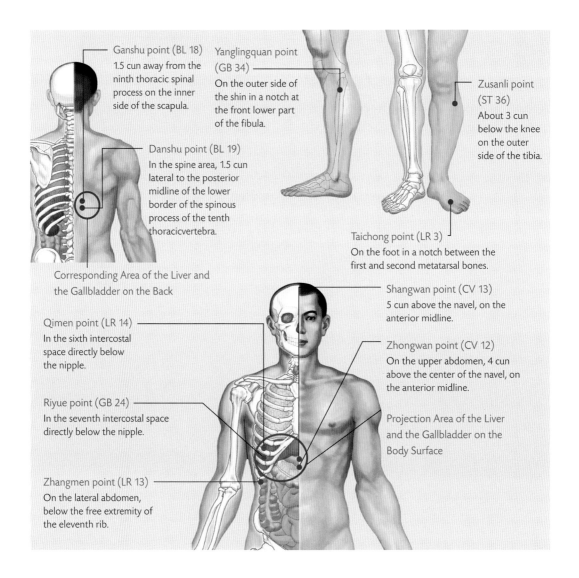

Ganshu point (BL 18)
1.5 cun away from the ninth thoracic spinal process on the inner side of the scapula.

Yanglingquan point (GB 34)
On the outer side of the shin in a notch at the front lower part of the fibula.

Zusanli point (ST 36)
About 3 cun below the knee on the outer side of the tibia.

Danshu point (BL 19)
In the spine area, 1.5 cun lateral to the posterior midline of the lower border of the spinous process of the tenth thoracicvertebra.

Taichong point (LR 3)
On the foot in a notch between the first and second metatarsal bones.

Corresponding Area of the Liver and the Gallbladder on the Back

Shangwan point (CV 13)
5 cun above the navel, on the anterior midline.

Qimen point (LR 14)
In the sixth intercostal space directly below the nipple.

Zhongwan point (CV 12)
On the upper abdomen, 4 cun above the center of the navel, on the anterior midline.

Riyue point (GB 24)
In the seventh intercostal space directly below the nipple.

Projection Area of the Liver and the Gallbladder on the Body Surface

Zhangmen point (LR 13)
On the lateral abdomen, below the free extremity of the eleventh rib.

Recommended Procedures

1. Projection Area of the Liver and the Gallbladder on the Body Surface, Qimen Point, Zhangmen Point and Riyue Point

Method: Use the flat-scraping to scrape the projection area on the right ribs, with stress on Qimen point, Zhangmen point and Riyue point on the right side.

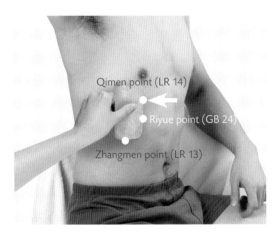

Qimen point (LR 14)
Riyue point (GB 24)
Zhangmen point (LR 13)

2. Shangwan Point and Zhongwan Point

Method: Use the surface-scraping to scrape from Shangwan point to Zhongwan point on the abdomen from up to down.

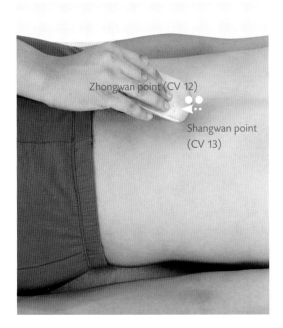

Zhongwan point (CV 12)
Shangwan point (CV 13)

3. Corresponding Area of the Liver and the Gallbladder on the Back, Ganshu Point and Danshu Point

Method: Use the flat-scraping to scrape the corresponding area from inside to outside. Use the surface-scraping to scrape Ganshu point and Danshu point on the back from up to down.

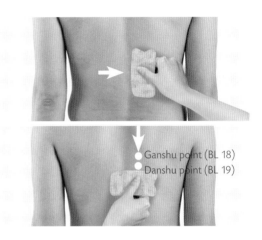

Ganshu point (BL 18)
Danshu point (BL 19)

4. Yanglingquan Point, Zusanli Point and Taichong Point

Method: Use the flat-pressing and kneading to press and knead Yanglingquan point on the right of the lower limb. Scrape Zusanli Point on both sides forcefully at a slow speed. Use the vertical-pressing and kneading to press and knead Taichong point on both sides.

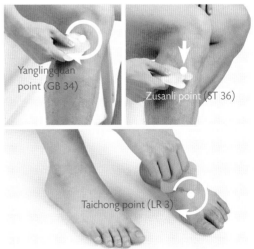

Yanglingquan point (GB 34)
Zusanli point (ST 36)
Taichong point (LR 3)

Chronic Gastritis

This is chronic inflammation of gastric mucosa or atrophic lesion caused by irritation of undesirable habits of diet, long-term gloomy thoughts and anger, smoking, alcoholic drinks or irritation from a certain kind of medicine. It is mostly featured by gastric distention after the meal, belching, decline of appetite, nausea and vomit, in a state of repeated attacks. In most cases, chronic gastritis resulting from helicobacter pylori does not show any symptom. The patient with gastritis of autoimmunity can be coupled with anaemia.

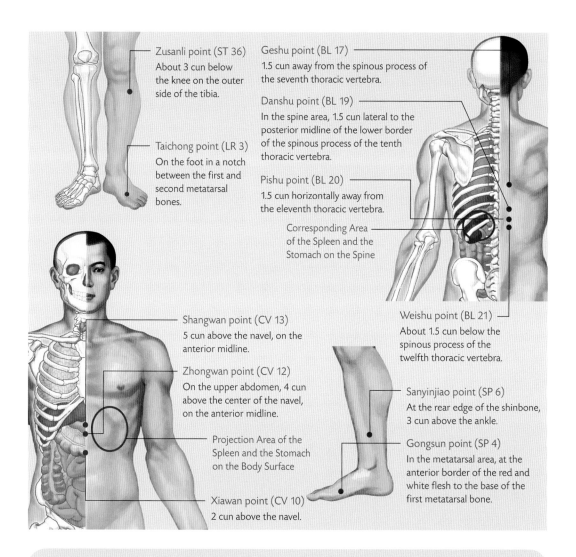

Zusanli point (ST 36)
About 3 cun below the knee on the outer side of the tibia.

Taichong point (LR 3)
On the foot in a notch between the first and second metatarsal bones.

Geshu point (BL 17)
1.5 cun away from the spinous process of the seventh thoracic vertebra.

Danshu point (BL 19)
In the spine area, 1.5 cun lateral to the posterior midline of the lower border of the spinous process of the tenth thoracic vertebra.

Pishu point (BL 20)
1.5 cun horizontally away from the eleventh thoracic vertebra.

Corresponding Area of the Spleen and the Stomach on the Spine

Shangwan point (CV 13)
5 cun above the navel, on the anterior midline.

Zhongwan point (CV 12)
On the upper abdomen, 4 cun above the center of the navel, on the anterior midline.

Projection Area of the Spleen and the Stomach on the Body Surface

Xiawan point (CV 10)
2 cun above the navel.

Weishu point (BL 21)
About 1.5 cun below the spinous process of the twelfth thoracic vertebra.

Sanyinjiao point (SP 6)
At the rear edge of the shinbone, 3 cun above the ankle.

Gongsun point (SP 4)
In the metatarsal area, at the anterior border of the red and white flesh to the base of the first metatarsal bone.

Therapy to Increase the Curative Effect
After getting up in early morning on an empty stomach, drink a glass of warm boiled water mixed with a small spoon of royal jelly and a big spoon of honey. Long-term intake will produce a certain effect of recuperation on gastric mucosa while serving to tonify spleen and reinforcing gastric motility.

Recommended Procedures

1. Projection Area of the Spleen and the Stomach on the Body Surface

Method: Use the flat-scraping to scrape the area.

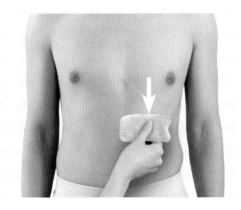

2. Corresponding Area of the Spleen and the Stomach on the Spine, Geshu Point, Danshu Point, Pishu Point and Weishu Point

Method: Use the surface-scraping to scrape the corresponding area from up to down. Use the dual-angle scraping to scrape Geshu point, Danshu point, Pishu point and Weishu point from up to down.

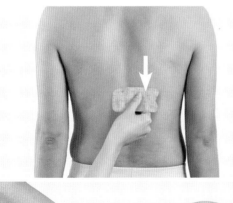

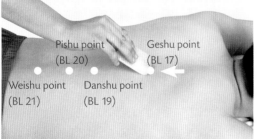

3. Shangwan Point, Zhongwan Point and Xiawan Point

Method: Use the surface-scraping to scrape Shangwan point, Zhongwan point and Xiawan point of Ren Meridian on the abdomen from up to down.

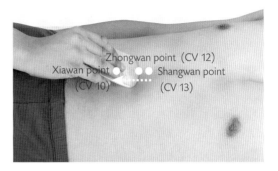

4. Zusanli Point, Sanyinjiao Point, Gongsun Point and Taichong Point

Method: Use the surface-scraping to scrape Zusanli point from up to down of Stomach Meridian, Sanyinjiao point and Gongsun point of Spleen Meridian. Use the vertical-pressing and kneading to press and knead Taichong point of Liver Meridian.

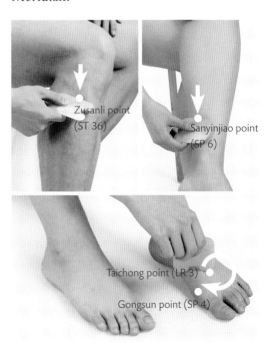

Chronic Enteritidis

It is mostly caused by the extension or repeated occurrence of acute enteritis, mainly marked by continual dull pain in the abdomen, abdominal distention, abdominal pain and diarrhea. It is aggravated after catching cold, eating oily food, emotional fluctuation, or fatigue. Over-tiredness, over-excitement, over-tension and undesirable nutrition can all be causes. Scraping therapy can enhance gastric and intestinal functions, easing the symptom.

The patient of chronic enteritis is weak in functions of digestion and absorption, food that can be easily digested or semi-liquid food with little residues is advised. The patient should eat less but more frequently to add nutrition and improve the symptom. If the patient dehydrates with low sodium, he/she may have more vegetable-leaf soups to supplement body fluid, salt and vitamin. The patient with too much gas and diarrhea should eat food with less sugar. Food which is apt to generate gas, such as potatoes, beans and milk, is not suggested.

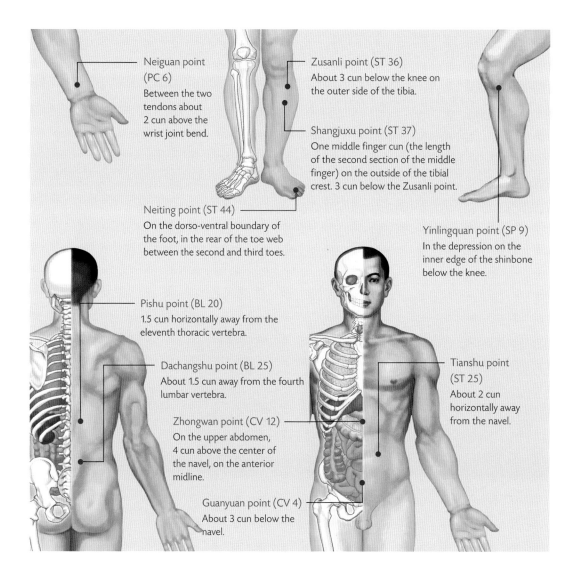

Neiguan point (PC 6)
Between the two tendons about 2 cun above the wrist joint bend.

Zusanli point (ST 36)
About 3 cun below the knee on the outer side of the tibia.

Shangjuxu point (ST 37)
One middle finger cun (the length of the second section of the middle finger) on the outside of the tibial crest. 3 cun below the Zusanli point.

Neiting point (ST 44)
On the dorso-ventral boundary of the foot, in the rear of the toe web between the second and third toes.

Yinlingquan point (SP 9)
In the depression on the inner edge of the shinbone below the knee.

Pishu point (BL 20)
1.5 cun horizontally away from the eleventh thoracic vertebra.

Dachangshu point (BL 25)
About 1.5 cun away from the fourth lumbar vertebra.

Tianshu point (ST 25)
About 2 cun horizontally away from the navel.

Zhongwan point (CV 12)
On the upper abdomen, 4 cun above the center of the navel, on the anterior midline.

Guanyuan point (CV 4)
About 3 cun below the navel.

Recommended Procedures

1. Zhongwan Point, Guanyuan Point and Tianshu Point

Method: Use the surface-scraping to scrape from Zhongwan point to Guanyuan point along the central line on the abdomen from up to down. Scraping should be done above and below the navel respectively. Then, use the angle-pressing and kneading to press and knead Zhongwan point, Guanyuan point and Tianshu point.

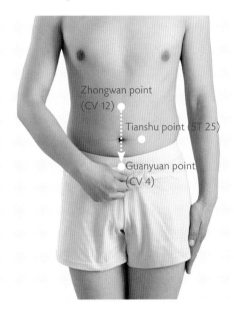

Zhongwan point (CV 12)
Tianshu point (ST 25)
Guanyuan point (CV 4)

2. Pishu Point and Dachangshu Point

Method: Use the surface-scraping to scrape from Pishu point to Dachangshu point on the back from up to down, until the skin turns red or *sha* appears.

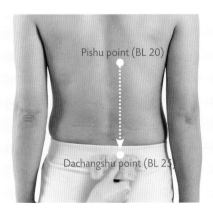

Pishu point (BL 20)
Dachangshu point (BL 25)

3. Yinlingquan Point, Zusanli Point, Shangjuxu Point and Neiting Point

Method: Use the surface-scraping to forcefully scrape Yinlingquan point on the inside of the lower limbs, Zusanli point on the outside of the lower limbs and Shangjuxu point respectively for 30 times. The appearance of *sha* is not necessary. Finally, use the corner of the scraping plate to scrape Neiting point in the sole, until *sha* appears.

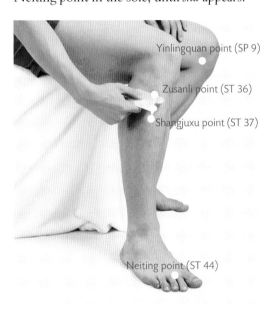

Yinlingquan point (SP 9)
Zusanli point (ST 36)
Shangjuxu point (ST 37)
Neiting point (ST 44)

4. Neiguan Point

Method: Use the surface-scraping to gently scrape Neiguan point on the inside of the upper limbs from up to down for 30 times, until *sha* appears.

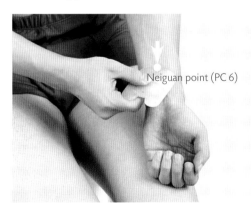

Neiguan point (PC 6)

Peptic Ulcer

It mainly refers to chronic ulcers taking place in the stomach and duodenum. There are quite many reasons for the formation of ulcers, which are chiefly caused by intrusion of acid gastric juice into the mucosa of the digestive tract. Scraping therapy can adjust the functions of gastric and intestinal digestion, restraining the secretion of gastric acid.

The patient of peptic ulcers had better not go to work or go to bed on an empty stomach. He/she should avoid or give up smoking, alcoholic drinks, spicy food, strong tea or coffee which are detrimental to the healing of ulcers.

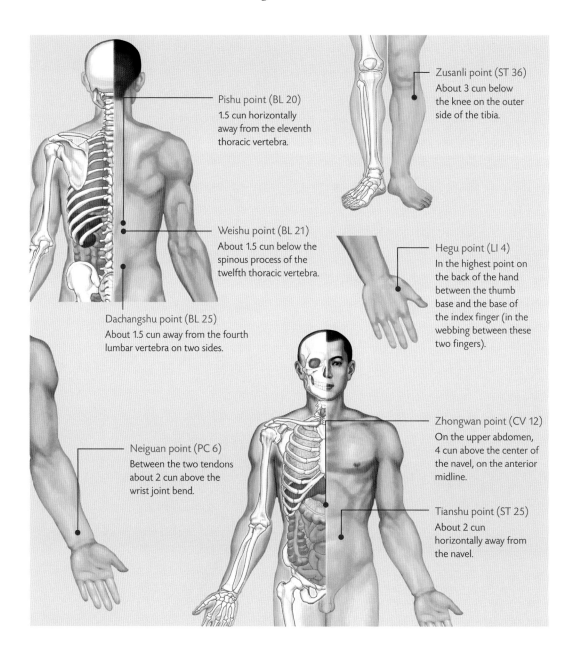

Pishu point (BL 20)
1.5 cun horizontally away from the eleventh thoracic vertebra.

Zusanli point (ST 36)
About 3 cun below the knee on the outer side of the tibia.

Weishu point (BL 21)
About 1.5 cun below the spinous process of the twelfth thoracic vertebra.

Hegu point (LI 4)
In the highest point on the back of the hand between the thumb base and the base of the index finger (in the webbing between these two fingers).

Dachangshu point (BL 25)
About 1.5 cun away from the fourth lumbar vertebra on two sides.

Neiguan point (PC 6)
Between the two tendons about 2 cun above the wrist joint bend.

Zhongwan point (CV 12)
On the upper abdomen, 4 cun above the center of the navel, on the anterior midline.

Tianshu point (ST 25)
About 2 cun horizontally away from the navel.

Recommended Procedures

1. Pishu Point, Weishu Point and Dachangshu Point

Method: Use the surface-scraping to sccrape from Pishu point to Dachangshu point on the back, until the skin is slightly red or *sha* appears.

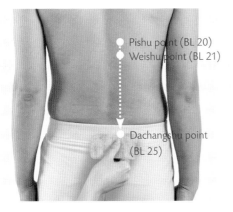

2. Neiguan Point and Hegu Point

Method: Use the angle-scraping to scrape Neiguan point on the inside of the forearm and Hegu point between the thumb and the index finger from up to down, until the skin is slightly red.

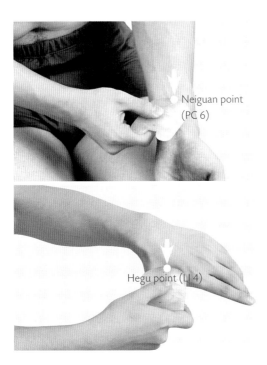

3. Zhongwan Point and Tianshu Point

Method: Use the surface-scraping to scrape Zhongwan point and Tianshu point on the abdomen from up to down respectively, until the skin is slightly red or *sha* appears.

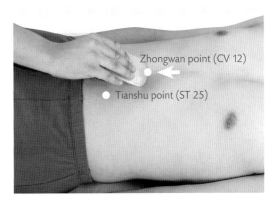

4. Zusanli Point

Method: Use the corner of the scraping plate to press and knead Zusanli point on the outside of the shin, until soreness and numbness are felt. Then, scrape it 15 times from up to down.

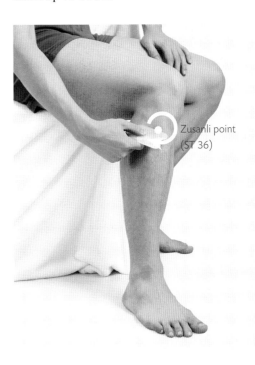

Urinary Incontinence

This refers to the loss of ability to discharge urine because of the damage to musculi sphincter vesicae or obstruction of nerve functions, resulting in the uncontrolled flow of urine, a disease that can take place among people of all ages. It is mainly marked by the outflow of urine when the abdominal pressure increases, such as cough, sneeze, climbing stairs or running.

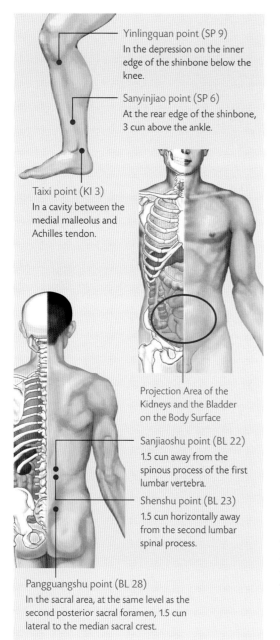

Yinlingquan point (SP 9)
In the depression on the inner edge of the shinbone below the knee.

Sanyinjiao point (SP 6)
At the rear edge of the shinbone, 3 cun above the ankle.

Taixi point (KI 3)
In a cavity between the medial malleolus and Achilles tendon.

Projection Area of the Kidneys and the Bladder on the Body Surface

Sanjiaoshu point (BL 22)
1.5 cun away from the spinous process of the first lumbar vertebra.

Shenshu point (BL 23)
1.5 cun horizontally away from the second lumbar spinal process.

Pangguangshu point (BL 28)
In the sacral area, at the same level as the second posterior sacral foramen, 1.5 cun lateral to the median sacral crest.

Recommended Procedures

1. Projection Area of the Kidneys and the Bladder on the Body Surface

Method: Use the surface-scraping to scrape the area until the skin turns red and feels heat.

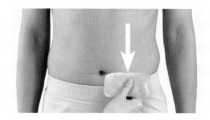

2. Sanjiaoshu Point, Shenshu Point and Pangguangshu Point

Method: Use the surface-scraping to scrape from Sanjiaoshu point, Shenshu point to Pangguangshu point.

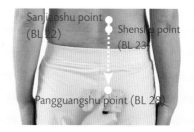

Sanjiaoshu point (BL 22)

Shenshu point (BL 23)

Pangguangshu point (BL 28)

3. Yinlingquan Point, Sanyinjiao Point and Taixi Point

Method: Use the surface-scraping to scrape from Yinlingquan point, Sanyinjiao point to Taixi point.

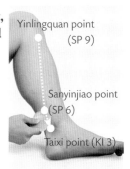

Yinlingquan point (SP 9)

Sanyinjiao point (SP 6)

Taixi point (KI 3)

Urine Retention

It is mainly marked by frequent discharge of urine, incomplete emptying and fullness and distention of the lower abdomen, etc. Long-time retention of urine will lead to urinary incontinence and urinary tract infection. Scraping therapy can reinforce the gasification function of the kidneys and the bladder while stimulating the bladder and the urinary system to promote the discharge of urine.

Recommended Procedures

1. Shenshu Point and Pangguangshu Point
Method: Use the surface-scraping to forcefully scrape from Shenshu point to Pangguangshu point on the back, until *sha* appears.

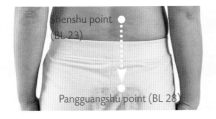

Shenshu point (BL 23)

Pangguangshu point (BL 28)

2. Guanyuan Point and Zhongji Point
Method: Use the surface-scraping to scrape from Guanyuan point to Zhongji point on the lower abdomen, until the skin turns red or *sha* appears.

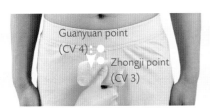

Guanyuan point (CV 4)

Zhongji point (CV 3)

3. Yinlingquan Point and Sanyinjiao Point
Method: Use the surface-scraping to scrape from Yinlingquan point to Sanyinjiao point on the inside of the lower limbs continuously, until the skin turns red or *sha* appears.

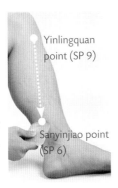

Yinlingquan point (SP 9)

Sanyinjiao point (SP 6)

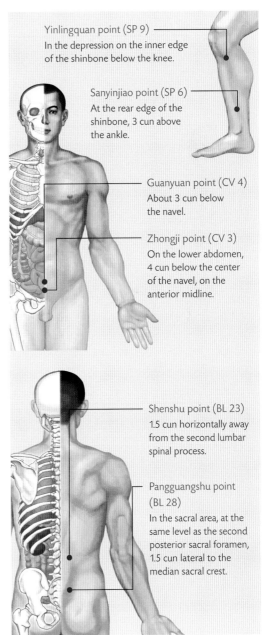

Yinlingquan point (SP 9)
In the depression on the inner edge of the shinbone below the knee.

Sanyinjiao point (SP 6)
At the rear edge of the shinbone, 3 cun above the ankle.

Guanyuan point (CV 4)
About 3 cun below the navel.

Zhongji point (CV 3)
On the lower abdomen, 4 cun below the center of the navel, on the anterior midline.

Shenshu point (BL 23)
1.5 cun horizontally away from the second lumbar spinal process.

Pangguangshu point (BL 28)
In the sacral area, at the same level as the second posterior sacral foramen, 1.5 cun lateral to the median sacral crest.

Chronic Nephritis

With a slow onset and long course, chronic nephritis has different manifestations. Some patients have no obvious symptoms, while some are marked by obvious hematuria, edema, high blood pressure, fatigue all over the body, abdominal distention and anaemia. According to Chinese medicine, it is mostly caused by the intrusion of exterior malignant elements, impairing spleen and stomach, reducing fluid in the body and upsetting gasification. In the course of treatment, applying scraping therapy at the same time can ease the symptom.

  The course of chronic nephritis lasts long so that scraping therapy should proceed with the course, mainly with the reinforcing method. The patient with insufficient kidney functions should try to avoid taking medicine which can impair kidney functions. In daily life, the patient should pay attention to controlling the amount of sodium salt in meals and eat low salt food.

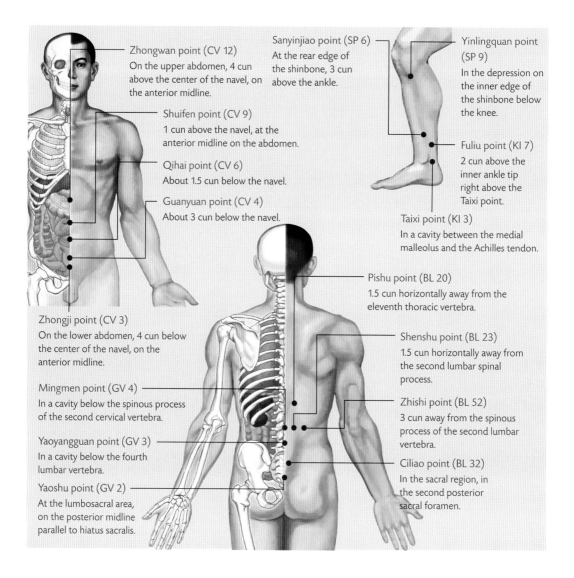

Zhongwan point (CV 12)
On the upper abdomen, 4 cun above the center of the navel, on the anterior midline.

Sanyinjiao point (SP 6)
At the rear edge of the shinbone, 3 cun above the ankle.

Yinlingquan point (SP 9)
In the depression on the inner edge of the shinbone below the knee.

Shuifen point (CV 9)
1 cun above the navel, at the anterior midline on the abdomen.

Qihai point (CV 6)
About 1.5 cun below the navel.

Guanyuan point (CV 4)
About 3 cun below the navel.

Fuliu point (KI 7)
2 cun above the inner ankle tip right above the Taixi point.

Taixi point (KI 3)
In a cavity between the medial malleolus and the Achilles tendon.

Zhongji point (CV 3)
On the lower abdomen, 4 cun below the center of the navel, on the anterior midline.

Pishu point (BL 20)
1.5 cun horizontally away from the eleventh thoracic vertebra.

Shenshu point (BL 23)
1.5 cun horizontally away from the second lumbar spinal process.

Mingmen point (GV 4)
In a cavity below the spinous process of the second cervical vertebra.

Yaoyangguan point (GV 3)
In a cavity below the fourth lumbar vertebra.

Zhishi point (BL 52)
3 cun away from the spinous process of the second lumbar vertebra.

Yaoshu point (GV 2)
At the lumbosacral area, on the posterior midline parallel to hiatus sacralis.

Ciliao point (BL 32)
In the sacral region, in the second posterior sacral foramen.

Recommended Procedures

1. Mingmen Point, Yaoyangguan Point and Yaoshu Point

Method: Use the surface-scraping to scrape from Mingmen point through Yaoyangguan point to Yaoshu point of Du Meridian on the back.

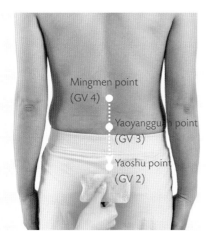

Mingmen point (GV 4)
Yaoyangguan point (GV 3)
Yaoshu point (GV 2)

2. Yinlingquan Point, Sanyinjiao Point, Fuliu Point and Taixi Point

Method: Use the surface-scraping to scrape from Yinlingquan point to Sanyinjiao point to Fuliu point and Taixi point along the inside of the shin.

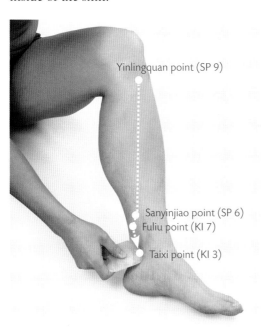

Yinlingquan point (SP 9)
Sanyinjiao point (SP 6)
Fuliu point (KI 7)
Taixi point (KI 3)

3. Pishu Point, Shenshu Point, Zhishi Point and Ciliao Point

Method: Use the surface-scraping to scrape from Pishu point of Bladder Meridian along both sides of the spine to Shenshu point, Zhishi point and Ciliao point.

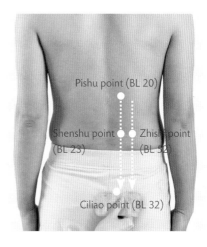

Pishu point (BL 20)
Shenshu point (BL 23)
Zhishi point (BL 52)
Ciliao point (BL 32)

4. Zhongwan Point, Shuifen Point, Qihai Point, Guanyuan Point and Zhongji Point

Method: Use the surface-scraping to scrape from Zhongwan point to Shuifen point, Qihai point, Guanyuan point and Zhongji point of Ren Meridian on the abdomen. The scraping is done above and below the navel separately.

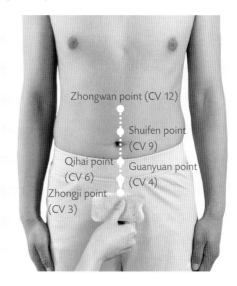

Zhongwan point (CV 12)
Shuifen point (CV 9)
Qihai point (CV 6)
Guanyuan point (CV 4)
Zhongji point (CV 3)

Urinary Calculus

It is divided into kidney stones, ureteral stones, bladder stones and urethral stones according to the place where stones are found. There is no symptom in terms of stones in the urethra. Stones in the ureter are marked by sharp pain in kidneys coupled with nausea and vomit. Hematuria takes place in a few patients and that upper urinary tract obstruction can be featured by anuresis. Long-term kidney stones can lead to insufficiency of kidney functions marked by a little urine and even no urine, decline of appetite, nausea and vomit. According to Chinese medicine, urinary calculus mainly results from accumulation of damp and heat in lower *jiao* (lower energizer) of the body as well as imbalance of the gasification in bladder. Scraping therapy can improve functions related to urination, easing the symptom.

Patients of urinary calculus should drink more water, with a daily amount of over 2000 ml and that the amount of urine should be the same as this amount. Appropriate physical exercise can benefit the expulsion of tiny stones. Strenuous exercise is forbidden. Those with urinary system infection should receive active medical treatment.

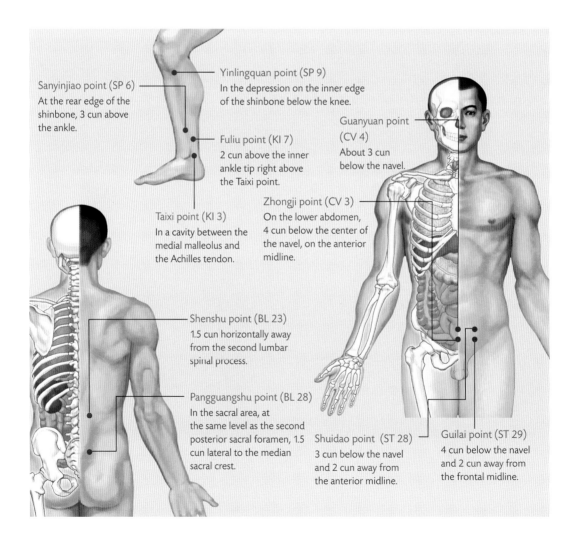

Sanyinjiao point (SP 6)
At the rear edge of the shinbone, 3 cun above the ankle.

Yinlingquan point (SP 9)
In the depression on the inner edge of the shinbone below the knee.

Fuliu point (KI 7)
2 cun above the inner ankle tip right above the Taixi point.

Guanyuan point (CV 4)
About 3 cun below the navel.

Taixi point (KI 3)
In a cavity between the medial malleolus and the Achilles tendon.

Zhongji point (CV 3)
On the lower abdomen, 4 cun below the center of the navel, on the anterior midline.

Shenshu point (BL 23)
1.5 cun horizontally away from the second lumbar spinal process.

Pangguangshu point (BL 28)
In the sacral area, at the same level as the second posterior sacral foramen, 1.5 cun lateral to the median sacral crest.

Shuidao point (ST 28)
3 cun below the navel and 2 cun away from the anterior midline.

Guilai point (ST 29)
4 cun below the navel and 2 cun away from the frontal midline.

Recommended Procedures

1. Shenshu Point and Pangguangshu Point

Method: Use the surface-scraping to scrape from Shenshu point to Pangguangshu point on both sides of the back.

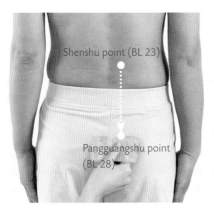

Shenshu point (BL 23)

Pangguangshu point (BL 28)

2. Yinlingquan Point, Sanyinjiao Point, Fuliu Point and Taixi Point

Method: Use the surface-scraping to scrape from Yinlingquan point to Sanyinjiao point, Fuliu point and Taixi point all the way along the inside of the shin.

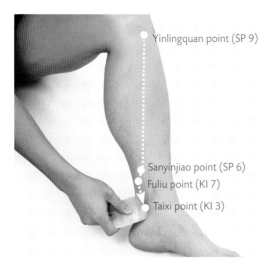

Yinlingquan point (SP 9)

Sanyinjiao point (SP 6)
Fuliu point (KI 7)
Taixi point (KI 3)

3. Guanyuan Point, Zhongji Point, Shuidao Point and Guilai Point

Method: Use the surface-scraping to scrape from Guanyuan point to Zhongji point of Ren Meridian on the abdomen, and from Shuidao point to Guilai point on both sides of Stomach Meridian.

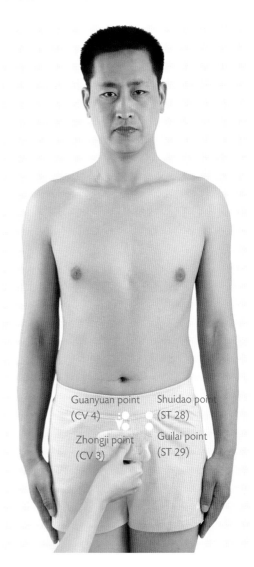

Guanyuan point (CV 4)   Shuidao point (ST 28)

Zhongji point (CV 3)   Guilai point (ST 29)

Therapies to Increase the Curative Effect

- Use palms to pat both sides of the kidney area and the lower abdomen several times a day.
- Use palms to rub and knead the kidney area on both sides until the area feels heat every morning and every evening.

Gout

This is caused by long-term disorder of purine metabolism, which leads to hyperuricemia and accumulation of lithic acid in joints, cartilage and kidneys, giving rise to inflammation.

In the early stage, the gout is marked by single-joint inflammation, mostly taking place in the first toe and the thumb, which can be red, swollen, hot and painful. Gradually, there will be joint-distention, deformation, stiffness and restriction over joint movement. Scraping therapy can stimulate main and collateral channels, smooth blood flow, promote the expulsion of lithic acid, so as to ease and eliminate the symptom.

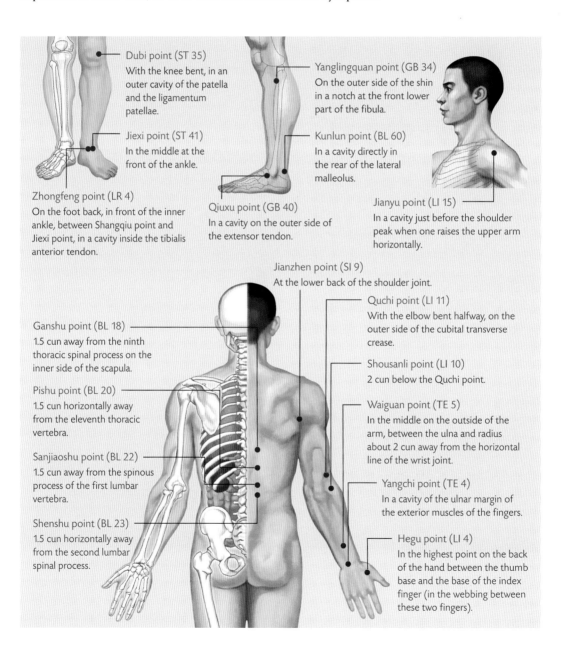

Dubi point (ST 35)
With the knee bent, in an outer cavity of the patella and the ligamentum patellae.

Jiexi point (ST 41)
In the middle at the front of the ankle.

Zhongfeng point (LR 4)
On the foot back, in front of the inner ankle, between Shangqiu point and Jiexi point, in a cavity inside the tibialis anterior tendon.

Yanglingquan point (GB 34)
On the outer side of the shin in a notch at the front lower part of the fibula.

Kunlun point (BL 60)
In a cavity directly in the rear of the lateral malleolus.

Qiuxu point (GB 40)
In a cavity on the outer side of the extensor tendon.

Jianyu point (LI 15)
In a cavity just before the shoulder peak when one raises the upper arm horizontally.

Jianzhen point (SI 9)
At the lower back of the shoulder joint.

Ganshu point (BL 18)
1.5 cun away from the ninth thoracic spinal process on the inner side of the scapula.

Pishu point (BL 20)
1.5 cun horizontally away from the eleventh thoracic vertebra.

Sanjiaoshu point (BL 22)
1.5 cun away from the spinous process of the first lumbar vertebra.

Shenshu point (BL 23)
1.5 cun horizontally away from the second lumbar spinal process.

Quchi point (LI 11)
With the elbow bent halfway, on the outer side of the cubital transverse crease.

Shousanli point (LI 10)
2 cun below the Quchi point.

Waiguan point (TE 5)
In the middle on the outside of the arm, between the ulna and radius about 2 cun away from the horizontal line of the wrist joint.

Yangchi point (TE 4)
In a cavity of the ulnar margin of the exterior muscles of the fingers.

Hegu point (LI 4)
In the highest point on the back of the hand between the thumb base and the base of the index finger (in the webbing between these two fingers).

Recommended Procedures

1. Ganshu Point, Pishu Point, Sanjiaoshu Point and Shenshu Point

Method: Use the surface-scraping to scrape from Ganshu point, to Pishu point, Sanjiaoshu point and Shenshu point on the back.

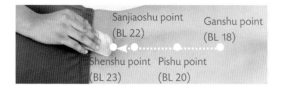

2. Jianyu Point, Jianzhen Point, Quchi Point, Shousanli Point, Waiguan Point, Yangchi Point and Hegu Point

Method: Use the angle-kneading to press, knead and scrape Jianyu point and Jianzhen point on the shoulder. Use the flat-scraping to scrape from Quchi point, to Shousanli point, Waiguan point and Yangchi point. Use the angle-kneading to press, knead and scrape Hegu point.

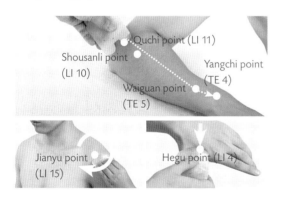

3. Yanglingquan Point, Dubi Point, Zhongfeng Point, Jiexi Point, Kunlun Point and Qiuxu Point

Method: Use the angle-kneading to press, knead and scrape Dubi point on lower limbs. Use the surface-scraping to scrape Yanglingquan point from up to down. Use the angle-kneading to press, knead and scrape Zhongfeng point, Jiexi point, Kunlun point and Qiuxu point on feet.

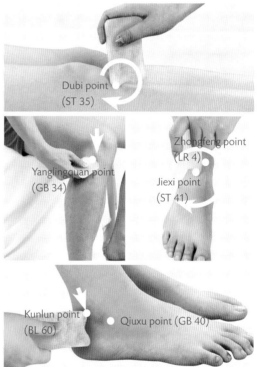

Expert Prompts

It is very important for the patient of the gout to control diet.

• Drink more water and eat more alkaline food, such as vegetables and fruits.

• It is a taboo to eat food rich in purines, such as inner organs of animals and beans, in addition to controlling the intake of energy, restricting the intake of fat and controlling weight.

• Reasonable cooking: The content of purines can be reduced if meat is boiled first and then cooked again after the soup is given up.

• When the gout is in acute period (manifested by red, swollen and heat pain in joints), it is advisable for the patient to eat food that can reduce internal heat, cool down the blood, eliminate swollen and stop pain. It is a taboo to eat irritating spicy food or those foods hot in nature. Smoking and alcoholic drinks are forbidden.

Anaemia

This refers to the fact that the total amount of red cells in the blood all over the body is less than the normal value. The patient of anaemia is generally marked by fatigue, sleepiness, weakness, and palpitation and short breath after activities. Some patients may suffer from heart failure. The anaemic patient can also be featured by dry skin, headache, dizziness, tinnitus, distraction, drowsiness, decline of appetite, abdominal distention, and nausea. According to Chinese medicine, anaemia is mainly caused by deficiency of spleen and kidneys. Scraping therapy plays an active role in smoothing the circulation of the vital energy and blood and regulating the functions of spleen and kidneys.

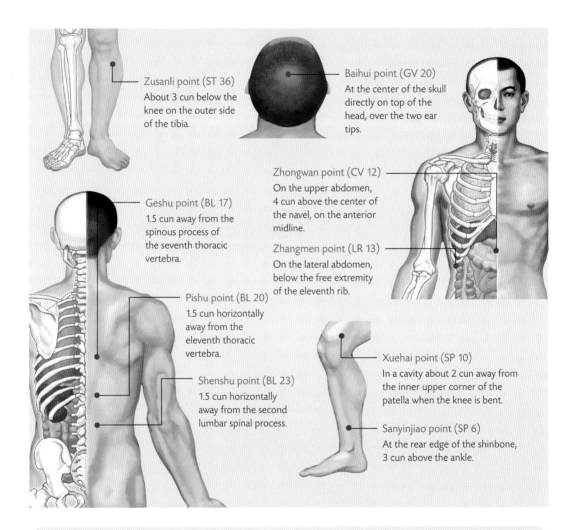

Zusanli point (ST 36)
About 3 cun below the knee on the outer side of the tibia.

Baihui point (GV 20)
At the center of the skull directly on top of the head, over the two ear tips.

Geshu point (BL 17)
1.5 cun away from the spinous process of the seventh thoracic vertebra.

Zhongwan point (CV 12)
On the upper abdomen, 4 cun above the center of the navel, on the anterior midline.

Zhangmen point (LR 13)
On the lateral abdomen, below the free extremity of the eleventh rib.

Pishu point (BL 20)
1.5 cun horizontally away from the eleventh thoracic vertebra.

Shenshu point (BL 23)
1.5 cun horizontally away from the second lumbar spinal process.

Xuehai point (SP 10)
In a cavity about 2 cun away from the inner upper corner of the patella when the knee is bent.

Sanyinjiao point (SP 6)
At the rear edge of the shinbone, 3 cun above the ankle.

Therapy to Increase the Curative Effect
Porridge with longans and red dates: 15-gram longans, five dates and 100-gram millet are boiled into porridge. Eat while it is still hot, twice to three times a week.

Recommended Procedures

1. Baihui Point

Method: Use the falt-pressing and kneading to press and knead Baihui point on the top of the head, until soreness, distention and warmth are felt.

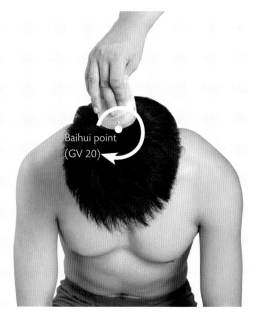

2. Zhongwan Point and Zhangmen Point

Method: Use the surface-scraping to scrape Zhongwan point on Ren Meridian on the abdomen from up to down, and Zhangmen point of Liver Meridian on both sides.

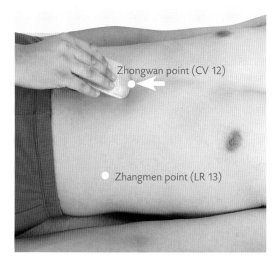

3. Geshu Point, Pishu Point and Shenshu Point

Method: Use the surface-scraping to scrape Geshu point, Pishu point and Shenshu point on both sides of the back.

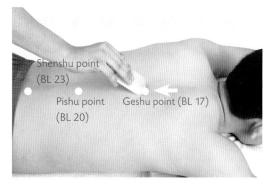

4. Xuehai Point, Sanyinjiao Point and Zusanli Point

Method: Use the flat-pressing and kneading to forcefully press and knead Xuehai point of Spleen Meridian on lower limbs, scrape Sanyinjiao point on the inside of the shin and Zusanli point of Stomach Meridian on the outside of the shin from up to down.

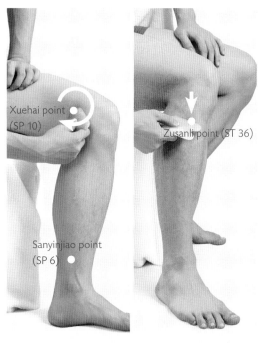

Hemorrhoids

They are vein mass caused by the varicose expansion of lower-end mucosa of the rectum and subcutaneous venous plexus of anal tubes because of the backflow obstruction. This disease is associated with sitting or standing at work for a long time, or shouldering heavy things, or long treks, or dysentery and diarrhea for a long time, constipation, or addiction to eating spicy and oily food.

Hemorrhoid is usually divided into internal, external and mixed ones. External hemorrhoid is marked by obvious symptoms, such as a little inflammatory secretion at the anus, distention and pain of anus. Internal hemorrhoid is not obvious in the early stage, but with bright blood which is not mixed with excrement.

Hemorrhoid is very apt to reoccur. Therefore, the patient should also pay attention to avoiding pathogenic factors in daily life even when medical treatment is rendered. The patient should drink more water, eat more food rich in dietary fibers, have regular bowel movement, cure constipation in time and avoid sitting or standing for a long time. The patient can often lift legs or contract anus to avoid the occurrence of hemorrhoid.

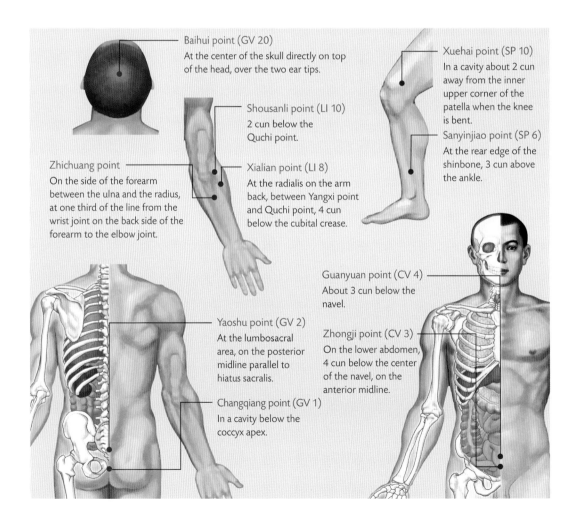

Baihui point (GV 20)
At the center of the skull directly on top of the head, over the two ear tips.

Xuehai point (SP 10)
In a cavity about 2 cun away from the inner upper corner of the patella when the knee is bent.

Shousanli point (LI 10)
2 cun below the Quchi point.

Sanyinjiao point (SP 6)
At the rear edge of the shinbone, 3 cun above the ankle.

Zhichuang point
On the side of the forearm between the ulna and the radius, at one third of the line from the wrist joint on the back side of the forearm to the elbow joint.

Xialian point (LI 8)
At the radialis on the arm back, between Yangxi point and Quchi point, 4 cun below the cubital crease.

Guanyuan point (CV 4)
About 3 cun below the navel.

Yaoshu point (GV 2)
At the lumbosacral area, on the posterior midline parallel to hiatus sacralis.

Zhongji point (CV 3)
On the lower abdomen, 4 cun below the center of the navel, on the anterior midline.

Changqiang point (GV 1)
In a cavity below the coccyx apex.

Recommended Procedures

1. Baihui Point

Method: Use the surface-scraping to scrape Baihui point on the top of the head, until soreness, distention and warmth are felt.

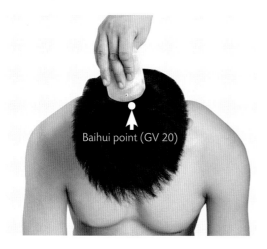

Baihui point (GV 20)

2. Guanyuan Point and Zhongji Point

Method: Use the surface-scraping to scrape from Guanyuan point to Zhongji point on the abdomen from up to down.

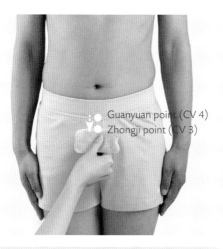

Guanyuan point (CV 4)
Zhongji point (CV 3)

Therapy to Increase the Curative Effect
5-gram immersed black fungus, and 30-gram dried persimmon slices are boiled for oral use once or twice a day. This prescription benefits the vital energy and nourishes yin, expels stasis and stops bleeding, suitable for stopping the bleeding of hemorrhoid.

3. Yaoshu Point and Changqiang Point

Method: Use the surface-scraping to scrape from Yaoshu point to Changqiang point of Bladder Meridian on the back.

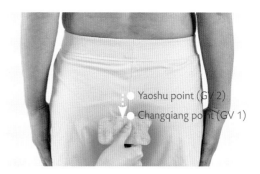

Yaoshu point (GV 2)
Changqiang point (GV 1)

4. Shousanli Point, Xialian Point, Zhichuang Point, Xuehai Point and Sanyinjiao Point

Method: Use the surface-scraping to scrape Shousanli point, Xialian point and Zhichuang point on upper limbs. Use the surface-scraping or flat-pressing and kneading to press and knead Xuehai point and Sanyinjiao point on lower limbs.

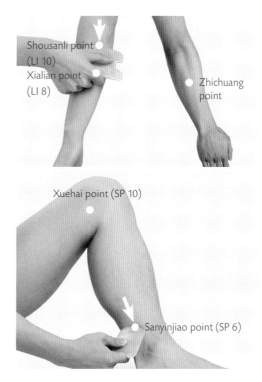

Shousanli point (LI 10)
Xialian point (LI 8)
Zhichuang point
Xuehai point (SP 10)
Sanyinjiao point (SP 6)

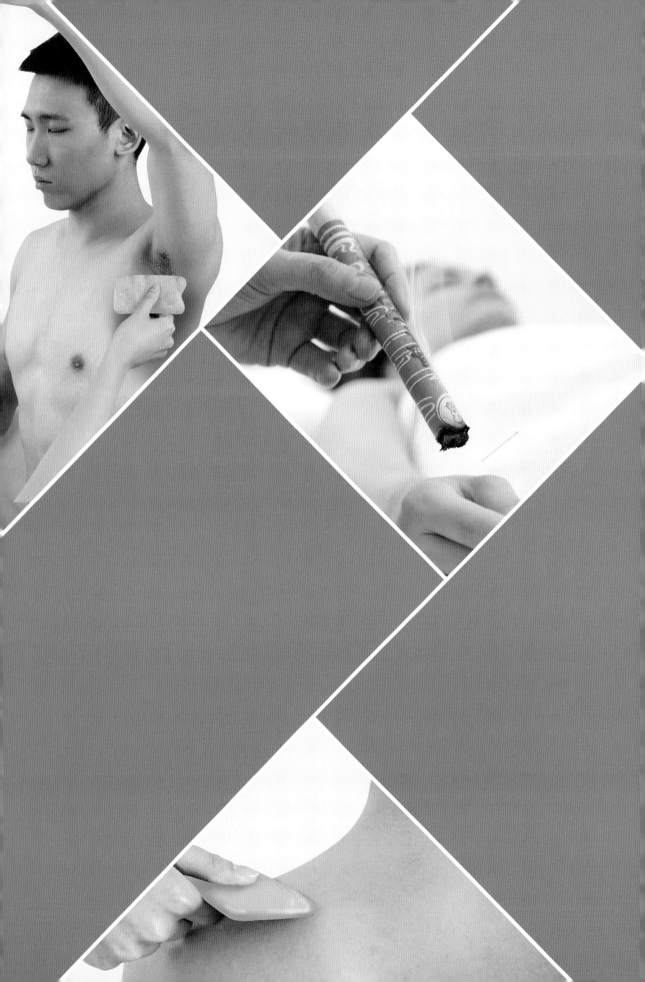

CHAPTER FIVE
Use *Gua Sha* to Expel Wind-Damp and Cold Toxin to Get Rid of Joint Problems

Wind, damp and the cold are all malignant elements in the Mother Nature. Various problems will occur if they intrude the human body, particularly the joints, inducing joint pain. Through smoothing vital energy and blood in main collateral channels, scraping therapy can expel the pathogenic wind, damp, and cold from the human body, thus eliminating joint pain.

Cervical Spondylosis

This refers to a series of pathological changes gradually taking place in cervical vertebra due to certain trauma and damage. It is generally marked by pain or numbness with pain in the neck, shoulders and arms, the upper part of shoulders, the upper chest and upper limbs, restricting neck movement. The pain often becomes worse because of fatigue or the cold. The area of pain is closely associated with the passage of channels. Scraping therapy produces an obvious effect on easing and reducing the symptom.

Apart from receiving scraping therapy, the person concerned should move the neck more and do neck exercise if working at the desk for a long time, which is conducive to easing the symptom or preventing the recurrence of pain. The patient with cervical spondylosis should pay attention to keeping the neck warm in daily life and setting the pillow at a height no more than 10 centimeters.

There are five kinds of cervical spondylosis, i.e., cervical spondylotic radiculopathy, cervical spondylotic myelopathy, sympathetic cervical spondylosis, vertebral artery type of cervical spondylosis and mixed type of cervical spondylosis. Among them, cervical spondylotic radiculopathy (it is mainly marked by weakness and heaviness in lower limbs and difficulty in walk) should not be directly scraped, but acupoints of other related areas can be scraped.

Recommended Procedures
1. Reflection Areas of the Cervical Vertebra and the Neck-Shoulder on the Hand Back
Method: Use the vertical-pressing and kneading to press and knead the areas and look for the points of pain to be pressed and kneaded emphatically.

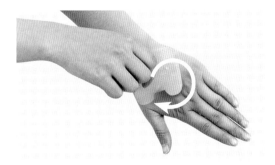

2. Reflection Area of the Cervical Vertebra on the Medial Foot

Method: Apply the scraping oil to the arch of the foot and use the surface-scraping to scrape the reflection area on the rear of the medial foot on the inside of the big toe. Scrape the points with nodules and pain emphatically and slowly.

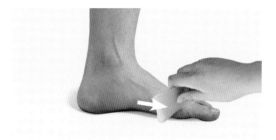

3. Fengfu Point, Shenzhu Point, Tianzhu Point, Dazhu Point, Fengchi Point and Jianjing Point

Method: Use the surface-scraping to scrape from Fengfu point to Shenzhu point of Du Meridian in the rear of the neck in separate sections from up to down. Use two corners of the scraping plate to scrape from Tianzhu point to Dazhu point of Bladder Meridian on both sides of the neck in separate sections from up to down. Use the single-angle scraping to scrape Fengchi point. Use the surface-scraping to scrape from Fengchi point to Jianjing point on both sides in separate sections, with stress on Jianjing point. Scrape the areas with pain, nodules, muscle tension or stiffness emphatically.

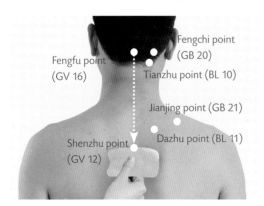

4. Waiguan Point, Zhongzhu Point, Yanglingquan Point and Xuanzhong Point

Method: Use the surface-scraping to scrape Waiguan point on upper limbs from up to down. Use the vertical-pressing and kneading to press and knead Zhongzhu point on the hand back. Use the surface-scraping to scrape from Yanglingquan point to Xuanzhong point from up to down.

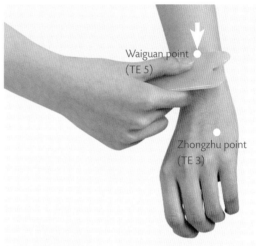

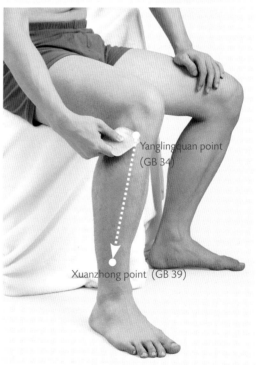

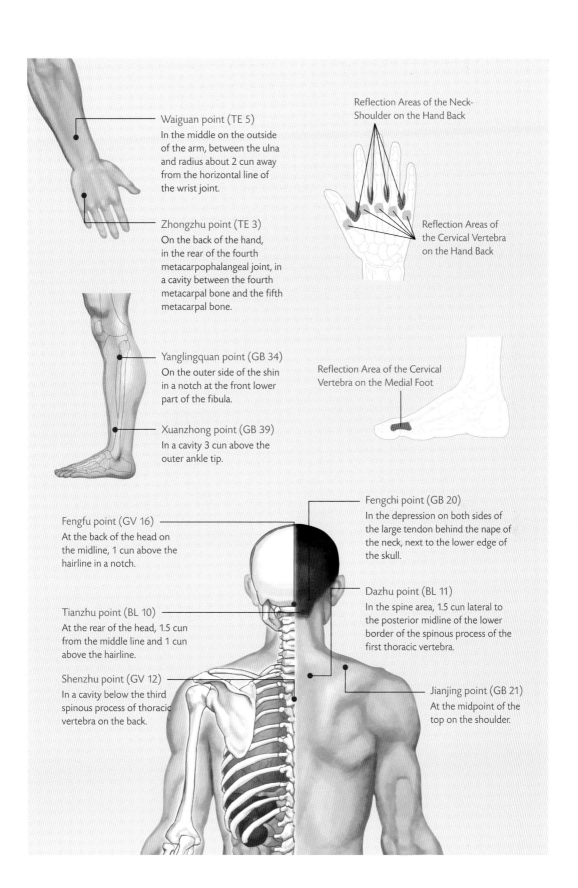

Waiguan point (TE 5)
In the middle on the outside of the arm, between the ulna and radius about 2 cun away from the horizontal line of the wrist joint.

Zhongzhu point (TE 3)
On the back of the hand, in the rear of the fourth metacarpophalangeal joint, in a cavity between the fourth metacarpal bone and the fifth metacarpal bone.

Reflection Areas of the Neck-Shoulder on the Hand Back

Reflection Areas of the Cervical Vertebra on the Hand Back

Yanglingquan point (GB 34)
On the outer side of the shin in a notch at the front lower part of the fibula.

Reflection Area of the Cervical Vertebra on the Medial Foot

Xuanzhong point (GB 39)
In a cavity 3 cun above the outer ankle tip.

Fengfu point (GV 16)
At the back of the head on the midline, 1 cun above the hairline in a notch.

Fengchi point (GB 20)
In the depression on both sides of the large tendon behind the nape of the neck, next to the lower edge of the skull.

Dazhu point (BL 11)
In the spine area, 1.5 cun lateral to the posterior midline of the lower border of the spinous process of the first thoracic vertebra.

Tianzhu point (BL 10)
At the rear of the head, 1.5 cun from the middle line and 1 cun above the hairline.

Shenzhu point (GV 12)
In a cavity below the third spinous process of thoracic vertebra on the back.

Jianjing point (GB 21)
At the midpoint of the top on the shoulder.

Scapulohumeral Periarthritis

This refers to a chronic and retrogressive pathological change in joint capsules and surrounding soft tissues, mainly marked by pain around shoulders and functional obstruction of physical movement. It is mostly caused by chronic strains, trauma of tendons, intrusion of the cold-damp, leading to the blockage of vital energy and blood circulation and the passage of main and collateral channels. The pain of shoulder joints is worse at night, in cloudy and damp weather or after labor work. Scraping therapy can smooth the vital energy, blood and meridians around the shoulders, easing pain.

Reinforcing the movement of shoulder joints can release the adhesion of these joints, avoid the contraction of muscles and promote the restoration of normal joint functions. The patient of shoulder periarthritis should pay attention to protecting shoulders in daily life and covering shoulders in sleep. The patient of stubborn shoulder periarthritis failing to be cured for a long time should be mindful of illness in endocrine system, such as diabetes, requiring further diagnosis. Scraping should be done gently when it comes to shoulder periarthritis caused by trauma.

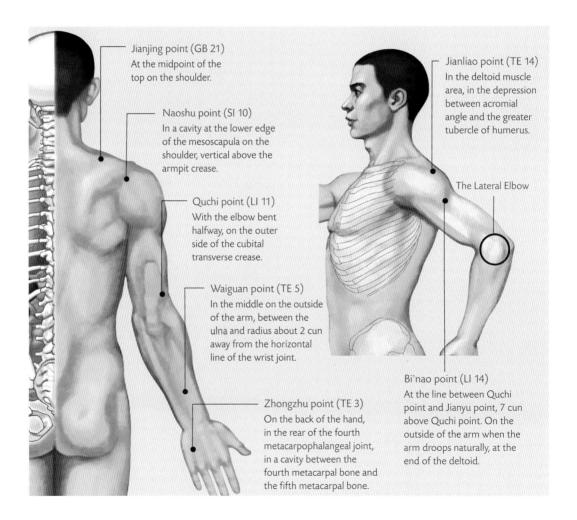

Jianjing point (GB 21)
At the midpoint of the top on the shoulder.

Naoshu point (SI 10)
In a cavity at the lower edge of the mesoscapula on the shoulder, vertical above the armpit crease.

Quchi point (LI 11)
With the elbow bent halfway, on the outer side of the cubital transverse crease.

Waiguan point (TE 5)
In the middle on the outside of the arm, between the ulna and radius about 2 cun away from the horizontal line of the wrist joint.

Zhongzhu point (TE 3)
On the back of the hand, in the rear of the fourth metacarpophalangeal joint, in a cavity between the fourth metacarpal bone and the fifth metacarpal bone.

Jianliao point (TE 14)
In the deltoid muscle area, in the depression between acromial angle and the greater tubercle of humerus.

The Lateral Elbow

Bi'nao point (LI 14)
At the line between Quchi point and Jianyu point, 7 cun above Quchi point. On the outside of the arm when the arm droops naturally, at the end of the deltoid.

Recommended Procedures

1. Quchi Point, Waiguan Point and Zhongzhu Point

Method: Use the single-angle scraping to scrape Quchi point and Waiguan point from up to down. Use the vertical-pressing and kneading to press and knead Zhongzhu point.

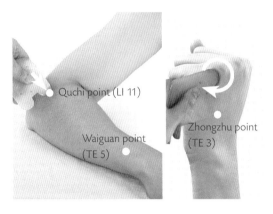

Quchi point (LI 11)

Waiguan point (TE 5)

Zhongzhu point (TE 3)

2. Jianjing Point and Naoshu Point

Method: Use the surface-scraping to scrape from Jianjing point to Naoshu point from inside to outside, with stress on areas with pain or nodules.

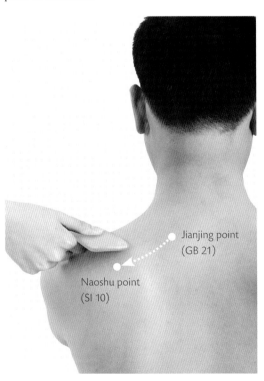

Jianjing point (GB 21)

Naoshu point (SI 10)

3. Jianliao Point and Bi'nao Point

Method: Use the surface-scraping to scrape from Jianliao point on the acromion to Bi'nao point at the root of the deltoid, with stress on areas with pain or nodules. Use the surface-scraping to scrape the lower part of the armpit, with stress on areas with pain or nodules.

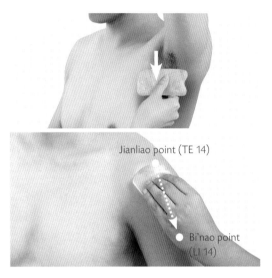

Jianliao point (TE 14)

Bi'nao point (LI 14)

4. Anterior Axillary Line, Posterior Axillary Line and the Lateral Elbow

Method: Use the single-angle scraping to scrape the anterior axillary line, the posterior axillary line and the lateral elbow, with stress on areas with pain or nodules.

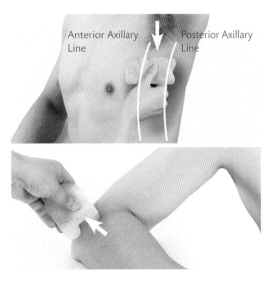

Anterior Axillary Line

Posterior Axillary Line

Rheumatic Arthritis

It is mainly marked by the pain of muscles and joints due to the intrusion of the pathogenic wind, cold and damp. The typical symptom is featured by mild or moderate fever, with mobile inflammation. It can occur repeatedly and becomes worse when the patient catches cold.

Scraping therapy can relax the muscles, stimulate the blood circulation, smooth main and collateral channels, while easing the pain. The recommended procedures of scraping are associated with shoulders, elbows, wrists, knees and ankles, which can be used as the case may be.

The patient of rheumatic arthritis should pay attention to avoiding catching cold, being caught in the rain or suffering from dampness, particularly keeping joints warm, avoiding wearing wet clothes, shoes and socks. During the active period of rheumatism, the patient should lie in bed for rest, avoid physical labor, and eat food rich in vitamin and low in fat and food that can be easily digested. The patient, after the activity of rheumatism is brought under control, should continue to lie in bed for 3 to 4 weeks and then begin to do physical exercise for rehabilitation, i.e., walking and jogging under the guidance of the doctor.

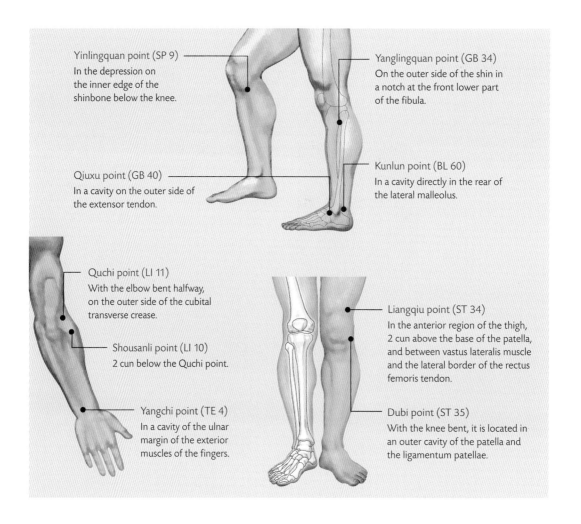

Yinlingquan point (SP 9)
In the depression on the inner edge of the shinbone below the knee.

Yanglingquan point (GB 34)
On the outer side of the shin in a notch at the front lower part of the fibula.

Qiuxu point (GB 40)
In a cavity on the outer side of the extensor tendon.

Kunlun point (BL 60)
In a cavity directly in the rear of the lateral malleolus.

Quchi point (LI 11)
With the elbow bent halfway, on the outer side of the cubital transverse crease.

Liangqiu point (ST 34)
In the anterior region of the thigh, 2 cun above the base of the patella, and between vastus lateralis muscle and the lateral border of the rectus femoris tendon.

Shousanli point (LI 10)
2 cun below the Quchi point.

Yangchi point (TE 4)
In a cavity of the ulnar margin of the exterior muscles of the fingers.

Dubi point (ST 35)
With the knee bent, it is located in an outer cavity of the patella and the ligamentum patellae.

Recommended Procedures

1. Scapular Area

Method: Use the surface-scraping to scrape scapular area from inside to outside, until *sha* appears. It is applicable to arthritis of scapular region.

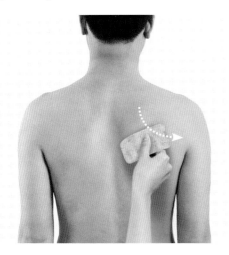

2. Quchi Point, Shousanli Point and Yangchi Point

Method: Use the single-angle scraping to scrape from Quchi point to Shousanli point on the elbow of upper limbs, until *sha* appears. Use the angle-scraping to scrape Yangchi point on the wrist from up to down, until *sha* appears. It is applicable to olenitis.

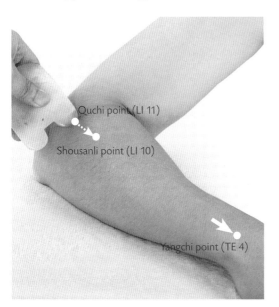

3. Liangqiu Point, Dubi Point, Yanglingquan Point and Yinlingquan Point

Method: Use the single-angle scraping to scrape from Liangqiu point to Dubi point on lower limbs, until *sha* appears. Use the surface-scraping to scrape Yanglingquan point and Yinlingquan point, until *sha* appears. It is applicable to gonitis.

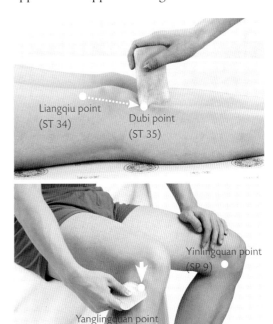

4. Kunlun Point and Qiuxu Point

Method: Use the single-angle scraping to scrape Kunlun point and Qiuxu point on the ankle from up to down, until *sha* appears. It is applicable to ankle arthritis.

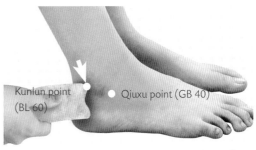

Other Methods of Expelling the Cold-Damp

• Moxibustion (fig. 54)

Moxibustion is also conducive to expelling the cold-damp as well as easing joint pain. The circulation of vital energy and blood will be condensed when they are caught in the cold and dispersed when they receive warmth. Through warm and hot stimulation of main and collateral channels and acupoints, moxibustion serves to warm up main and collateral channels as well as disperse the cold and stasis to reinforce the circulation of vital energy and blood in the human body, which is particularly effective to symptoms of the cold-damp. Moxibustion can deal with various joint pains caused by blood stasis due to the intrusion of the cold and obstruction of main and collateral channels. It will be more effective if sliced ginger or sliced garlic is applied to the area of pain or the related acupoints together with moxibustion.

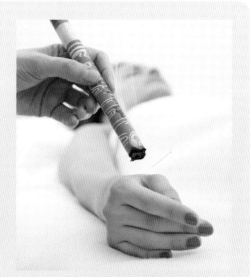

Fig. 54 Moxibustion can expel the cold and dampness.

• Cupping (fig. 55)

Cupping can dredge main and collateral channels as well as the circulation of vital energy and blood, serving to reduce distention, stop pain, adjust the balance between yin and yang, expel wind, toxin, cold and damp, which is very suitable for those suffering from joint pain due to the cold-damp. The area to be cupped is generally chosen at the place of joint pain. Cupping is generally done twice to three times a week, and once a week in winter since cupping of higher frequency will impair yang energy. Fire cupping is better than suction cupping. Cupping is not advisable if the patient is weak in yang energy or with weak physique.

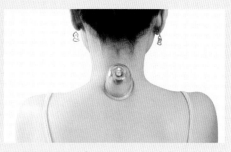

Fig. 55 Cupping therapy can expel the cold and dampness.

• Appropriate Exercise (fig. 56)

Expelling sweat through doing physical exercise is a very good way to get rid of cold-damp, as it can invigorate inner organs of the human body and speed up the expulsion of dampness. In particular, do not turn on the air-conditioner and the fan so as to discharge sweat. Otherwise, too much dampness plus the intrusion of the cold is very apt to result in the pain in muscles and joints. Such physical exercises "with quick breath and sweat" of an appropriate extent as jogging, quick walk, swimming, yoga and *taijiquan* (a kind of Chinese traditional shadow boxing) are the best for expelling the cold-damp in the body.

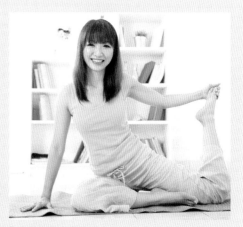

Fig. 56 Appropriate exercise with sweat can expel the cold and dampness.

Elbow Joint Pain

It is mostly caused by partial stasis of vital energy and blood, the obstruction of channels and malnutrition of tendons and bones due to trauma and strains of elbows or the intrusion of wind, the cold and the damp. Treatment should not only target at easing the pain, but also at restoring the functions of elbow joints. Scraping therapy can expel the wind and damp, promote the flow of the vital energy and blood as well as main and collateral channels, playing an active role in easing the pain and restoring joint functions.

Apart from trauma, elbow joint pain is largely due to external humeral epicondylitis which is commonly called "tennis elbow." This illness tends to develop slowly, being apt to be overlooked and that it will be troublesome to treat it if it lasts for a long time. Therefore, anyone with an obvious feeling of it should go to the hospital for timely examination.

Recommended Procedures

1. Zhouliao Point
Method: Use the surface-scraping to scrape Zhouliao point from up to down, until *sha* appears.

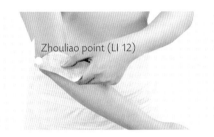

Zhouliao point (LI 12)

2. Shaohai Point
Method: Use the surface-scraping to scrape Shaohai point from up to down, until *sha* appears.

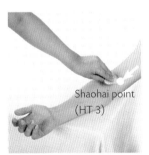

Shaohai point (HT 3)

3. Shousanli Point
Method: Use the surface-scraping to scrape Shousanli point from up to down, until *sha* appears.

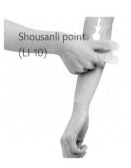

Shousanli point (LI 10)

Zhouliao point (LI 12)
On the outside of the arm, with the elbow bent, 1 cun above the Quchi point at the edge of the humerus.

Shaohai point (HT 3)
At the anterior cubital region, parallel with the cubital crease, at the front edge of the medial epicondyle of the humerus.

Shousanli point (LI 10)
2 cun below the Quchi point.

Therapy to Increase the Curative Effect
Before going to bed every night, pour some superior mature vinegar on a dry towel to wrap the elbow joint and wrap a layer of plastic wrap or a piece of plastic cloth to fix it. Keeping doing it for several days will ease the pain to a certain extent.

Wrist Pain

This is mostly caused by over-tiredness at work and tendon injury due to accumulated fatigue or intrusion of the cold, resulting in the stasis of vital energy and blood and failure to nurture tendons. People in modern times often use the mouse and keep the wrist in one posture for a long time, also constituting an important factor for the wrist pain. Scraping therapy can expel the cold, the damp, smooth main and collateral channels, regulate vital energy and blood, improve partial circulation, repair damaged tissues, so as to ease and cure wrist pain.

Recommended Procedures

1. Waiguan Point

Method: Use the surface-scraping to scrape Waiguan point from up to down, until the skin turns red. The appearance of *sha* is not necessary.

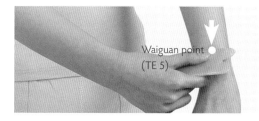

2. Yangchi Point and Yanggu Point

Method: Use the angle-scraping to scrape Yangchi point and Yanggu point from up to down, until *sha* appears. Or use the single-angle pressing and kneading to press and knead these two points, until soreness and distention are felt.

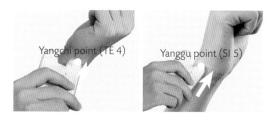

3. Wangu Point

Method: Use the single-angle pressing and kneading to press and knead Wangu point, until soreness and distention are felt.

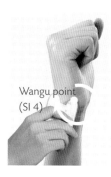

Wangu point (SI 4)

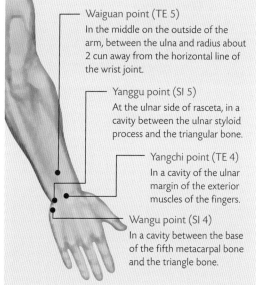

Waiguan point (TE 5)
In the middle on the outside of the arm, between the ulna and radius about 2 cun away from the horizontal line of the wrist joint.

Yanggu point (SI 5)
At the ulnar side of rasceta, in a cavity between the ulnar styloid process and the triangular bone.

Yangchi point (TE 4)
In a cavity of the ulnar margin of the exterior muscles of the fingers.

Wangu point (SI 4)
In a cavity between the base of the fifth metacarpal bone and the triangle bone.

Therapy to Increase the Curative Effect
Moxibustion can be an auxiliary means of treatment if the patient feels cold and painful in the wrist, i.e., light the moxa stick and direct it at Wangu point, Yanggu point and Yangchi point for 10 minutes respectively. Then, the patient will feel warm in the wrist along with the reduction of pain. Do it once every day and the pain will be obviously eased in a week.

Ankle Joint Pain

It is mostly caused by joint sprain. The harm to meridians in the ankle, the blockage of the vital energy and blood circulation and meridians, the energy stagnation and blood stasis after the injury will lead to partial bruising, pain and obstruction of joint movement to varying degrees.

The pain will be obvious when one walks since the ankle bears huge pressure of the human body. It cannot be overlooked even if the injury is not serious and without obvious pain, because the delay of treatment will result in a long cycle of recovery. Scraping therapy is conducive to restoring joint functions while removing blood stasis, reducing distention and stopping pain.

Don't use massage or scraping therapy to treat ankle sprain at the beginning. The sprain should be relieved by cold compression first for 2 to 3 days, and 3 to 5 times each day. Those therapies can be exerted after the pain and distention are slightly eased. The patient with obvious distention should raise the affected limb for a rest to facilitate the reduction of swelling.

Recommended Procedures

1. Jiexi Point and Kunlun Point

Method: Use the angle-pressing and kneading to gently press and knead Jiexi point and Kunlun point.

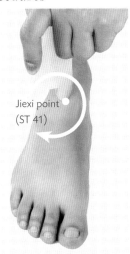

Jiexi point (ST 41)

2. The Surrounding Area of the Related Acupoints

Method: If the ankle distention is very serious or its skin is broken, making it difficult to scrape or press and knead, the operator may gently scrape the surrounding area of the related acupoints.

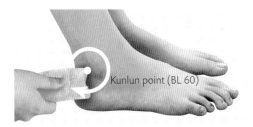

Kunlun point (BL 60)

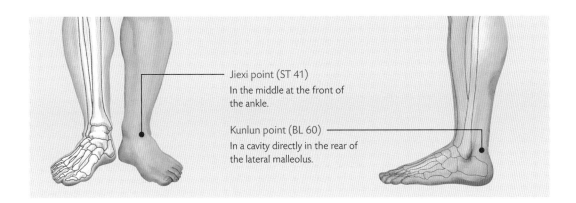

Jiexi point (ST 41)
In the middle at the front of the ankle.

Kunlun point (BL 60)
In a cavity directly in the rear of the lateral malleolus.

Knee Joint Pain

Knee joint pain reflects many kinds of diseases, such as rheumatic arthritis, rheumatoid arthritis, knee ligaments injuries, meniscus injury of knee joints, hyperosteogeny of knee joints and periarticular fibrositis. Rheumatism, strains, excessive movement and obesity are all major factors for causing knee joint pain. Scraping therapy can smooth main and collateral channels, vital energy and blood in the related area and ease pain.

It is not advisable to scrape the joints when the knee joint pain in impaired tissues attacks within 24 hours, nor is it advisable to scrape the affected areas in the case of serious damage to ligaments or joint swelling with fluid accumulated inside. It is acceptable to scrape acupoints at the far end or the reflection areas of knee joints on hands and feet.

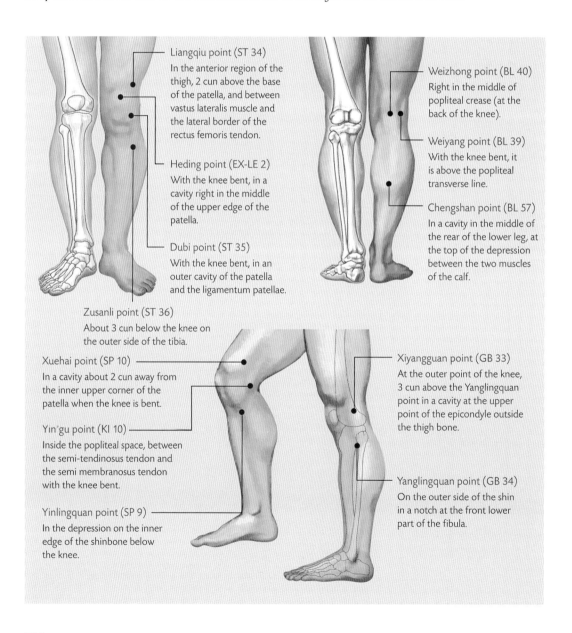

Liangqiu point (ST 34)
In the anterior region of the thigh, 2 cun above the base of the patella, and between vastus lateralis muscle and the lateral border of the rectus femoris tendon.

Heding point (EX-LE 2)
With the knee bent, in a cavity right in the middle of the upper edge of the patella.

Dubi point (ST 35)
With the knee bent, in an outer cavity of the patella and the ligamentum patellae.

Zusanli point (ST 36)
About 3 cun below the knee on the outer side of the tibia.

Xuehai point (SP 10)
In a cavity about 2 cun away from the inner upper corner of the patella when the knee is bent.

Yin'gu point (KI 10)
Inside the popliteal space, between the semi-tendinosus tendon and the semi membranosus tendon with the knee bent.

Yinlingquan point (SP 9)
In the depression on the inner edge of the shinbone below the knee.

Weizhong point (BL 40)
Right in the middle of popliteal crease (at the back of the knee).

Weiyang point (BL 39)
With the knee bent, it is above the popliteal transverse line.

Chengshan point (BL 57)
In a cavity in the middle of the rear of the lower leg, at the top of the depression between the two muscles of the calf.

Xiyangguan point (GB 33)
At the outer point of the knee, 3 cun above the Yanglingquan point in a cavity at the upper point of the epicondyle outside the thigh bone.

Yanglingquan point (GB 34)
On the outer side of the shin in a notch at the front lower part of the fibula.

Recommended Procedures

1. Dubi Point and Heding Point

Method: Use the corner of the scraping plate to press Dubi point on both knees. Use the surface-scraping to scrape from the upper part of the Heding point toward the lower part of the knee.

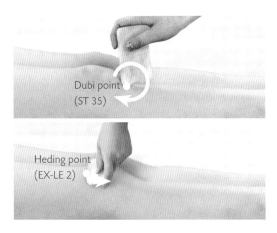

Dubi point (ST 35)

Heding point (EX-LE 2)

2. Liangqiu Point, Zusanli Point, Xiyangguan Point and Yanglingquan Point

Method: Use the surface-scraping to scrape Liangqiu point on the upper part outside the knee and Zusanli point on the lower part of the knee, and then from Xiyangguan point to Yanglingquan point.

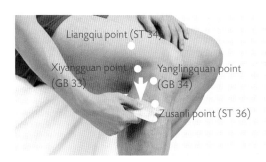

Liangqiu point (ST 34)

Xiyangguan point (GB 33)   Yanglingquan point (GB 34)

Zusanli point (ST 36)

3. Xuehai Point and Yinlingquan Point

Method: Use the surface-scraping to scrape Xuehai point on the upper part on the inside of the knee and Yinlingquan point on the lower part on the inside of the knee.

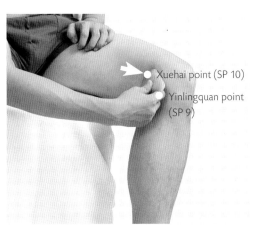

Xuehai point (SP 10)

Yinlingquan point (SP 9)

4. Weizhong Point, Weiyang Point, Yin'gu Point and Chengshan Point

Method: Use the surface-scraping to scrape Weizhong point, Weiyang point, Yin'gu point and Chengshan point on the rear side of lower limbs from up to down.

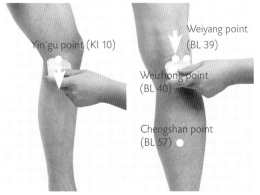

Yin'gu point (KI 10)

Weiyang point (BL 39)

Weizhong point (BL 40)

Chengshan point (BL 57)

Therapy to Increase the Curative Effect

Salt-ironing therapy: 500-gram salt and 120-gram fennel are fried hot together on a pan, half of which is enclosed in a piece of cloth to wrap the area of pain. The other half will be used when the first half becomes cool. The cool half can be fried again. Such salt-ironing is repeatedly applied for several days, and once every day. This can expel the wind and remove the cold, serving to deal with various kinds of joint pains caused by rheumatic arthritis while also producing a curative effect on rheumatic waist pain.

Heel Pain

This is germ-free inflammation caused by acute or chronic damage. The heel is an important bearing point for supporting the whole body. Heel pain can be caused by bearing weight and walking for a long time, or by injury, strains and intrusion of the cold-damp into main and collateral channels. According to Chinese medicine, chronic heel pain is also associated with weak liver and kidney functions, malnutrition of muscles and bones as well as excessive strains among old people. Scraping therapy can expel stasis and obstruction of main and collateral channels or stasis of vital energy and blood, nurturing tendons, bones and muscles so as to eliminate pain.

First of all, shoes of appropriate size should be chosen to prevent and ease heel pain. In daily life, feet can be immersed in warm water or treated with hot compression. Over-tiredness, walking or standing for a long time should be avoided. It is easy for people with flatfeet to suffer from heel pain. So, they should pay more attention to excessive movement in order to avoid harm to plantar fascia and that they had better wear corrective shoes.

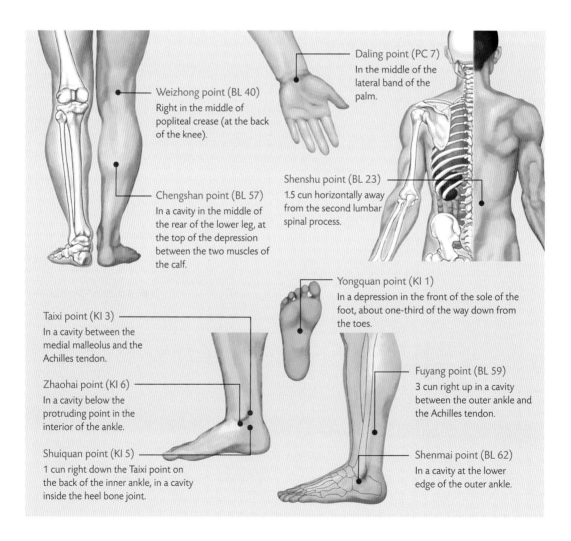

Daling point (PC 7)
In the middle of the lateral band of the palm.

Weizhong point (BL 40)
Right in the middle of popliteal crease (at the back of the knee).

Shenshu point (BL 23)
1.5 cun horizontally away from the second lumbar spinal process.

Chengshan point (BL 57)
In a cavity in the middle of the rear of the lower leg, at the top of the depression between the two muscles of the calf.

Yongquan point (KI 1)
In a depression in the front of the sole of the foot, about one-third of the way down from the toes.

Taixi point (KI 3)
In a cavity between the medial malleolus and the Achilles tendon.

Fuyang point (BL 59)
3 cun right up in a cavity between the outer ankle and the Achilles tendon.

Zhaohai point (KI 6)
In a cavity below the protruding point in the interior of the ankle.

Shuiquan point (KI 5)
1 cun right down the Taixi point on the back of the inner ankle, in a cavity inside the heel bone joint.

Shenmai point (BL 62)
In a cavity at the lower edge of the outer ankle.

Recommended Procedures

1. Daling Point

Method: Use the surface-scraping to scrape Daling point of Pericardium Meridian on the upper limb of the affected side from up to down.

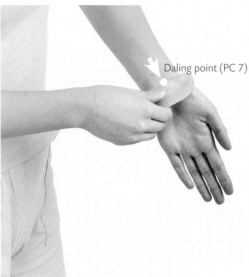

Daling point (PC 7)

2. Weizhong Point, Chengshan Point, Fuyang Point and Shenmai Point

Method: Use the surface-scraping to scrape from Weizhong point to Chengshan point, Fuyang point and Shenmai point of Bladder Meridian on the lower limb of the affected side from up to down.

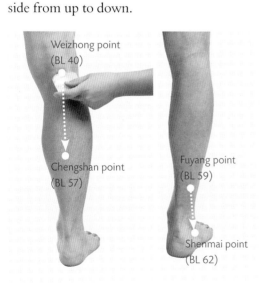

Weizhong point (BL 40)

Chengshan point (BL 57)

Fuyang point (BL 59)

Shenmai point (BL 62)

3. Taixi Point, Shuiquan Point and Zhaohai Point

Method: Use the flat-pressing and kneading to press and knead Taixi point, Shuiquan point and Zhaohai point of the affected side on the foot.

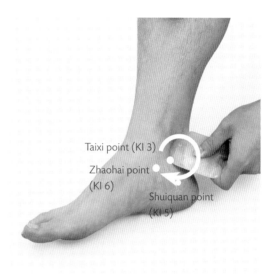

Taixi point (KI 3)

Zhaohai point (KI 6)

Shuiquan point (KI 5)

4. Shenshu Point and Yongquan Point

Method: Use the surface-scraping to scrape Shenshu point on the back from up to down. Use the single-angle scraping to scrape Yongquan point of the affected side in the sole.

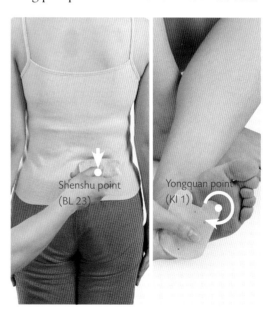

Shenshu point (BL 23)

Yongquan point (KI 1)

Lumbar Disc Protrusion

This refers to a series of symptoms marked by the distention and protrusion of the intervertebral disc from the damaged fiber rings, irritating or pressing the spinal cord and the nerve root. The symptoms are mainly featured by radiating pain or numbness in the waist and lower limbs. There will be more pain when the patient stands, walks, coughs, sneezes or forcefully discharges excrement. The pain will be reduced when the patient bends at hips or knees or rests in bed.

According to Chinese medicine, this disease is mostly associated with trauma, strains, and the intrusion of the pathogenic wind, cold, damp and heat, as well as the disharmony between *ying*-energy and *wei*-energy, harm to the vital energy and blood in main and collateral channels, or liver-kidney insufficiency. Scraping therapy can help to smooth vital energy and blood in main and collateral channels, easing the pain.

When lumbar disc protrusion is in the acute period, it is not advisable to scrape acupoints or apply other kinds of techniques around the waist, but acupoints on lower limbs can be chosen. The patient of lumbar disc protrusion is not supposed to stand or sit for a long time, nor should he/she lift heavy things or bend the waist forcefully. He/she should keep warm and avoid catching the cold while paying attention to resting in flat-board bed on his/her back.

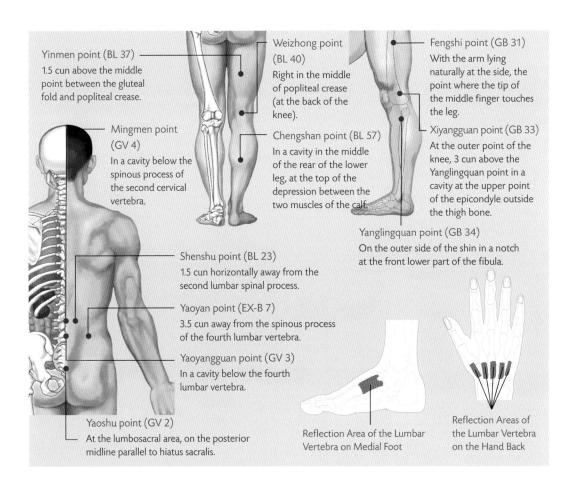

Yinmen point (BL 37)
1.5 cun above the middle point between the gluteal fold and popliteal crease.

Mingmen point (GV 4)
In a cavity below the spinous process of the second cervical vertebra.

Weizhong point (BL 40)
Right in the middle of popliteal crease (at the back of the knee).

Chengshan point (BL 57)
In a cavity in the middle of the rear of the lower leg, at the top of the depression between the two muscles of the calf.

Fengshi point (GB 31)
With the arm lying naturally at the side, the point where the tip of the middle finger touches the leg.

Xiyangguan point (GB 33)
At the outer point of the knee, 3 cun above the Yanglingquan point in a cavity at the upper point of the epicondyle outside the thigh bone.

Yanglingquan point (GB 34)
On the outer side of the shin in a notch at the front lower part of the fibula.

Shenshu point (BL 23)
1.5 cun horizontally away from the second lumbar spinal process.

Yaoyan point (EX-B 7)
3.5 cun away from the spinous process of the fourth lumbar vertebra.

Yaoyangguan point (GV 3)
In a cavity below the fourth lumbar vertebra.

Yaoshu point (GV 2)
At the lumbosacral area, on the posterior midline parallel to hiatus sacralis.

Reflection Area of the Lumbar Vertebra on Medial Foot

Reflection Areas of the Lumbar Vertebra on the Hand Back

Recommended Procedures

1. Reflection Areas of the Lumbar Vertebra on the Hand Back and on Medial Foot

Method: Use the surface-scraping to scrape the areas. The operator should find the point of pain and scrape it slowly and emphatically.

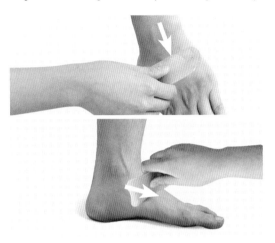

2. Mingmen Point, Yaoyangguan Point, Shenshu Point, Yaoshu Point and Yaoyan Point

Method: Use the surface-scraping to scrape from Mingmen point to Yaoyangguan point from up to down. Then, use the surface-scraping to scrape from Shenshu point to Yaoshu point from up to down. Use the angle-pressing and kneading to press and knead Yaoyan point on both sides, until soreness and distention are felt.

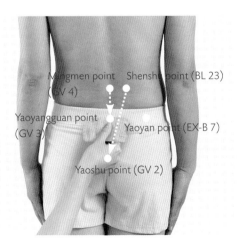

3. Yinmen Point, Weizhong Point and Chengshan Point

Method: Use the surface-scraping to scrape Yinmen point, Weizhong point and Chengshan point from up to down.

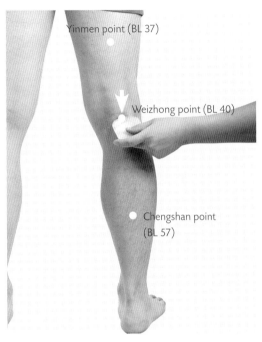

4. Fengshi Point, Xiyangguan Point and Yanglingquan Point

Method: Use the surface-scraping to scrape from Fengshi point to Xiyangguan point from up to down. Use the angle-scraping to scrape Yanglingquan point.

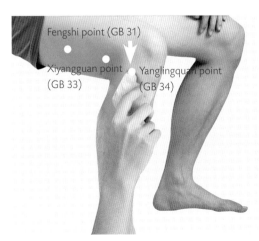

Lumbar Hyperosteogeny

It is mainly seen among old people. Along with the aging, decline and aging of physiological functions take place. Retrogressive intervertebral disc loses fluid, the centrum is not stable, the protruding nucleus pulposus pushes up the bone membrane of the posterior longitudinal ligament and generates new bones, forming bony spurs or hyperosteogeny.

The patient with hyperosteogeny should try to avoid fierce physical exercise, but physical exercise of appropriate extent is necessary. Timely treatment is needed if joints are injured. Controlling weight is also very helpful in easing the symptom.

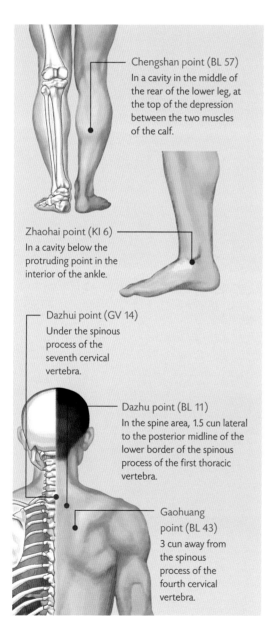

Chengshan point (BL 57)
In a cavity in the middle of the rear of the lower leg, at the top of the depression between the two muscles of the calf.

Zhaohai point (KI 6)
In a cavity below the protruding point in the interior of the ankle.

Dazhui point (GV 14)
Under the spinous process of the seventh cervical vertebra.

Dazhu point (BL 11)
In the spine area, 1.5 cun lateral to the posterior midline of the lower border of the spinous process of the first thoracic vertebra.

Gaohuang point (BL 43)
3 cun away from the spinous process of the fourth cervical vertebra.

Recommended Procedures

1. Dazhui Point, Dazhu Point and Gaohuang Point
Method: Use the surface-scraping to scrape Dazhui point, Dazhu point and Gaohuang point from up to down, until the skin turns red or *sha* appears.

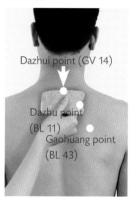

Dazhui point (GV 14)

Dazhu point (BL 11)

Gaohuang point (BL 43)

2. Chengshan Point
Method: Use the surface-scraping to scrape Chengshan point from up to down, until the skin turns red or *sha* appears.

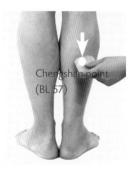

Chengshan point (BL 57)

3. Zhaohai Point
Method: Use the angle-scraping to scrape Zhaohai point from up to down, until the skin turns red or *sha* appears.

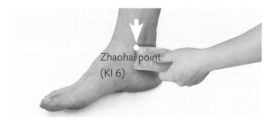

Zhaohai point (KI 6)

Ankylosing Spondylitis

As a chronic inflammatory illness, it mainly intrudes the spine and the soft tissues beside it. In the early stage, the patient has no obvious discomfort. As the illness progresses, there will be such symptoms as pain in the waist, back, neck, buttocks and hips as well as restriction over the movement. It will be obvious at night or early in the morning and it will be eased after the movement.

In daily life, the patient of ankylosing spondylitis should pay attention to keeping proper standing and sitting postures. If feeling stiff in the spine after getting up in the morning, the patient is advised to breathe in and out deeply, expand the chest and straighten up the back to ease the symptom.

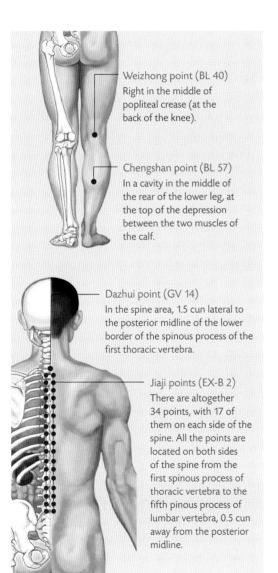

Weizhong point (BL 40)
Right in the middle of popliteal crease (at the back of the knee).

Chengshan point (BL 57)
In a cavity in the middle of the rear of the lower leg, at the top of the depression between the two muscles of the calf.

Dazhui point (GV 14)
In the spine area, 1.5 cun lateral to the posterior midline of the lower border of the spinous process of the first thoracic vertebra.

Jiaji points (EX-B 2)
There are altogether 34 points, with 17 of them on each side of the spine. All the points are located on both sides of the spine from the first spinous process of thoracic vertebra to the fifth pinous process of lumbar vertebra, 0.5 cun away from the posterior midline.

Recommended Procedures

1. Dazhui Point and Jiaji Points

Method: Use the surface-scraping to scrape Dazhui point from up to down. Use the dual-angle scraping to scrape Jiaji points from up to down, until the skin turns red or *sha* appears.

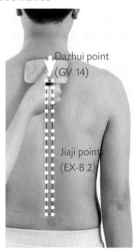

Dazhui point (GV 14)

Jiaji point (EX-B 2)

2. Weizhong Point and Chengshan Point

Method: Use the surface-scraping to scrape from Weizhong point to Chengshan point, until the skin turns red or *sha* appears.

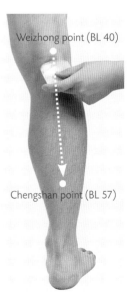

Weizhong point (BL 40)

Chengshan point (BL 57)

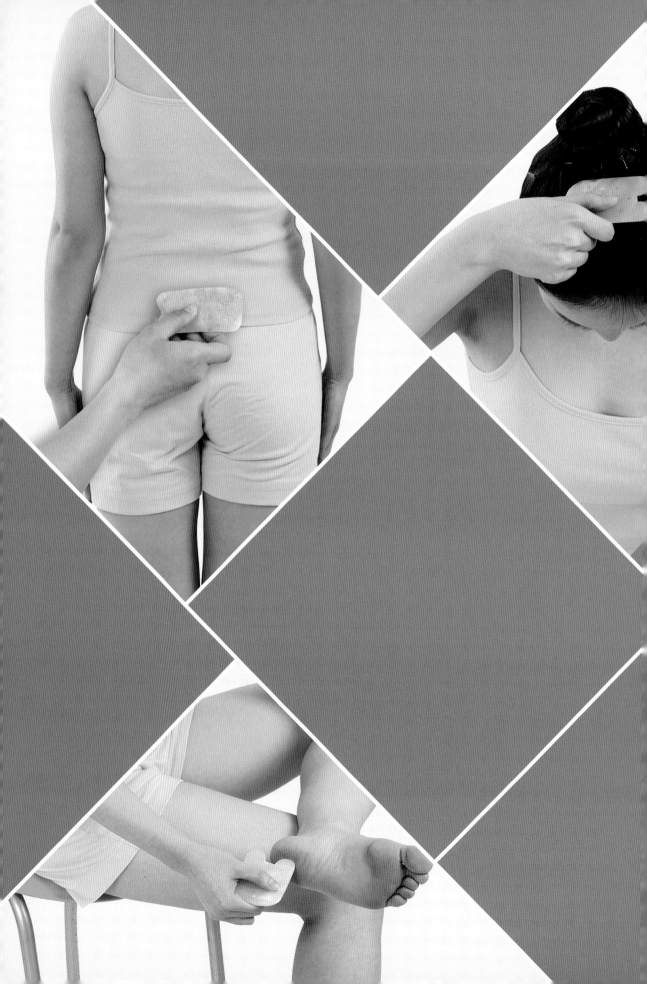

CHAPTER SIX
Use *Gua Sha* to Expel Male and Female Diseases

Scraping therapy can adjust yin and yang because many diseases of men and women are caused by the imbalance between yin and yang. In the course of medical treatment, scraping therapy as an auxiliary means is very helpful in expelling illness.

Premature Ejaculation

This refers to immediate sperm ejaculation before entering the vagina or as soon as the penis enters the vagina and then slumped, which is a symptom of failure to have sex intercourse. According to Chinese medicine, this is caused by too excessive sex intercourse or frequent masturbation, leading to the weakness of kidney meridian, insufficiency of kidney yin, or weak physique, asthenic spermatorrhea for a long time, weakness of kidney energy and harm to yin and yang.

The mental factor is also an important reason for premature ejaculation. Therefore, mental adjustment should also be paid attention to in the course of treatment, i.e., avoid a malicious cycle of mentality due to the failure in sex intercourse.

The patient of premature ejaculation had better eat more food which can tonify kidneys, warm up yang, induce astringency and stop spermatorrhea, such as walnut kernel, gorgon fruit, sheep bones and chicken. It is a taboo to eat raw and food cold in nature.

Recommended Procedures

1. Mingmen Point and Zhishi Point
Method: Use the surface-scraping to scrape Mingmen point and Zhishi point from up to down, 10 to 15 times respectively.

2. Shenshu Point and Pangguangshu Point
Method: Use the surface-scraping to scrape from Shenshu point to Pangguangshu point from up to down 10 to 15 times.

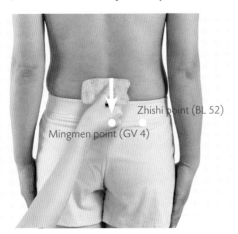

Zhishi point (BL 52)
Mingmen point (GV 4)

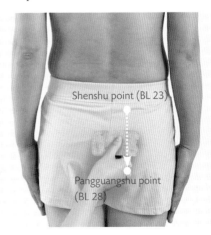

Shenshu point (BL 23)
Pangguangshu point (BL 28)

3. Guanyuan Point

Method: Use the surface-scraping to scrape Guanyuan point from up to down 10 to 15 times, and use the corner of the scraping plate to knead it in whirls for 30 times, until *sha* appears.

4. Sanyinjiao Point and Taixi Point

Method: Use the surface-scraping to scrape Sanyinjiao point from up to down for 30 times. Use the single-angle scraping to scrape, press and knead Taixi point for 30 times, until *sha* appears.

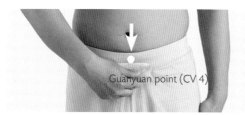

Guanyuan point (CV 4)

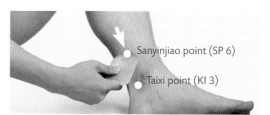

Sanyinjiao point (SP 6)

Taixi point (KI 3)

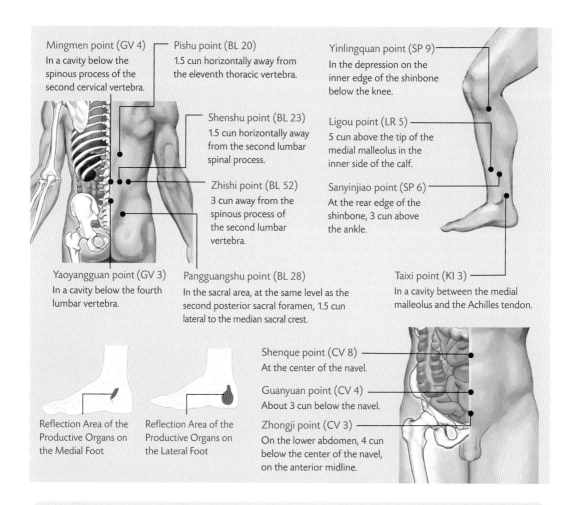

Mingmen point (GV 4)
In a cavity below the spinous process of the second cervical vertebra.

Pishu point (BL 20)
1.5 cun horizontally away from the eleventh thoracic vertebra.

Yinlingquan point (SP 9)
In the depression on the inner edge of the shinbone below the knee.

Shenshu point (BL 23)
1.5 cun horizontally away from the second lumbar spinal process.

Ligou point (LR 5)
5 cun above the tip of the medial malleolus in the inner side of the calf.

Zhishi point (BL 52)
3 cun away from the spinous process of the second lumbar vertebra.

Sanyinjiao point (SP 6)
At the rear edge of the shinbone, 3 cun above the ankle.

Yaoyangguan point (GV 3)
In a cavity below the fourth lumbar vertebra.

Pangguangshu point (BL 28)
In the sacral area, at the same level as the second posterior sacral foramen, 1.5 cun lateral to the median sacral crest.

Taixi point (KI 3)
In a cavity between the medial malleolus and the Achilles tendon.

Shenque point (CV 8)
At the center of the navel.

Guanyuan point (CV 4)
About 3 cun below the navel.

Reflection Area of the Productive Organs on the Medial Foot

Reflection Area of the Productive Organs on the Lateral Foot

Zhongji point (CV 3)
On the lower abdomen, 4 cun below the center of the navel, on the anterior midline.

Therapy to Increase the Curative Effect
200-gram mutton and 30-gram Chinese wolfberries are simmered with water into soup for oral use.

Impotence

This refers to the failure to complete sex intercourse due to erectile dysfunction, though the man has the sexual desire, but cannot erect, or slumps quickly after managing to erect for a very short time. Male erection is a complex process which is associated with nerves, hormones and sentiments. In clinical practice, impotence is most commonly seen among men with liver or kidney illness, weak physique and the particularly people with kidney deficiency. Scraping therapy can improve the sex dysfunctions to a certain extent.

Most cases of impotence are caused by mental factors. Patients of organic impotence are also often influenced by mental factors. Therefore, it is very important to adjust mentality in curing impotence.

Recommended Procedures

1. Reflection Areas of the Productive Organs on the Medial and Lateral Foot
Method: Use the flat-pressing and kneading to press and knead the areas.

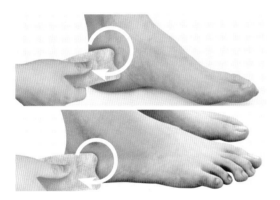

2. Shenque Point, Guanyuan Point and Zhongji Point
Method: Use the flat-pressing and kneading to press and knead Shenque point. Then, use the surface-scraping to scrape from Guanyuan point to Zhongji point below the navel from up to down, then press and knead Guanyuan point and Zhongji point for 30 times respectively.

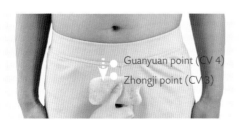

3. Pishu Point, Shenshu Point, Mingmen Point and Yaoyangguan Point
Method: Use the surface-scraping to scrape Pishu point, Shenshu point, Mingmen point and Yaoyangguan point on the back from up to down.

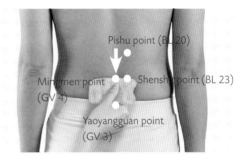

Pishu point (BL 20)
Mingmen point (GV 4)
Shenshu point (BL 23)
Yaoyangguan point (GV 3)

4. Yinlingquan Point, Ligou Point and Sanyinjiao Point
Method: Use the surface-scraping to scrape Yinlingquan point, Ligou apoint and Sanyinjiao point on the inside of the lower limbs from up to down.

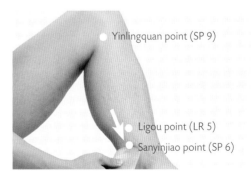

Yinlingquan point (SP 9)
Ligou point (LR 5)
Sanyinjiao point (SP 6)

Spermatorrhea

This refers to a kind of male illness marked by automatic discharge of sperms without having sex intercourse. Generally, it is a normal physiological phenomenon for an adult man to have spermatorrhea for no more than once a week. If it is more than once a week or several times a day coupled with low spirits, waist soreness, weak legs, palpitation and short breath, then, it is pathological spermatorrhea. According to Chinese medicine, spermatorrhea is mostly due to weak kidneys failing to control sperms, or heart-kidney imbalance, or downward flow of damp-heat.

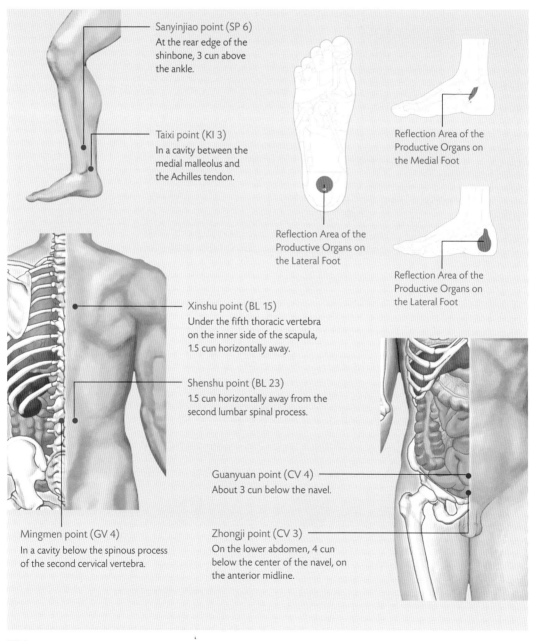

Sanyinjiao point (SP 6)
At the rear edge of the shinbone, 3 cun above the ankle.

Taixi point (KI 3)
In a cavity between the medial malleolus and the Achilles tendon.

Reflection Area of the Productive Organs on the Medial Foot

Reflection Area of the Productive Organs on the Lateral Foot

Reflection Area of the Productive Organs on the Lateral Foot

Xinshu point (BL 15)
Under the fifth thoracic vertebra on the inner side of the scapula, 1.5 cun horizontally away.

Shenshu point (BL 23)
1.5 cun horizontally away from the second lumbar spinal process.

Guanyuan point (CV 4)
About 3 cun below the navel.

Mingmen point (GV 4)
In a cavity below the spinous process of the second cervical vertebra.

Zhongji point (CV 3)
On the lower abdomen, 4 cun below the center of the navel, on the anterior midline.

Recommended Procedures

1. Reflection Areas of the Productive Organs on Medial and Lateral Foot and in the Sole

Method: Use the flat-pressing and kneading or the angle-pressing and kneading to press and knead the areas.

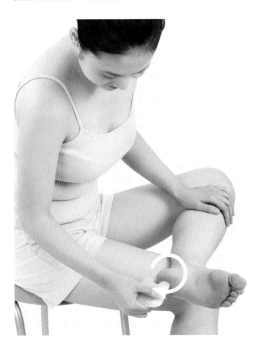

2. Xinshu Point, Mingmen Point and Shenshu Point

Method: Use the surface-scraping to scrape Xinshu point, Mingmen point and Shenshu point on the waist and the back from up to down.

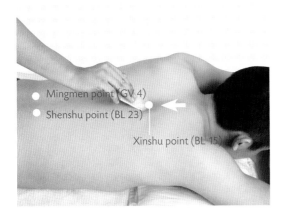

3. Guanyuan Point and Zhongji Point

Method: Use the surface-scraping to scrape from Guanyuan point to Zhongji point on the lower abdomen from up to down.

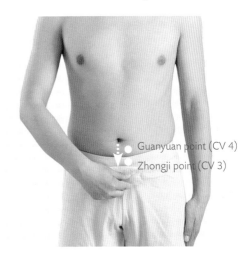

Guanyuan point (CV 4)
Zhongji point (CV 3)

4. Taixi Point and Sanyinjiao Point

Method: Use the surface-scraping to scrape Sanyinjiao point on the inside of the shin for 30 times. Use the angle-pressing and kneading to press and knead Taixi point with some force, until soreness, numbness and distention are felt.

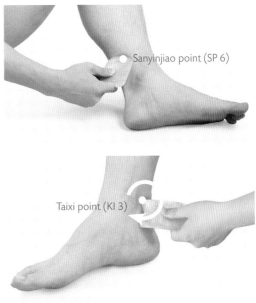

Sanyinjiao point (SP 6)

Taixi point (KI 3)

Mingmen point (GV 4)
Shenshu point (BL 23)
Xinshu point (BL 15)

Prostatitis

Prostatitis and prostatic hyperplasia are common diseases with the prostate gland, generally marked by frequent micturition, urgent urination and white secretions flowing out of the urethral opening after urine is discharged. It is mostly caused by the damp and heat in the lower energizer and disorder of gasification. Scraping therapy can smooth vital energy and blood, adjust functions of various endocrine glands and smooth the bladder.

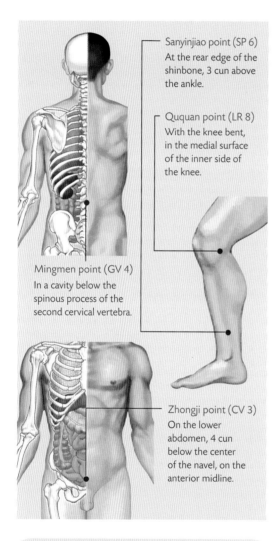

Sanyinjiao point (SP 6)
At the rear edge of the shinbone, 3 cun above the ankle.

Ququan point (LR 8)
With the knee bent, in the medial surface of the inner side of the knee.

Mingmen point (GV 4)
In a cavity below the spinous process of the second cervical vertebra.

Zhongji point (CV 3)
On the lower abdomen, 4 cun below the center of the navel, on the anterior midline.

Therapy to Increase the Curative Effect
White gourd and coix seed soup: 350-gram sliced white gourd and 50-gram coix seeds are boiled into soup with an appropriate amount of white sugar for oral use, once every day.

Recommended Procedures

1. Mingmen Point
Method: Use the surface-scraping to gently scrape Mingmen point 30 times from up to down, until the skin turns red.

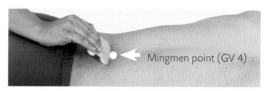

Mingmen point (GV 4)

2. Zhongji Point
Method: Use the surface-scraping to scrape Zhongji point 30 times from up to down with moderate force, until the skin turns red.

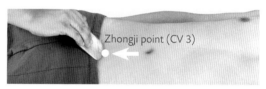

Zhongji point (CV 3)

3. Ququan Point and Sanyinjiao Point
Method: Use the surface-scraping to scrape Ququan point and Sanyinjiao point 10 to 15 times respectively from up to down with force, until *sha* appears.

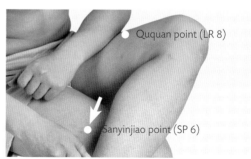

Ququan point (LR 8)

Sanyinjiao point (SP 6)

Hyperplasia of Prostate Gland

This is a benign pathological change in the prostate gland marked by slow onset of discharging urine, fine urinary streams, shortened range of urinary shot and urinary dripping after urine is discharged. Frequent micturition takes place at night first, followed by frequent micturition even in the daytime. Frequent micturition becomes more serious in the late stage due to the reduction of effective capacity in the bladder.

Generally, benign hyperplasia of the prostate gland enjoys favorable prognosis after treatment. Without treatment, it will seriously affect the quality of life. Chronic lower urinary tract obstruction may lead to the failure of kidney functions, which can threaten the life.

Recommended Procedures

1. Reflection Areas of the Productive Organs on the Medial and Lateral Foot
Method: Use the flat-pressing and kneading to press and knead the areas.

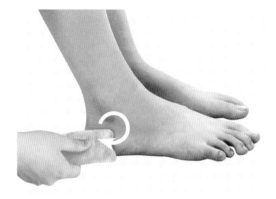

2. Corresponding Area of the Productive Organs on the Spine
Method: Use the surface-scraping and the dual-angle scraping to scrape the area.

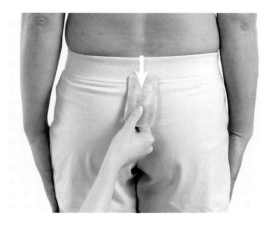

3. Shuidao Point and Guilai Point
Method: Use the surface-scraping to scrape from Shuidao point to Guilai point on the abdomen from up to down.

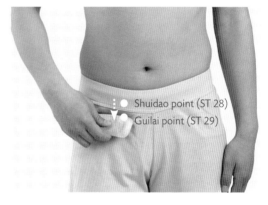

Shuidao point (ST 28)
Guilai point (ST 29)

4. Yinlingquan Point, Sanyinjiao Point, Fuliu Point and Taixi Point
Method: Use the surface-scraping to scrape Yinlingquan point, Sanyinjiao point, Fuliu point and Taixi point on the inside of the lower limbs.

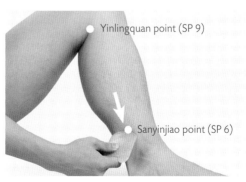

Yinlingquan point (SP 9)
Sanyinjiao point (SP 6)

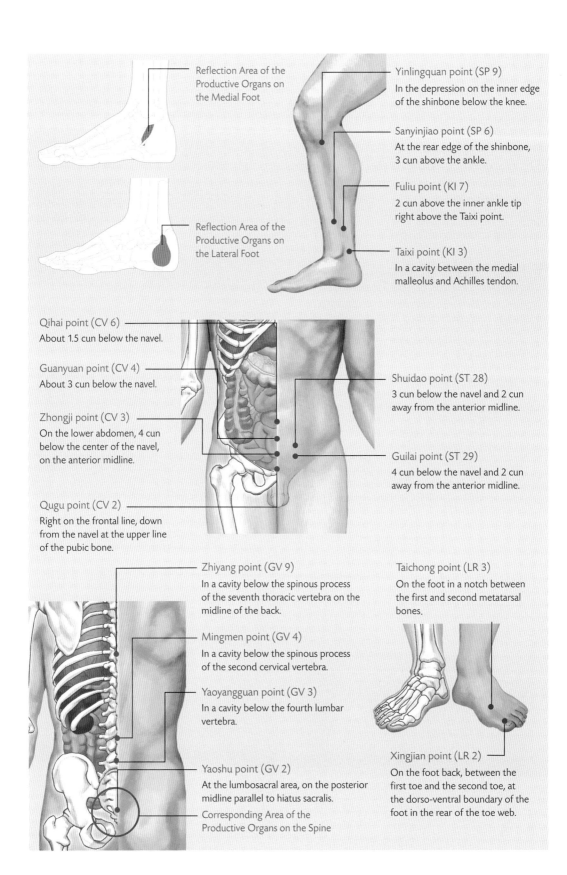

Reflection Area of the Productive Organs on the Medial Foot

Reflection Area of the Productive Organs on the Lateral Foot

Yinlingquan point (SP 9)
In the depression on the inner edge of the shinbone below the knee.

Sanyinjiao point (SP 6)
At the rear edge of the shinbone, 3 cun above the ankle.

Fuliu point (KI 7)
2 cun above the inner ankle tip right above the Taixi point.

Taixi point (KI 3)
In a cavity between the medial malleolus and Achilles tendon.

Qihai point (CV 6)
About 1.5 cun below the navel.

Guanyuan point (CV 4)
About 3 cun below the navel.

Zhongji point (CV 3)
On the lower abdomen, 4 cun below the center of the navel, on the anterior midline.

Qugu point (CV 2)
Right on the frontal line, down from the navel at the upper line of the pubic bone.

Shuidao point (ST 28)
3 cun below the navel and 2 cun away from the anterior midline.

Guilai point (ST 29)
4 cun below the navel and 2 cun away from the anterior midline.

Zhiyang point (GV 9)
In a cavity below the spinous process of the seventh thoracic vertebra on the midline of the back.

Mingmen point (GV 4)
In a cavity below the spinous process of the second cervical vertebra.

Yaoyangguan point (GV 3)
In a cavity below the fourth lumbar vertebra.

Yaoshu point (GV 2)
At the lumbosacral area, on the posterior midline parallel to hiatus sacralis.

Corresponding Area of the Productive Organs on the Spine

Taichong point (LR 3)
On the foot in a notch between the first and second metatarsal bones.

Xingjian point (LR 2)
On the foot back, between the first toe and the second toe, at the dorso-ventral boundary of the foot in the rear of the toe web.

Male Infertility

This refers to a man at the normal age of childbearing with normal sex life, failing to enable the wife to be pregnant though no contraceptive measures are taken in a year or longer than that. Scraping therapy is conducive to stimulating kidney functions and restoring male functions of childbearing.

There are quite many syndromes of male infertility. The following steps 1 to 3 lay stress on stimulating kidneys to help restore male functions of childbearing. Long-term depression leading to infertility is seen quite often. Step 4 serves to adjust the health of people of this kind. Concrete reasons for infertility require diagnosis by doctors for symptomatic treatment.

Recommended Procedures

1. Corresponding Area of the Productive Organs on the Spine
Method: Use the surface-scraping and the dual-angle scraping to scrape the area.

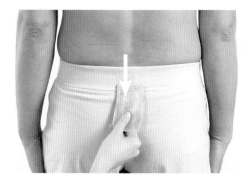

2. Zhiyang Point, Mingmen Point, Yaoyangguan Point and Yaoshu Point
Method: Use the surface-scraping to scrape Zhiyang point, Mingmen point, Yaoyangguan point and Yaoshu point along the spine.

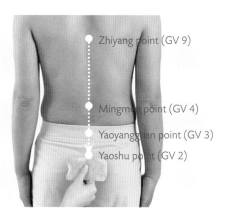

Zhiyang point (GV 9)
Mingmen point (GV 4)
Yaoyangguan point (GV 3)
Yaoshu point (GV 2)

3. Qihai Point, Guanyuan Point, Zhongji Point and Qugu Point
Method: Use the surface-scraping to scrape from Qihai point to Guanyuan point, Zhongji point and Qugu point on the lower abdomen.

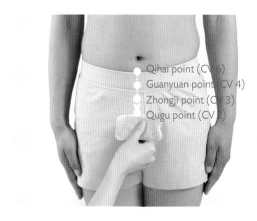

Qihai point (CV 6)
Guanyuan point (CV 4)
Zhongji point (CV 3)
Qugu point (CV 2)

4. Taichong Point and Xingjian Point
Method: Use the corner of the scraping plate to vertically press and knead Taichong point and Xingjian point, until soreness and distention are felt (it is applicable to those of infertility often under depression).

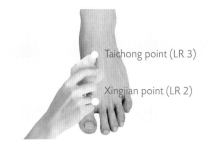

Taichong point (LR 3)
Xingjian point (LR 2)

Female Infertility

This refers to a woman at the age of childbearing still failing to be pregnant despite having normal sex life without taking contraceptive measures in a year of longer than that. Infertility includes primary infertility (without pregnancy after marriage) and secondary infertility (had pregnancy after marriage).

There are many reasons for infertility, such as diseases in the system of reproduction, malnutrition and weak physique. Therefore, infertility requires all-round physical checkup for targeted treatment, instead of blindly relying on so-called folk prescription. In daily life, paying attention to physical exercise, reinforcing physique, improving anaemia and malnutrition, giving up smoking and alcoholic drinks are all conducive to restoring the ability of fertility among women of infertility.

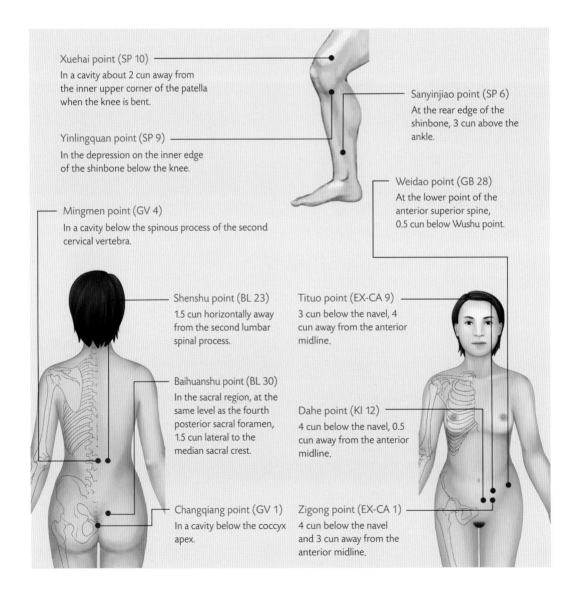

Xuehai point (SP 10)
In a cavity about 2 cun away from the inner upper corner of the patella when the knee is bent.

Sanyinjiao point (SP 6)
At the rear edge of the shinbone, 3 cun above the ankle.

Yinlingquan point (SP 9)
In the depression on the inner edge of the shinbone below the knee.

Weidao point (GB 28)
At the lower point of the anterior superior spine, 0.5 cun below Wushu point.

Mingmen point (GV 4)
In a cavity below the spinous process of the second cervical vertebra.

Shenshu point (BL 23)
1.5 cun horizontally away from the second lumbar spinal process.

Tituo point (EX-CA 9)
3 cun below the navel, 4 cun away from the anterior midline.

Baihuanshu point (BL 30)
In the sacral region, at the same level as the fourth posterior sacral foramen, 1.5 cun lateral to the median sacral crest.

Dahe point (KI 12)
4 cun below the navel, 0.5 cun away from the anterior midline.

Changqiang point (GV 1)
In a cavity below the coccyx apex.

Zigong point (EX-CA 1)
4 cun below the navel and 3 cun away from the anterior midline.

Recommended Procedures

1. Mingmen Point and Changqiang Point

Method: Use the surface-scraping to scrape from Mingmen point to Changqiang point, until the skin turns red (the appearance of *sha* is not necessary).

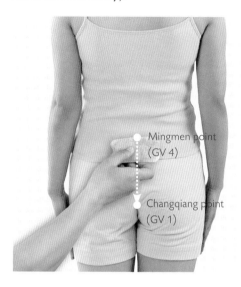

Mingmen point (GV 4)

Changqiang point (GV 1)

2. Shenshu Point and Baihuanshu Point

Method: Use the surface-scraping to scrape from Shenshu point to Baihuanshu point, until the skin turns red (the appearance of *sha* is not necessary).

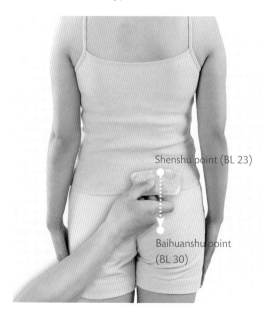

Shenshu point (BL 23)

Baihuanshu point (BL 30)

3. Xuehai Point, Yinlingquan Point and Sanyinjiao Point

Method: Use the surface-scraping to scrape Xuehai point, Yinlingquan point and Sanyinjiao point on the inside of the lower limbs from up to down, until the skin turns red (the appearance of *sha* is not necessary).

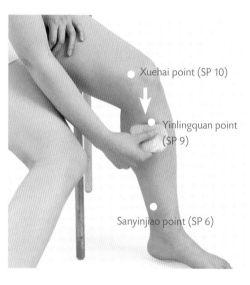

Xuehai point (SP 10)

Yinlingquan point (SP 9)

Sanyinjiao point (SP 6)

4. Weidao Point, Tituo Point, Zigong Point and Dahe Point

Method: Use the surface-scraping to scrape Weidao point, Tituo point, Zigong point and Dahe point from up to down, until the skin turns red (the appearance of *sha* is not necessary).

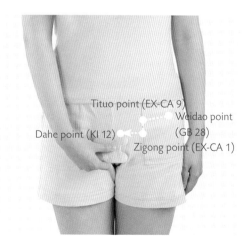

Tituo point (EX-CA 9)

Weidao point (GB 28)

Dahe point (KI 12)

Zigong point (EX-CA 1)

Irregular Menstruation

This is a common disease among women, generally marked by abnormality of the cycle of menstruation or the amount of bleeding. In the period of menstruation, women can suffer from abdominal pain and related symptoms all over the body. The reasons are likely to be organic lesion or abnormality of functions. Irregular menstruation can also be caused by the neglect of nurturing health, depression, anxiety, anger, being caught in the cold rain, and eating raw and cold food.

Mental stimulation and fluctuating emotions are important elements for irregular menstruation, requiring the regulation of emotions. During the period of menstruation, it's better not to eat raw, cold, sour or spicy food. Drink more hot water and keep the bowel movement smooth. Taking appropriate amount of dates, motherwort, angelica and haws can invigorate blood and adjust menstruation to a certain extent.

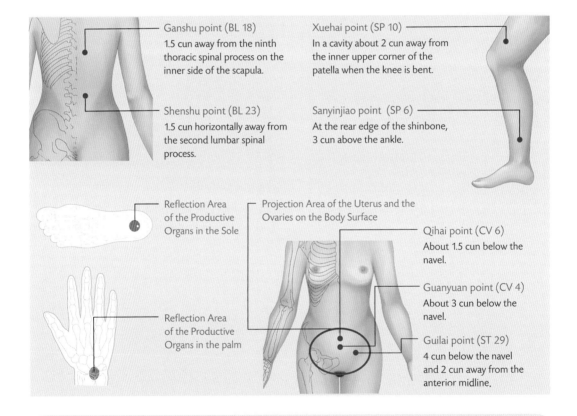

Ganshu point (BL 18)
1.5 cun away from the ninth thoracic spinal process on the inner side of the scapula.

Xuehai point (SP 10)
In a cavity about 2 cun away from the inner upper corner of the patella when the knee is bent.

Shenshu point (BL 23)
1.5 cun horizontally away from the second lumbar spinal process.

Sanyinjiao point (SP 6)
At the rear edge of the shinbone, 3 cun above the ankle.

Reflection Area of the Productive Organs in the Sole

Projection Area of the Uterus and the Ovaries on the Body Surface

Qihai point (CV 6)
About 1.5 cun below the navel.

Guanyuan point (CV 4)
About 3 cun below the navel.

Reflection Area of the Productive Organs in the palm

Guilai point (ST 29)
4 cun below the navel and 2 cun away from the anterior midline.

Therapies to Increase the Curative Effect
• Angelica tea for adjusting menstruation: 2-gram black tea and 10-gram washed angelica are put into the boiling water for five minutes as tea to be drunk, once every day.
• Haw and brown sugar beverage: 5-gram raw haws and 40-gram brown sugar are boiled as hot beverage, drink once every day. It is suitable for women with small amount of bleeding during the period of menstruation, but not suitable for those of large amount of bleeding.

Recommended Procedures

1. Reflection Area of the Productive Organs in the Palm and the Sole
Method: Use the angle-pressing and kneading to press and knead the areas.

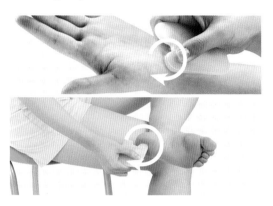

2. Projection Area of the Uterus and the Ovary on Body Surface
Method: Use the surface-scraping to scrape the area on the lower abdomen from up to down, which can be coupled with cupping.

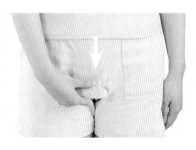

3. Qihai Point, Guanyuan Point and Guilai Point
Method: Use the surface-scraping to scrape Qihai point, Guanyuan point and Guilai point on the lower abdomen from up to down.

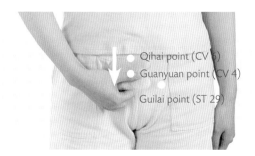

Qihai point (CV 6)
Guanyuan point (CV 4)
Guilai point (ST 29)

4. Ganshu Point and Shenshu Point
Method: Use the surface-scraping to scrape from Ganshu point to Shenshu point on the waist and back from up to down.

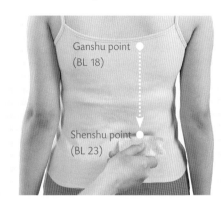

Ganshu point (BL 18)

Shenshu point (BL 23)

5. Xuehai Point and Sanyinjiao Point
Method: Use the surface-scraping to scrape Xuehai point and Sanyinjiao point on the inside of the lower limbs from up to down.

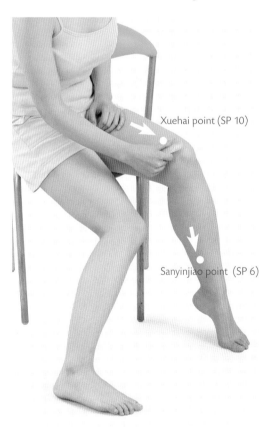

Xuehai point (SP 10)

Sanyinjiao point (SP 6)

Dysmenorrhea

This refers to the pain in the lower abdomen or the waist and even in the lumbosacral area before and after menstruation. It attacks together with the cycle of menstruation. Women of serious cases may suffer from nausea, vomit, dripping cold sweat, cold hands and even coma. According to Chinese medicine, dysmenorrhea is mostly caused by stasis of vital energy and blood or stasis of the cold-damp. Scraping therapy has a better effect on primary dysmenorrhea without organic lesion.

Too much pressure at work, over-fatigue and tension can also result in over-sensitivity of women to the pain. The neglect of keeping the abdomen warm is also a major factor leading to dysmenorrhea. Catching cold in the period of menstruation will contract blood vessels in the uterus and pelvic cavity, resulting in the disorder of ovary functions, the sharp reduction of the amount of menstruation and even amenorrhea.

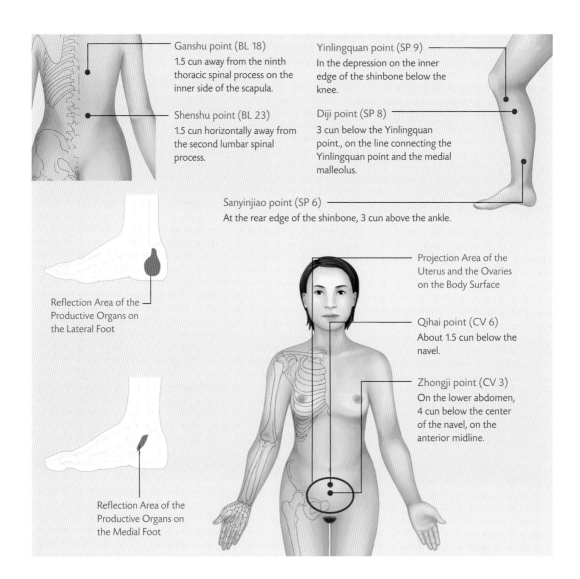

Ganshu point (BL 18)
1.5 cun away from the ninth thoracic spinal process on the inner side of the scapula.

Shenshu point (BL 23)
1.5 cun horizontally away from the second lumbar spinal process.

Yinlingquan point (SP 9)
In the depression on the inner edge of the shinbone below the knee.

Diji point (SP 8)
3 cun below the Yinlingquan point., on the line connecting the Yinlingquan point and the medial malleolus.

Sanyinjiao point (SP 6)
At the rear edge of the shinbone, 3 cun above the ankle.

Reflection Area of the Productive Organs on the Lateral Foot

Reflection Area of the Productive Organs on the Medial Foot

Projection Area of the Uterus and the Ovaries on the Body Surface

Qihai point (CV 6)
About 1.5 cun below the navel.

Zhongji point (CV 3)
On the lower abdomen, 4 cun below the center of the navel, on the anterior midline.

Recommended Procedures

1. Reflection Areas of the Productive Organs on the Medial and Lateral Foot
Method: Use the angle-pressing and kneading to press and knead the areas.

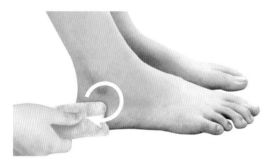

2. Projection Area of the Uterus and the Ovary on the Body Surface
Method: Use the surface-scraping to scrape the area on the lower abdomen from up to down, which can be coupled with cupping.

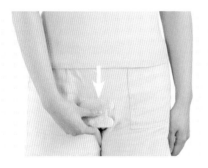

3. Qihai Point and Zhongji Point
Method: Use the surface-scraping to scrape from Qihai point to Zhongji point on the lower abdomen from up to down.

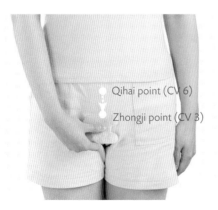

Qihai point (CV 6)
Zhongji point (CV 3)

4. Ganshu Point and Shenshu Point
Method: Use the surface-scraping to scrape from Ganshu point to Shenshu point on the waist and back from up to down.

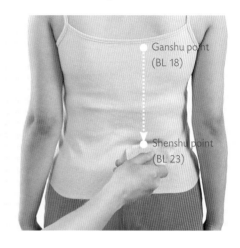

Ganshu point (BL 18)
Shenshu point (BL 23)

5. Yinlingquan Point, Diji Point and Sanyinjiao Point
Method: Use the surface-scraping to scrape from Yinlingquan point to Diji point and Sanyinjiao point on the inside of the lower limbs from up to down.

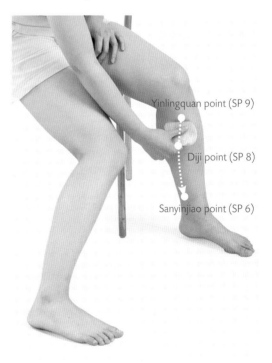

Yinlingquan point (SP 9)
Diji point (SP 8)
Sanyinjiao point (SP 6)

Amenorrhea

There are two kinds of amenorrhea, primary amenorrhea and secondary amenorrhea. Those of more than 16 years old without menstruation fall into the category of primary amenorrhea. After the first menstruation, those whose menstruation stops for more than 3 months fall into the category of secondary amenorrhea (with such factors as the period of pregnancy, the period of breast-feeding and the period of menopause excluded). According to Chinese medicine, amenorrhea can be caused by the congenital insufficiency of kidney energy, acquired liver-kidney deficiency, or mental irritation, anger, stasis of liver energy or catching cold during the period of menstruation.

Menstruation results from the fall-off of endometria periodically due to periodic adjustment of hypothalamus, hypohysis and ovarian axis. Organic or functional changes of any link will be likely to result in amenorrhea. Other kinds of organic and functional abnormality related to endocrine glands are also likely to affect menstruation to the extent of leading to amenorrhea. Therefore, attention should be paid to making identification once amenorrhea takes place, trying to find out the pathogenesis to facilitate treatment.

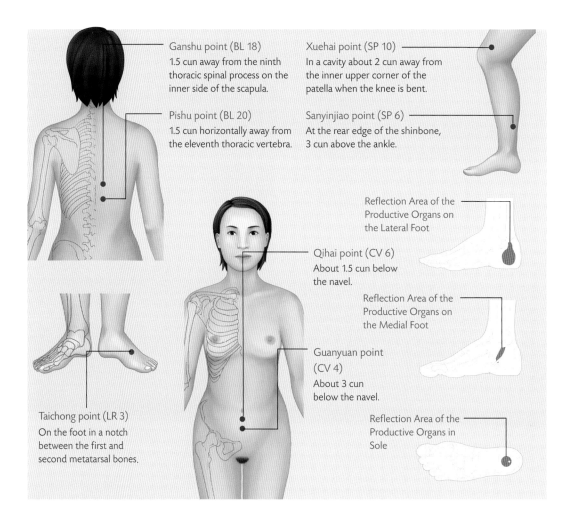

Ganshu point (BL 18)
1.5 cun away from the ninth thoracic spinal process on the inner side of the scapula.

Xuehai point (SP 10)
In a cavity about 2 cun away from the inner upper corner of the patella when the knee is bent.

Pishu point (BL 20)
1.5 cun horizontally away from the eleventh thoracic vertebra.

Sanyinjiao point (SP 6)
At the rear edge of the shinbone, 3 cun above the ankle.

Reflection Area of the Productive Organs on the Lateral Foot

Qihai point (CV 6)
About 1.5 cun below the navel.

Reflection Area of the Productive Organs on the Medial Foot

Guanyuan point (CV 4)
About 3 cun below the navel.

Taichong point (LR 3)
On the foot in a notch between the first and second metatarsal bones.

Reflection Area of the Productive Organs in Sole

Recommended Procedures

1. Reflection Areas of the Productive Organs on the Medial and the Lateral Foot and in Sole

Method: Use the angle-pressing and kneading to press and knead the areas, with stress on the point of pain.

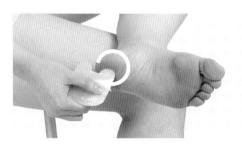

2. Qihai Point and Guanyuan Point

Method: Use the surface-scraping to scrape from Qihai point to Guanyuan point on the lower abdomen from up to down. Use the corner of the scraping plate to press and knead these two acupoints for 30 times respectively.

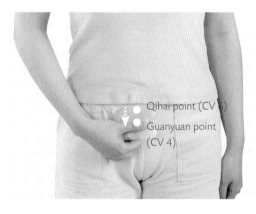

Qihai point (CV 6)
Guanyuan point (CV 4)

> **Therapy to Increase the Curative Effect**
> Sliced ginger fried with cuttlefish: 50-gram peeled-off and sliced ginger and 200-gram washed and sliced cuttlefish are fried in oil with salt added. This dish serves to supplement blood and smooth the main and collateral channels, helpful as an auxiliary treatment to the women with amenorrhea due to deficiency of blood.

3. Pishu Point and Ganshu Point

Method: Use the surface-scraping to scrape Pishu point and Ganshu point on the waist and back from up to down.

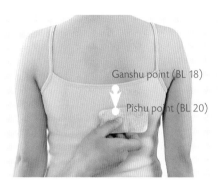

Ganshu point (BL 18)
Pishu point (BL 20)

4. Xuehai Point, Sanyinjiao Point and Taichong Point

Method: Use the surface-scraping to scrape Xuehai point and Sanyinjiao point on the inside of the lower limbs from up to down. Then, use the angle-pressing and kneading to press and knead Taichong point on the foot-back 15 to 30 times, until soreness and distention are felt.

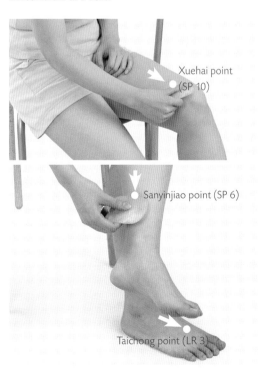

Xuehai point (SP 10)
Sanyinjiao point (SP 6)
Taichong point (LR 3)

Abnormal Leukorrhea

A small amount of white and viscous liquid secreted from the vagina is called leukorrhea. It is called "leukorrheal disease" if leukorrhea continues with a big amount, bad smell and abnormal color as well as symptoms all over the body. According to Chinese medicine, this disease is mostly due to the downward flow of damp-heat or weakness in vital energy and blood, leading to disorder of Belt Channel and imbalance between Chong Meridian and Ren Meridian.

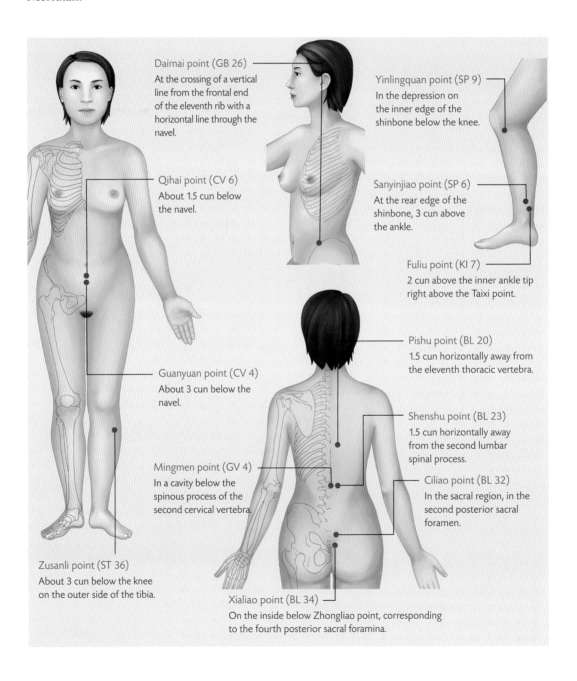

Daimai point (GB 26)
At the crossing of a vertical line from the frontal end of the eleventh rib with a horizontal line through the navel.

Qihai point (CV 6)
About 1.5 cun below the navel.

Guanyuan point (CV 4)
About 3 cun below the navel.

Mingmen point (GV 4)
In a cavity below the spinous process of the second cervical vertebra.

Zusanli point (ST 36)
About 3 cun below the knee on the outer side of the tibia.

Yinlingquan point (SP 9)
In the depression on the inner edge of the shinbone below the knee.

Sanyinjiao point (SP 6)
At the rear edge of the shinbone, 3 cun above the ankle.

Fuliu point (KI 7)
2 cun above the inner ankle tip right above the Taixi point.

Pishu point (BL 20)
1.5 cun horizontally away from the eleventh thoracic vertebra.

Shenshu point (BL 23)
1.5 cun horizontally away from the second lumbar spinal process.

Ciliao point (BL 32)
In the sacral region, in the second posterior sacral foramen.

Xialiao point (BL 34)
On the inside below Zhongliao point, corresponding to the fourth posterior sacral foramina.

Recommended Procedures

1. Qihai Point, Guanyuan Point and Daimai Point

Method: Use the surface-scraping to scrape from Qihai point to Guanyuan point on the lower abdomen from up to down as well as Daimai point on both sides.

2. Pishu Point, Shenshu Point, Mingmen Point, Ciliao Point and Xialiao Point

Method: Use the surface-scraping to scrape from Pishu point to Shenshu point on both sides of the waist and back from up to down. Then, use the surface-scraping to scrape Mingmen point, Ciliao point and Xialiao point respectively.

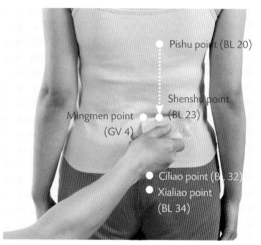

3. Yinlingquan Point, Sanyinjiao Point, Zusanli Point and Fuliu Point

Method: Use the surface-scraping to scrape from Yinlingquan point to Sanyinjiao point. Then, use the flat-pressing and kneading to press and knead Zusanli point and Fuliu point.

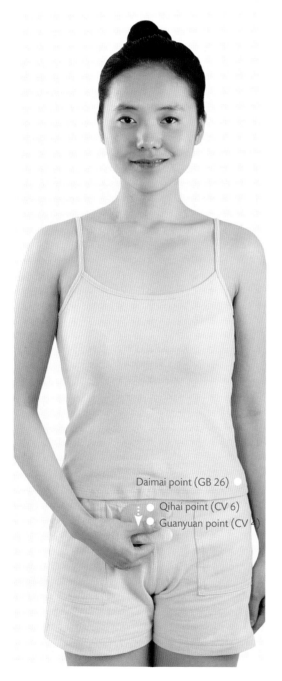

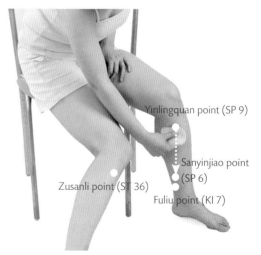

Uterine Prolapse

This refers to the fact that uterus descends or falls off along vagina from its normal position. It is often marked by soreness and pain in the lumbosacral area and the feeling of tenesmus in the lower abdomen, vagina and perineal area. Such a feeling will be more obvious after physical labor but will be eased after resting in bed. Those of serious cases will suffer from difficulties in discharging urine, or frequent urination and the increase of leukorrhea.

Menopause is the period of high frequency of occurrence in terms of uterine prolapse. Women in this period should pay particular attention to avoiding being over-tired, keeping a happy mood, expelling tension and anxiety, being mindful of doing physical exercise to an appropriate extent and adhering to lifting anal muscles (forcefully contracting anal muscles for 10 minutes each time, several times a day) to prevent tissues from being too loosened or declining too early.

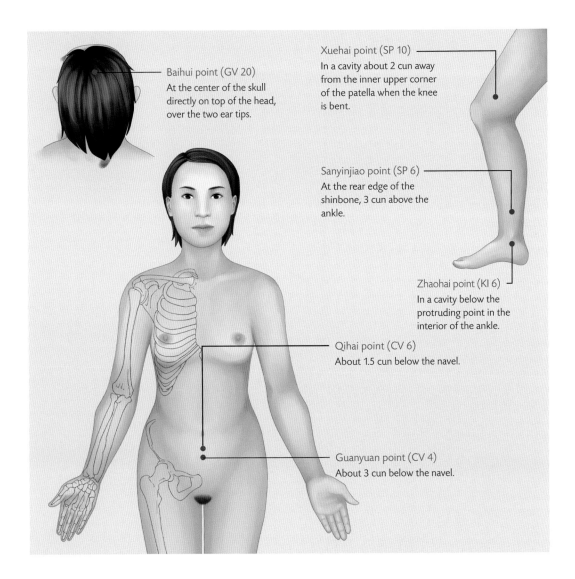

Baihui point (GV 20)
At the center of the skull directly on top of the head, over the two ear tips.

Xuehai point (SP 10)
In a cavity about 2 cun away from the inner upper corner of the patella when the knee is bent.

Sanyinjiao point (SP 6)
At the rear edge of the shinbone, 3 cun above the ankle.

Zhaohai point (KI 6)
In a cavity below the protruding point in the interior of the ankle.

Qihai point (CV 6)
About 1.5 cun below the navel.

Guanyuan point (CV 4)
About 3 cun below the navel.

Recommended Procedures

1. Baihui Point

Method: Use the edge of the scraping plate to scrape Baihui point with increasing force, until soreness, distention and numbness are felt on the top of the head.

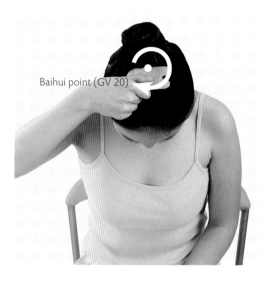

Baihui point (GV 20)

2. Qihai Point and Guanyuan Point

Method: Use the surface-scraping to scrape from Qihai point to Guanyuan point on the lower abdomen from up to down, until the skin turns red or *sha* appears.

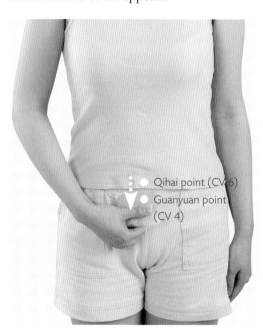

Qihai point (CV 6)
Guanyuan point (CV 4)

3. Xuehai Point, Sanyinjiao Point and Zhaohai Point

Method: Use the corner of the scraping plate to press and knead Xuehai point 20 to 30 times, until soreness and distention are felt. Use the surface-scraping to scrape Sanyinjiao point and Zhaohai point from up to down. The appearance of *sha* is not necessary.

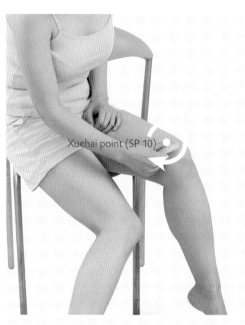

Xuehai point (SP 10)

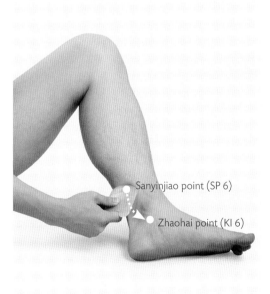

Sanyinjiao point (SP 6)
Zhaohai point (KI 6)

Uterine Fibroid

This is benign uterine tumor caused by cellular proliferation of smooth muscles in uterus, marked by too much menstruation and secondary anaemia, generally without obvious symptoms on the part of the patient. Pain in the lower abdomen or bearing-down pain takes place according to the area and size of the fibroid. There are more incidences of abortion after pregnancy. The fibroid presses the bladder and rectum and even leads to urine retention and constipation.

With uterine fibroid confirmed, the patient should go to the hospital for check-up once a month. Follow-up check-up can be done once every half year if the size of the fibroid expands slowly or remains the same. Surgical operation should be considered if the fibroid expands obviously, so as to prevent serious bleeding or compression over inner organs in the abdomen.

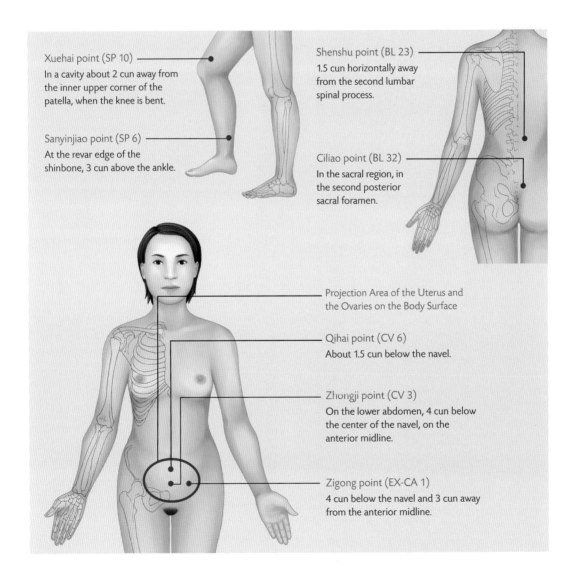

Xuehai point (SP 10)
In a cavity about 2 cun away from the inner upper corner of the patella, when the knee is bent.

Sanyinjiao point (SP 6)
At the revar edge of the shinbone, 3 cun above the ankle.

Shenshu point (BL 23)
1.5 cun horizontally away from the second lumbar spinal process.

Ciliao point (BL 32)
In the sacral region, in the second posterior sacral foramen.

Projection Area of the Uterus and the Ovaries on the Body Surface

Qihai point (CV 6)
About 1.5 cun below the navel.

Zhongji point (CV 3)
On the lower abdomen, 4 cun below the center of the navel, on the anterior midline.

Zigong point (EX-CA 1)
4 cun below the navel and 3 cun away from the anterior midline.

Recommended Procedures

1. Projection Area of the Uterus and the Ovaries on the Body Surface, Qihai Point, Zhongji Point, and Zigong Point

Method: Use the surface-scraping to scrape the projection area on the lower abdomen, with stress on Qihai point, Zhongji point and Zigong point.

2. Shenshu Point and Ciliao Point

Method: Use the surface-scraping to scrape Shenshu point and Ciliao point on both sides of the back from up to down.

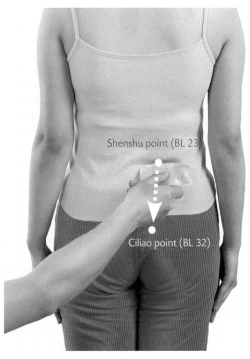

Shenshu point (BL 23)

Ciliao point (BL 32)

3. Xuehai Point and Sanyinjiao Point

Method: Use the surface-scraping to scrape Xuehai point and Sanyinjiao point on both sides of the Spleen Meridian on lower limbs from up to down.

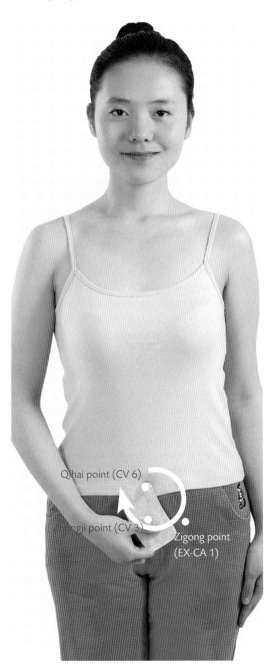

Qihai point (CV 6)

Zhongji point (CV 3)

Zigong point (EX-CA 1)

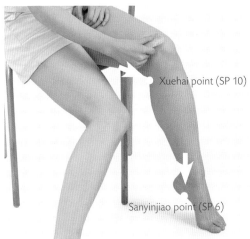

Xuehai point (SP 10)

Sanyinjiao point (SP 6)

Chronic Pelvic Inflammation

This refers to chronic inflammation in female productive organs and surrounding connective tissues, often resulting from incomplete treatment of acute pelvic inflammation and the delay of the disease-course. It is mainly marked by the bearing-down pain in the lower abdomen or soreness and pain in the lumbosacral area coupled with low fever, a big amount of leukorrhea and irregular menstruation. Scraping therapy is conducive to promoting the circulation of vital energy and blood and eliminating inflammation.

When acute pelvic inflammation or chronic pelvic inflammation attacks, there will be diffuse peritonitis, septicemia and infectious shock, which should be treated in time. During the period of treatment, attention should be paid to personal hygiene and persistent physical exercise to reinforce physique.

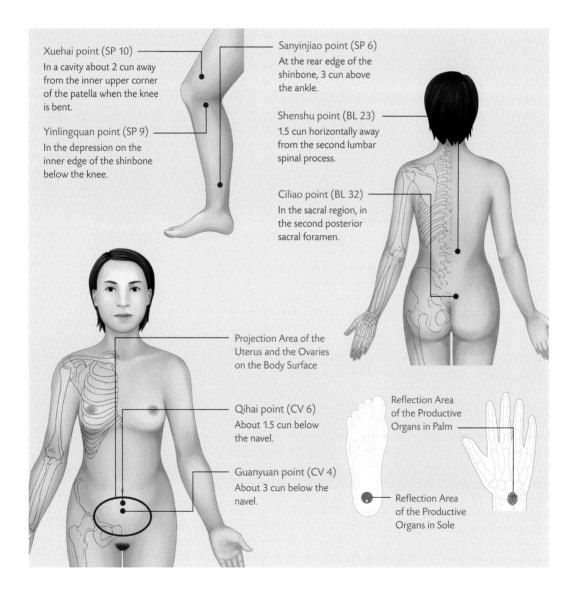

Xuehai point (SP 10)
In a cavity about 2 cun away from the inner upper corner of the patella when the knee is bent.

Yinlingquan point (SP 9)
In the depression on the inner edge of the shinbone below the knee.

Sanyinjiao point (SP 6)
At the rear edge of the shinbone, 3 cun above the ankle.

Shenshu point (BL 23)
1.5 cun horizontally away from the second lumbar spinal process.

Ciliao point (BL 32)
In the sacral region, in the second posterior sacral foramen.

Projection Area of the Uterus and the Ovaries on the Body Surface

Qihai point (CV 6)
About 1.5 cun below the navel.

Guanyuan point (CV 4)
About 3 cun below the navel.

Reflection Area of the Productive Organs in Palm

Reflection Area of the Productive Organs in Sole

Recommended Procedures

1. Projection Area of the Uterus and the Ovaries on the Body Surface
Method: Use the surface-scraping to scrape the area from up to down.

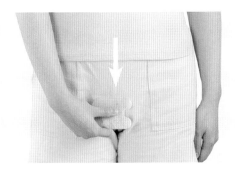

2. Reflection Areas of the Productive Organs in Palm and Sole
Method: Use the angle-pressing and kneading to press and knead the areas.

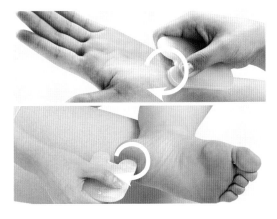

3. Qihai Point and Guanyuan Point
Method: Use the surface-scraping to scrape from Qihai point to Guanyuan point on the lower abdomen from up to down, until the skin turns red.

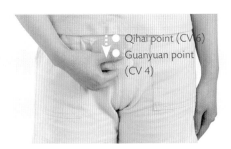

Qihai point (CV 6)
Guanyuan point (CV 4)

4. Shenshu Point and Ciliao Point
Method: Use the surface-scraping to scrape from Shenshu point to Ciliao point on the waist and back from up to down.

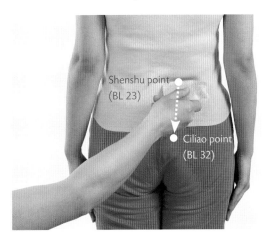

Shenshu point (BL 23)
Ciliao point (BL 32)

5. Xuehai Point, Yinlingquan Point and Sanyinjiao Point
Method: Use the surface-scraping to scrape Xuehai point, Yinlingquan point and Sanyinjiao point respectively on the inside of the lower limbs from up to down.

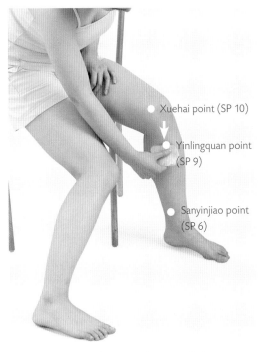

Xuehai point (SP 10)
Yinlingquan point (SP 9)
Sanyinjiao point (SP 6)

Acute Mastitis

This is acute pyogenic inflammation of mammary glands caused by germ infection, mostly taking place in women in the breast-feeding period. It is marked by breast distending pain possibly with fester flowing out, coupled with fever, fear of the cold and weakness all over the body. Scraping therapy can expel toxin and stasis, which is conducive to eliminating inflammation.

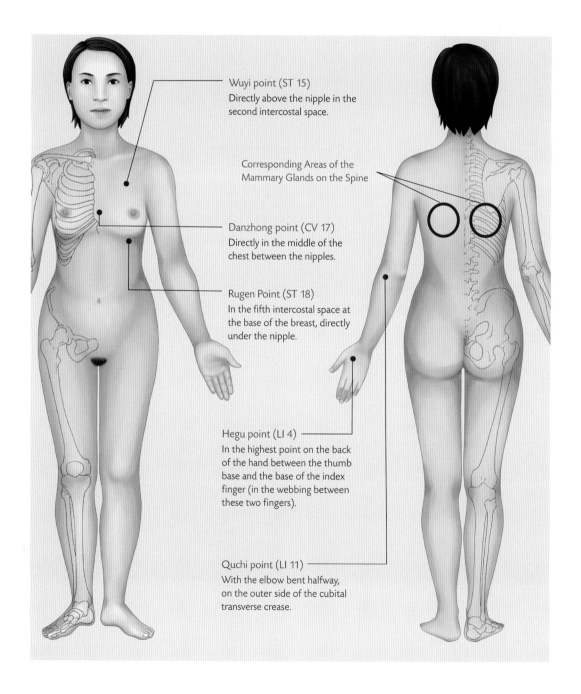

Wuyi point (ST 15)
Directly above the nipple in the second intercostal space.

Corresponding Areas of the Mammary Glands on the Spine

Danzhong point (CV 17)
Directly in the middle of the chest between the nipples.

Rugen Point (ST 18)
In the fifth intercostal space at the base of the breast, directly under the nipple.

Hegu point (LI 4)
In the highest point on the back of the hand between the thumb base and the base of the index finger (in the webbing between these two fingers).

Quchi point (LI 11)
With the elbow bent halfway, on the outer side of the cubital transverse crease.

Recommended Procedures

1. Corresponding Areas of the Mammary Glands on the Spine
Method: Use the surface-scraping to scrape the area from up to down.

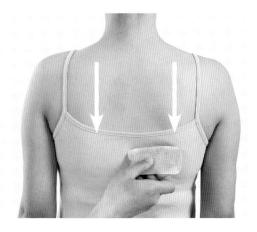

2. Danzhong Point, Wuyi Point and Rugen Point
Method: Use the angle-scraping to scrape Danzhong point from up to down. Then, gently scrape Wuyi point and Rugen point from inside to outside.

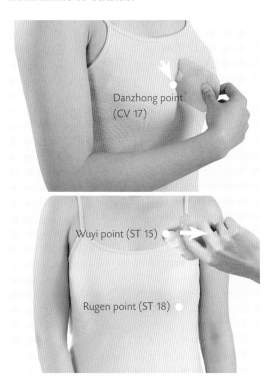

Danzhong point (CV 17)

Wuyi point (ST 15)

Rugen point (ST 18)

3. Quchi Point and Hegu Point
Method: Use the surface-scraping to scrape Quchi point on upper limbs from up to down. Use the single-angle pressing and kneading to press and knead Hegu point forcefully, until soreness and numbness are felt.

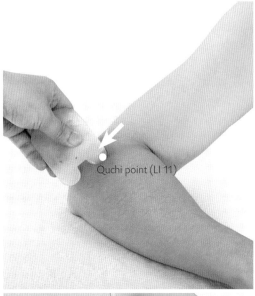

Quchi point (LI 11)

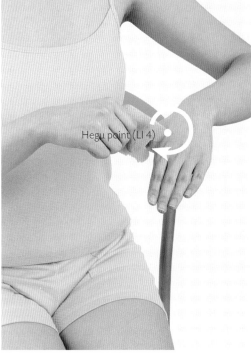

Hegu point (LI 4)

Hyperplasia of Mammary Glands

This is the commonest disease among females, often taking place in young and middle-aged women, with the conspicuous symptom of breast distending pain as well as lumps within breasts. According to Chinese medicine, main reasons for it are depression, stasis of vital energy, disorder of spleen functions, damp and phlegm, over-work and consumption of vital energy, etc. Scraping therapy can adjust and smooth vital energy circulation to a certain extent, preventing and treating hyperplasia of mammary glands.

Undesirable psychological factors such as excessive tension, irritation, apprehension and sorrow will lead nervous to break down, aggravating the imbalance of endocrine and causing hyperplasia. Therefore, women of this disease should try to avoid radical change of emotions and try to be pleasant. Active and outgoing moods are conducive to the elimination and recovery of hyperplasia. The early-stage symptoms of the tumor of mammary glands are similar to those of hyperplasia. Therefore, timely check-up is required to specify its nature for timely treatment.

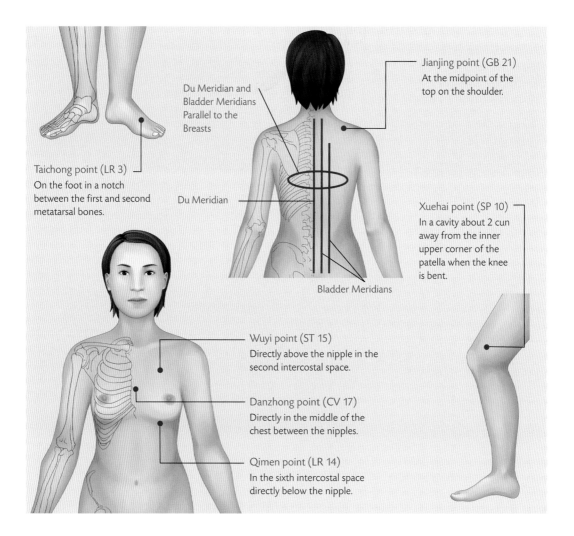

Jianjing point (GB 21)
At the midpoint of the top on the shoulder.

Du Meridian and Bladder Meridians Parallel to the Breasts

Taichong point (LR 3)
On the foot in a notch between the first and second metatarsal bones.

Du Meridian

Bladder Meridians

Xuehai point (SP 10)
In a cavity about 2 cun away from the inner upper corner of the patella when the knee is bent.

Wuyi point (ST 15)
Directly above the nipple in the second intercostal space.

Danzhong point (CV 17)
Directly in the middle of the chest between the nipples.

Qimen point (LR 14)
In the sixth intercostal space directly below the nipple.

Recommended Procedures

1. Du Meridian and Bladder Meridians

Method: Use the surface-scraping to scrape Du Meridian and Bladder Meridians parallel to the breasts on the back from up to down.

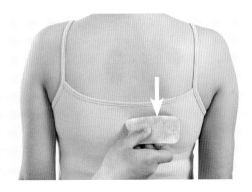

2. Danzhong Point, Wuyi Point and Qimen Point

Method: Use the angle-scraping to scrape Danzhong point on the chest from up to down. Then gently scrape Wuyi point and Qimen point from inside to outside.

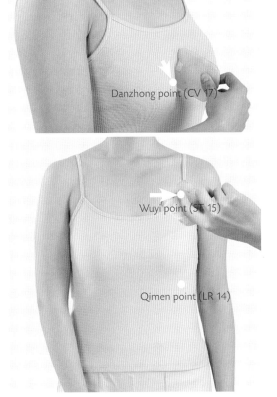

Danzhong point (CV 17)

Wuyi point (ST 15)

Qimen point (LR 14)

3. Jianjing Point

Method: Use the surface-scraping to scrape Jianjing point on the shoulder from inside to outside with considerable force, until *sha* appears.

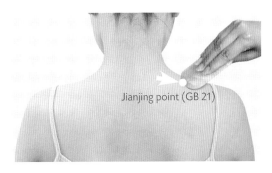

Jianjing point (GB 21)

4. Xuehai Point and Taichong Point

Method: Use the surface-scraping to scrape Xuehai point on lower limbs from up to down. Then, use the vertical-pressing and kneading to press and knead Taichong point on the foot back, until soreness and distention are felt.

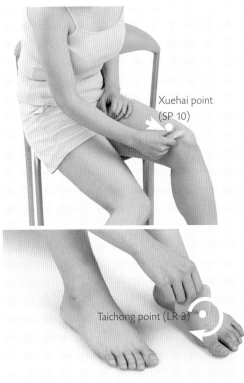

Xuehai point (SP 10)

Taichong point (LR 3)

Female's Climacteric Syndrome

Generally, climacteric takes place at the age from 45 to 50 for females, including the period of time before and after menopause. Before and after menopause, there will be fluctuation and reduction of sex hormone among these women. Therefore, a series of physical and mental symptoms arising from it are called climacteric syndrome. Generally speaking, these symptoms include disorder of menstruation, dizziness, tinnitus, palpitation, insomnia, decline of memory, easy excitement, agitation, fluctuating mood, frequent urination, red face, weakness and soreness in the waist, fatigue and obesity, etc.

During the period of menopause, women are apt to suffer from high blood pressure, coronary heart disease and tumor, periodical physical check-up is necessary. In this period, they are also apt to be marked by bone rarefaction. Therefore, they should pay attention to supplementing calcium, strictly controlling weight, setting restriction over irritating food and eating less salty food, so as to achieve diet balance.

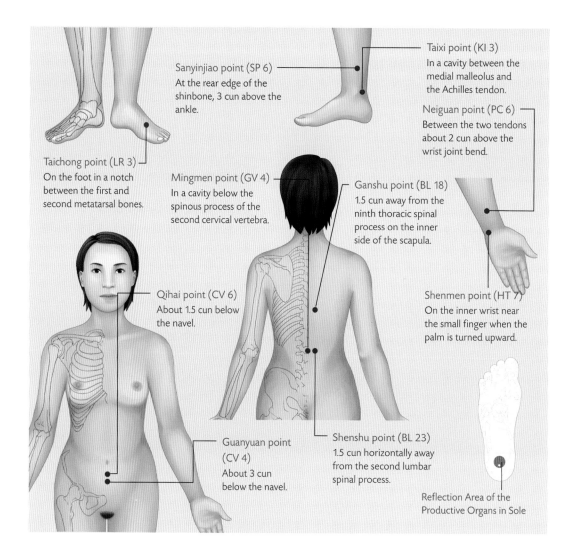

Sanyinjiao point (SP 6)
At the rear edge of the shinbone, 3 cun above the ankle.

Taixi point (KI 3)
In a cavity between the medial malleolus and the Achilles tendon.

Neiguan point (PC 6)
Between the two tendons about 2 cun above the wrist joint bend.

Taichong point (LR 3)
On the foot in a notch between the first and second metatarsal bones.

Mingmen point (GV 4)
In a cavity below the spinous process of the second cervical vertebra.

Ganshu point (BL 18)
1.5 cun away from the ninth thoracic spinal process on the inner side of the scapula.

Qihai point (CV 6)
About 1.5 cun below the navel.

Shenmen point (HT 7)
On the inner wrist near the small finger when the palm is turned upward.

Guanyuan point (CV 4)
About 3 cun below the navel.

Shenshu point (BL 23)
1.5 cun horizontally away from the second lumbar spinal process.

Reflection Area of the Productive Organs in Sole

Recommended Procedures

1. Reflection Area of the Productive Organs in Sole

Method: Use the angle-pressing and kneading to press and knead the area.

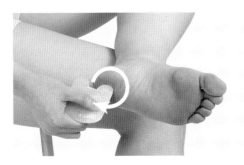

2. Neiguan Point and Shenmen Point

Method: Use the flat-scraping to scrape Neiguan point on the inside of the upper limbs. Then, use the corner of the scraping plate to press and knead Shenmen point on the wrist for 20 to 30 times.

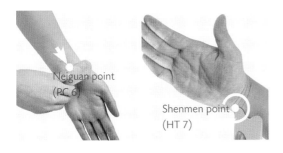

Neiguan point (PC 6)

Shenmen point (HT 7)

3. Qihai Point and Guanyuan Point

Method: Use the flat-scraping to scrape from Qihai point to Guanyuan point on the lower abdomen from up to down, until the skin turns red.

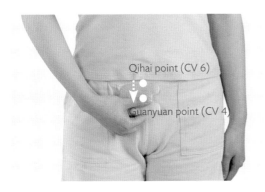

Qihai point (CV 6)

Guanyuan point (CV 4)

4. Ganshu Point, Shenshu Point and Mingmen Point

Method: Use the surface-scraping to scrape Ganshu point, Shenshu point and Mingmen point on the waist and back from up to down.

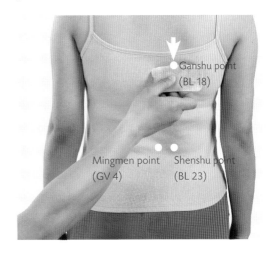

Ganshu point (BL 18)

Mingmen point (GV 4)

Shenshu point (BL 23)

5. Sanyinjiao Point, Taixi Point and Taichong Point

Method: Use the flat-scraping to scrape Sanyinjiao point on the inside of the lower limbs, until the skin turns red. Then, use the corner of the scraping plate to forcefully scrape Taixi point 30 times. Finally, use the vertical-pressing and kneading to press and knead Taichong point, until soreness and numbness are felt.

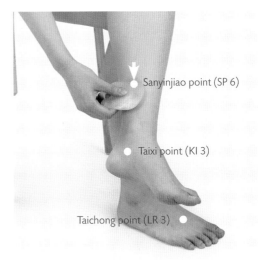

Sanyinjiao point (SP 6)

Taixi point (KI 3)

Taichong point (LR 3)

INDEX

B

Baihuanshu point 240, 241
Baihui point 44, 62, 80, 81, 84, 85, 106–109, 154, 155, 167, 168, 174, 175, 206–209, 250, 251
Bi'nao point 214, 215

C

Changqiang point 154, 155, 208, 209, 240, 241
Chengqi point 122, 169, 170
Chengshan point 150, 151, 169, 171, 222–229
Chize point 48, 49, 66, 67, 70, 71, 127, 128, 172, 173, 176, 177, 180–185
Ciliao point 200, 201, 248, 249, 252–255
Cuanzhu point 116–119, 122, 169, 170, 174, 175, 178, 179

D

Dachangshu point 12, 15, 100–103, 120, 121, 194–197
Dadun point 50, 51
Dahe point 240, 241
Daimai point 248, 249
Daling point 13, 89, 162, 163, 224, 225
Danshu point 76, 77, 110, 111, 118, 119, 129, 138, 139, 186, 187, 190–193
Danzhong point 27, 41, 45, 68, 69, 78, 79, 156, 157, 160–163, 165, 166, 184, 185, 188, 189, 256–259
Dazhong point 54, 55
Dazhu point 70–73, 172, 173, 180, 181, 184, 185, 212, 213, 228
Dazhui point 27, 66, 67, 72–75, 93–95, 106, 107, 112, 113, 130, 136, 137, 140, 141, 146–149, 154, 155, 160, 161, 167, 168, 172, 173, 176, 177, 184–189, 228, 229
Dicang point 142, 143, 169, 170
Diji point 101, 186, 187, 244, 245
Dingchuan point 172, 173, 184, 185
Dubi point 150, 151, 204, 205, 216, 217, 222, 223

E

E'ni point 96
Erjian point 88
Ermen point 82, 83

F

Feishu point 15, 65, 66, 70–75, 120, 121, 126, 154, 155, 172, 173, 176, 177, 182, 183
Feiyang point 54, 55
Fengchi point 41, 44, 65, 66, 74, 75, 80, 81, 106, 107, 112–117, 130, 140, 141, 145–147, 167, 168, 174–177, 212, 213
Fengfu point 93, 106, 107, 112, 113, 136, 137, 146, 147, 167, 168, 176, 177, 212, 213
Fenglong point 52, 53, 123, 140, 141, 156, 157, 162–165, 169, 171, 184, 185, 188, 189
Fengmen point 74, 75, 146, 147, 172, 173, 180, 181
Fengshi point 27, 140, 154, 155, 169, 171, 226, 227
Fuliu 200–203, 237, 238, 248, 249
Fuyang point 224, 225

G

Ganshu point 76, 77, 82, 83, 110, 111, 118, 119, 126, 129, 136–139, 144, 145, 178, 179, 186, 187, 190, 191, 204, 205, 242–247, 260, 261
Gaohuang point 78, 79, 182, 183, 228
Geshu point 97, 134–137, 165, 166, 184–187, 192, 193, 206, 207
Gongsun point 94, 95, 123, 164, 165, 192, 193
Guangming point 50, 51, 178, 179
Guanyuan point 12, 96, 156, 157, 162, 163, 194, 195, 199–203, 208, 209, 232–235, 238, 239, 242, 243, 246–251, 254, 255, 260, 261
Guilai point 202, 203, 237, 238, 242, 243

H

Heding point 222, 223
Hegu point 42, 66, 67, 69, 84–88, 93, 134, 135, 138, 139, 142, 143, 146, 147, 174–177, 196, 197, 204, 205, 256, 257
Houxi point 27, 112, 113
Huantiao point 150, 151, 169, 171
Hunmen point 110, 111, 129

J

Jiache point 86–88, 142, 143, 169, 170
Jiaji points 45, 111, 148, 149, 167, 168, 188, 189, 229

Jianjing point   106, 107, 112, 113, 146, 147, 154, 155, 212–215, 258, 259
Jianliao point   214, 215
Jianshi point   76, 77, 160, 161
Jianyu point   146, 147, 169, 170, 204, 205, 214
Jianzhen point   41, 169, 170, 204, 205
Jiexi point   169, 171, 204, 205, 221
Jingming point   118, 119, 178, 179
Jueyinshu point   78, 79, 160–163
Juque point   78, 79, 160–163

K

Kongzui point   68, 69
Kouheliao point   176, 177
Kunlun point   142, 143, 204, 205, 216, 217, 221

L

Laogong point   13, 89, 162, 163
Laozhen point   112, 113
Liangqiu point   216, 217, 222, 223
Lianquan point   169, 170
Lieque point   27, 70, 71, 84, 85, 174–177, 180, 181
Ligou point   232, 233

M

Mingmen point   148–151, 200, 201, 226, 227, 231–236, 238–241, 248, 249, 260, 261

N

Naoshu point   214, 215
Neiguan point   42, 62, 78, 79, 93, 96, 108, 109, 160, 161, 164, 165, 184, 185, 194–197, 260, 261
Neiting point   13, 88, 89, 138, 139, 142, 143, 158, 180, 181, 194, 195

P

Pangguangshu point   198, 199, 202, 203, 231, 232
Pishu point   15, 76, 77, 91, 92, 94, 95, 100, 101, 114, 115, 120, 121, 158, 159, 165, 166, 176, 177, 186, 187, 192–197, 200, 201, 204–207, 232, 233, 246–249

Q

Qianzheng point   142, 143
Qihai point   94–96, 98–101, 134, 135, 158, 159, 162, 163, 200, 201, 238, 239, 242–255, 260, 261

Qimen point   76, 77, 110, 111, 186–191, 258, 259
Qiuxu point   186, 187, 204, 205, 216, 217
Quchi point   12, 48, 49, 66, 67, 72, 73, 102, 127, 128, 130, 131, 136–141, 146, 147, 154, 155, 164, 165, 169, 170, 204, 205, 208, 214–217, 219, 256, 257
Qugu point   238, 239
Ququan point   50, 51, 150, 151, 186, 187, 236
Quze point   184, 185

R

Renying point   180, 181
Riyue point   186–191
Rugen point   256, 257

S

Sanjiaoshu point   94, 95, 188, 189, 198, 204, 205
Sanyinjiao point   52, 53, 82, 83, 123, 131, 133, 136–139, 156–159, 174, 175, 186, 187, 192, 193, 198–203, 206–209, 232–238, 240–255, 260, 261
Shangjuxu point   100, 101, 123, 194, 195
Shangwan point   98, 99, 190–193
Shangyang point   48, 49, 127, 128
Shangyingxiang point   174, 175
Shaochong point   46, 47
Shaohai point   46, 47, 219
Shaoshang point   48, 49, 66, 127, 128, 180–183
Shaoze point   46, 47
Shendao point   108, 109
Shenmai point   224, 225
Shenmen point   108, 109, 260, 261
Shenque point   159, 232, 233
Shenshu point   82, 83, 106–109, 126, 144, 145, 148, 149, 156–159, 165, 166, 178, 179, 184, 185, 198–207, 224–227, 231–235, 240–245, 248, 249, 252–255, 260, 261
Shentang point   78, 79, 160, 161
Shenting point   114, 115
Shenzhu point   106, 107, 130, 186, 187, 212, 213
Shousanli point   102, 103, 130, 131, 136, 137, 140, 141, 204, 205, 208, 209, 216, 217, 219
Shuidao point   202, 203, 237, 238
Shuifen point   200, 201
Shuiquan point   224, 225
Sishencong points   80, 81, 106–108

T

Taichong point   76, 77, 84, 85, 110, 111, 154, 155, 180, 181, 186–193, 238, 239, 246, 247, 258–261

Taixi point 82, 83, 86, 87, 96, 154, 155, 158, 160, 161, 198, 200–203, 224, 225, 232, 234, 235, 237, 238, 248, 260, 261

Taiyang point 43, 80, 81, 84, 85, 114–117, 142, 143

Taiyuan point 49, 78, 79, 158, 172–175, 182–185

Taodao point 140, 141

Tianshu point 12, 27, 94, 95, 98–103, 156, 157, 194–197

Tiantu point 45, 172, 173, 180, 181, 184, 185

Tianzhu point 108, 109, 146, 147, 212, 213

Tiaokou point 176, 177

Tinggong point 27, 82, 83

Tinghui point 82, 83

Tituo point 240, 241

Tongziliao point 118, 119, 122, 178, 179

Touwei point 43, 44, 80, 81, 84, 85, 114, 115

W

Waiguan point 138, 139, 169, 170, 204, 205, 212–215, 220

Wangu point 220

Weidao point 240, 241

Weishu point 15, 91, 92, 97, 120, 121, 186, 187, 192, 193, 196, 197

Weiyang point 222, 223

Weizhong point 54, 55, 150, 151, 169, 171, 222–227, 229

Wuyi point 256–259

X

Xiaguan point 86–88

Xialian point 208, 209

Xialiao point 248, 249

Xiaohai point 46, 47, 124, 125

Xiawan point 98, 99, 192, 193

Ximen point 160–165

Xingjian point 86, 87, 238, 239

Xinshu point 23, 78, 79, 106–109, 114, 115, 154, 155, 160–163, 165, 166, 188, 189, 234, 235

Xiyanggguan point 150, 151, 222, 223, 226, 227

Xuanshu point 94, 95, 188, 189

Xuanzhong point 186, 187, 212, 213

Xuehai point 124, 125, 136–139, 144, 164, 165, 206–209, 222, 223, 240–243, 246, 247, 250–255, 258, 259

Y

Yamen point 93, 169, 170

Yangbai point 142, 143, 169, 170

Yangchi point 158, 159, 204, 205, 216, 217, 220

Yangfu point 178, 179

Yanggang point 129, 158, 159

Yanggu point 124, 220

Yanglao point 142, 143, 178, 179

Yanglaodian point 178, 179

Yanglingquan point 50, 51, 134, 135, 140, 141, 150, 151, 169, 171, 186–191, 204, 205, 212, 213, 216, 217, 222, 223, 226, 227

Yaoshu point 200, 201, 208, 209, 226, 227, 238, 239

Yaoyan point 226, 227

Yaoyanggguan point 148, 149, 167, 168, 200, 201, 226, 227, 232, 233, 238, 239

Yin'gu point 54, 55, 222, 223

Yingxiang point 142, 143, 174–177

Yinlingquan point 52, 53, 101, 123, 131, 138, 139, 150, 151, 174, 175, 186, 187, 194, 195, 198, 199, 200–203, 216, 217, 222, 223, 232, 233, 237, 238, 240, 241, 244, 245, 248, 249, 254, 255

Yinmen point 169, 171, 226, 227

Yintang point 27, 114, 115, 174–177

Yishe point 158, 159

Yongquan point 62, 133, 224, 225

Yuji point 180–183

Yunmen point 70, 71, 182, 183

Yuyao point 118, 119

Z

Zhangmen point 94, 95, 186–191, 206, 207

Zhaohai point 224, 225, 228, 250, 251

Zhichuang point 208, 209

Zhigou point 12, 68, 69, 102, 103, 169, 170

Zhishi point 150, 151, 184, 185, 200, 201, 231, 232

Zhiyang point 160, 161, 184–187, 238, 239

Zhizheng point 124, 125

Zhongdu point 140, 141

Zhongfeng point 204, 205

Zhongfu point 45, 65, 66, 70, 71, 172, 173, 182–185

Zhongji point 199–203, 208, 209, 232–236, 238, 239, 244, 245, 252, 253

Zhongting point 165, 166

Zhongwan point 68, 69, 94, 95, 100, 101, 156–159, 188–197, 200, 201, 206, 207

Zhongzhu point 112, 113, 212–215

Zhouliao point 219

Zigong point 240, 241, 252, 253

Zusanli point 13, 42, 52, 53, 62, 89, 94, 95, 100, 101, 123–125, 134, 135, 154–159, 162–165, 169, 171, 176, 177, 184, 185, 188–197, 206, 207, 222, 223, 248, 249